Mastocytosis

Editor

CEM AKIN

IMMUNOLOGY AND ALLERGY CLINICS OF NORTH AMERICA

www.immunology.theclinics.com

Consulting Editor
RAFEUL ALAM

May 2014 • Volume 34 • Number 2

ELSEVIER

1600 John F. Kennedy Boulevard • Suite 1800 • Philadelphia, Pennsylvania, 19103-2899

http://www.theclinics.com

IMMUNOLOGY AND ALLERGY CLINICS OF NORTH AMERICA Volume 34, Number 2

May 2014 ISSN 0889–8561, ISBN-13: 978-0-323-29709-7

Editor: Jessica McCool
Developmental Editor: Stephanie Carter

Immunology and Allergy Clinics of North America (ISSN 0889–8561) is published quarterly by Elsevier Inc., 360 Park Avenue South, New York, NY 10010-1710. Months of issue are February, May, August, and November. Periodicals postage paid at New York, NY and additional mailing offices. Subscription prices are $320.00 per year for US individuals, $454.00 per year for US institutions, $150.00 per year for US students and residents, $395.00 per year for Canadian individuals, $220.00 per year for Canadian students, $577.00 per year for Canadian institutions, $445.00 per year for international individuals, $577.00 per year for international institutions, $220.00 per year for international students. To receive student/resident rate, orders must be accompanied by name of affiliated institution, date of term, and the *signature* of program/residency coordinator on institution letterhead. Orders will be billed at individual rate until proof of status is received. Foreign air speed delivery is included in all *Clinics* subscription prices. All prices are subject to change without notice. **POSTMASTER**: Send address changes to *Immunology and Allergy Clinics of North America,* Elsevier Health Sciences Division, Subscription Customer Service, 3251 Riverport Lane, Maryland Heights, MO 63043. **Customer Service: 1-800-654-2452 (U.S. and Canada); 314-447-8871 (outside U.S. and Canada). Fax: 314-447-8029. E-mail: journalscustomerservice-usa@elsevier.com (for print support); journalsonlinesupport-usa@elsevier.com (for online support).**

Reprints. For copies of 100 or more, of articles in this publication, please contact the Commercial Reprints Department, Elsevier Inc., 360 Park Avenue South, New York, New York 10010-1710. Tel. 212-633-3874, Fax: 212-633-3820, E-mail: reprints@elsevier.com.

Immunology and Allergy Clinics of North America is covered in MEDLINE/PubMed (Index Medicus), Current Contents/Life Sciences, Science Citation Index, ISI/BIOMED, Chemical Abstracts, and EMBASE/Excerpta Medica.

Contributors

CONSULTING EDITOR

RAFEUL ALAM, MD, PhD
Professor and Chief, Division of Allergy and Immunology, National Jewish Health and University of Colorado Denver, Denver, Colorado

EDITOR

CEM AKIN, MD, PhD
Associate Professor of Medicine, Harvard Medical School; Director, Mastocytosis Center, Brigham and Women's Hospital, Boston, Massachusetts

AUTHORS

SILVANO ADAMI, MD
Rheumatology Section, Department of Medicine, University of Verona, Verona, Italy

CEM AKIN, MD, PhD
Associate Professor of Medicine, Harvard Medical School; Director, Mastocytosis Center, Brigham and Women's Hospital, Boston, Massachusetts

IVAN ALVAREZ-TWOSE, MD
Mastocytosis Unit of Castilla La-Mancha, Hospital Virgen del Valle; Spanish Network on Mastocytosis (REMA), Toledo, Spain

MICHEL AROCK, PharmD, PhD
Molecular Oncology and Pharmacology, LBPA CNRS UMR8113, Ecole Normale Supérieure de Cachan, Cachan, France

SIHAM BIBI, PhD
Molecular Oncology and Pharmacology, LBPA CNRS UMR8113, Ecole Normale Supérieure de Cachan, Cachan, France

CARSTEN BINDSLEV-JENSEN, MD, PhD, DMSc
Professor, Head, Department of Dermatology and Allergy Centre, Mastocytosis Centre Odense University Hospital, MastOUH, Odense University Hospital, Odense, Denmark

PATRIZIA BONADONNA, MD
Allergy Unit, Azienda Ospedaliera Universitaria Integrata of Verona, Verona, Italy

FABIENNE BRENET, PhD
Signaling, Hematopoiesis and Mechanism of Oncogenesis, Inserm, U1068, CRCM; Institut Paoli-Calmettes; Aix-Marseille University, UM 105; CNRS, UMR7258, CRCM, Marseille, France

KNUT BROCKOW, MD
Associated Professor, Department of Dermatology and Allergy Biederstein, Technische Universität München, Munich, Germany

SIGURD BROESBY-OLSEN, MD
Department of Dermatology and Allergy Centre, Mastocytosis Centre Odense University Hospital (MastOUH), Odense University Hospital, Odense, Denmark

JOSEPH BUTTERFIELD, MD, FAAAAI
Professor of Medicine, Mayo Clinic College of Medicine; Cochair, Program of Excellence in Mast Cell and Eosinophil Disorders, Division of Allergic Disease, Department of Internal Medicine, Rochester, Minnesota

MARIANA C. CASTELLS, MD, PhD
Division of Rheumatology, Immunology, and Allergy, Department of Medicine, Brigham and Women's Hospital, Harvard Medical School, Boston, Massachusetts

GLENN CRUSE, PhD
Mast Cell Biology Section, Laboratory of Allergic Diseases, National Institute of Allergy and Infectious Diseases (NIAID), National Institutes of Health, Bethesda, Maryland

GANDHI DAMAJ, MD
Faculty of Medicine et AP-HP Necker-Enfants Malades, Mastocytosis Reference Center, Paris; Clinical Hematology Department, Hôpital Sud, CHU Amiens, Ave René Laënnec - Salouël, Amiens, France

LEONA A. DOYLE, MD
Department of Pathology, Brigham and Women's Hospital, Harvard Medical School, Boston, Massachusetts

PATRICE DUBREUIL, PhD
Signaling, Hematopoiesis and Mechanism of Oncogenesis, Inserm, U1068, CRCM; Institut Paoli-Calmettes; Aix-Marseille Université, UM 105; CNRS, UMR7258, CRCM, Marseille, France; Faculté de Médecine et AP-HP Necker-Enfants Malades, Centre de Référence des Mastocytoses, Paris, France

LUIS ESCRIBANO, MD, PhD
Spanish Network on Mastocytosis (REMA), Toledo; Servicio General de Citometría, Departamento de Medicina, Centro de Investigación del Cáncer (IBMCC-CSIC/USAL and IBSAL), Universidad de Salamanca, Salamanca; Centro de Estudios de Mastocitosis de Castilla La Mancha, Hospital Virgen del Valle, Toledo, Spain

RAPHAËL GAILLARD, MD, PhD
Laboratoire de "Physiopathologie des maladies Psychiatriques", Centre de Psychiatrie et Neurosciences, U894, INSERM, Université Paris Descartes, Sorbonne Paris Cité; Service de Psychiatrie, Faculté de M\xE9decine Paris Descartes, Centre Hospitalier Sainte-Anne, Université Paris Descartes, Sorbonne Paris Cité, Paris, France

ANDRÉS C. GARCÍA-MONTERO, PhD
Spanish Network on Mastocytosis (REMA), Toledo; Departments of Cytometry and Medicine, Centro de Investigación del Cáncer, (IBMCC-CSIC/USAL and IBSAL) University of Salamanca, Salamanca, Spain

DAVIDE GATTI, MD
Rheumatology Section, Department of Medicine, University of Verona, Verona, Italy

SOPHIE GEORGIN-LAVIALLE, MD, PhD
Laboratory of Cellular and Molecular Mechanisms of Hematological Disorders and Therapeutical Implications; Paris Descartes – Sorbonne Paris Cité University, Imagine Institute; CNRS ERL 8254; Laboratory of Excellence GR-Ex; Service d'Hématologie clinique, Assistance Publique-Hôpitaux de Paris, Hôpital Necker; Service de médecine Interne, Hôpital Tenon, Assistance Publique-Hôpitaux de Paris, Université Pierre et Marie Curie, Paris, France

DAVID B.K. GOLDEN, MD, PhD
Division of Allergy-Immunology, Johns Hopkins University, Baltimore, Maryland

PHILIP M. HANSBRO, PhD
Priority Research Centre for Asthma and Respiratory Disease, Hunter Medical Research Institute and University of Newcastle, Newcastle, Australia

OLIVIER HERMINE, MD, PhD
Clinical Hematology Department, Faculty of Medicine and AP-HP Necker-Enfants Malades, Paris Descartes University; Faculty of Medicine et AP-HP Necker-Enfants Malades, Mastocytosis Reference Center; Laboratory of Cellular and Molecular Mechanisms of Hematological Disorders and Therapeutical Implications; Paris Descartes – Sorbonne Paris Cité University, Imagine Institute; CNRS ERL 8254; Laboratory of Excellence GR-Ex; Service d'Hématologie clinique, Assistance Publique-Hôpitaux de Paris, Hôpital Necker, Paris, France

JASON L. HORNICK, MD, PhD
Director of Surgical Pathology, Department of Pathology, Brigham and Women's Hospital, Harvard Medical School, Boston, Massachusetts

HANS-PETER HORNY, MD
Institute of Pathology, Ludwig-Maximilians-Universität, Munich, Germany

LUCA IDOLAZZI, MD
Rheumatology Section, Department of Medicine, University of Verona, Verona, Italy

MARÍA JARA-ACEVEDO, MSc
Spanish Network on Mastocytosis (REMA), Toledo; Departments of Cytometry and Medicine, Centro de Investigación del Cáncer, (IBMCC-CSIC/USAL and IBSAL) University of Salamanca, Salamanca, Spain

SYLVIE JEANNINGROS, MSc
Molecular Oncology and Pharmacology, LBPA CNRS UMR8113, Ecole Normale Supérieure de Cachan, Cachan, France

PHILIP M. KLUIN, MD, PhD
Department of Pathology and Medical Biology, University Medical Center Groningen, University of Groningen, Groningen, The Netherlands

JOHANNA C. KLUIN-NELEMANS, MD, PhD
Department of Hematology, University Medical Center Groningen, University of Groningen, Groningen, The Netherlands

ANNA KOVALSZKI, MD
Clinical Director, Division of Allergy and Inflammation, Department of Medicine, Beth Israel Deaconess Medical Center, Harvard Medical School, Boston, Massachusetts

FLORENT LANGENFELD, PhD
Molecular Oncology and Pharmacology, LBPA CNRS UMR8113, Ecole Normale Supérieure de Cachan, Cachan, France

CARLA LOMBARDO, MD
Allergy Unit, Azienda Ospedaliera Universitaria Integrata of Verona, Verona, Italy

ALMUDENA MATITO, MD, PhD
Mastocytosis Unit of Castilla La-Mancha, Hospital Virgen del Valle; Spanish Network on Mastocytosis (REMA), Toledo, Spain

MARCUS MAURER, MD
Department of Dermatology and Allergy, Interdisciplinary Mastocytosis Center Charité, Charité-Universitätsmedizin Berlin, Berlin, Germany

ANDREA MAYADO, PhD
Spanish Network on Mastocytosis (REMA), Toledo; Servicio General de Citometría, Departamento de Medicina, Centro de Investigación del Cáncer (IBMCC-CSIC/USAL and IBSAL), Universidad de Salamanca, Salamanca, Spain

DEAN D. METCALFE, MD
Mast Cell Biology Section, Laboratory of Allergic Diseases, National Institute of Allergy and Infectious Diseases (NIAID), National Institutes of Health, Bethesda, Maryland

JOSE MARIO T. MORGADO, MSc
Instituto de Estudios de Mastocitosis de Castilla La Mancha; Spanish Network on Mastocytosis (REMA), Toledo, Spain

DANIELA S. MOURA, PhD
Laboratory of Cellular and Molecular Mechanisms of Hematological Disorders and Therapeutical Implications; Paris Descartes – Sorbonne Paris Cité University, Imagine Institute; CNRS ERL 8254; Laboratory of Excellence GR-Ex; Service d'Hématologie clinique, Assistance Publique-Hôpitaux de Paris, Hôpital Necker, Paris, France

MAREK NIEDOSZYTKO, MD, PhD
Department of Allergology, Medical University of Gdansk, Gdańsk, Poland

ANA OLIVERA, PhD
Mast Cell Biology Section, Laboratory of Allergic Diseases, National Institute of Allergy and Infectious Diseases (NIAID), National Institutes of Health, Bethesda, Maryland

ALBERTO ORFAO, MD, PhD
Spanish Network on Mastocytosis (REMA), Toledo; Servicio General de Citometría, Departamento de Medicina, Centro de Investigación del Cáncer (IBMCC-CSIC/USAL and IBSAL), Universidad de Salamanca, Salamanca, Spain

GIOVANNI ORSOLINI, MD
Rheumatology Section, Department of Medicine, University of Verona, Verona, Italy

JOANNE N.G. OUDE ELBERINK, MD, PhD
Department of Allergology, Groningen Research Institute for Asthma and COPD, University Medical Center Groningen, University of Groningen, Groningen, The Netherlands

OMAR PERBELLINI, MD
Section of Hematology, Department of Medicine, University of Verona, Verona, Italy

ALICIA PRIETO-GARCÍA, MD, PhD
Allergy Service, Hospital Universitario Gregorio Marañón, Instituto de Investigación Sanitaria Gregorio Marañón, Madrid, Spain

MAURIZIO ROSSINI, MD
Rheumatology Section, Department of Medicine, University of Verona, Verona, Italy

LAURA SÁNCHEZ-MUÑOZ, MD, PhD
Instituto de Estudios de Mastocitosis de Castilla La Mancha; Spanish Network on Mastocytosis (REMA), Toledo, Spain

DONATELLA SCHENA, MD
Dermatology Section, Department of Medicine, University of Verona, Verona, Italy

FRANK SIEBENHAAR, MD
Department of Dermatology and Allergy, Interdisciplinary Mastocytosis Center Charité, Charité-Universitätsmedizin Berlin, Berlin, Germany

KARL SOTLAR, MD
Institute of Pathology, Ludwig-Maximilians-Universität, Munich, Germany

ERINN SOUCIE, PhD
Signaling, Hematopoiesis and Mechanism of Oncogenesis, Inserm, U1068, CRCM; Institut Paoli-Calmettes; Aix-Marseille University, UM 105; CNRS, UMR7258, CRCM, Marseille, France

RICHARD L. STEVENS, PhD
Division of Rheumatology, Immunology, and Allergy, Department of Medicine, Brigham and Women's Hospital, Harvard Medical School, Boston, Massachusetts

CRISTINA TEODOSIO, PhD
Spanish Network on Mastocytosis (REMA), Toledo; Servicio General de Citometría, Departamento de Medicina, Centro de Investigación del Cáncer (IBMCC-CSIC/USAL and IBSAL), Universidad de Salamanca, Salamanca, Spain

GAIA TRIPI, MD
Rheumatology Section, Department of Medicine, University of Verona, Verona, Italy

PETER VALENT, MD
Professor, Division of Hematology and Hemostaseology, Department of Internal Medicine I, Ludwig Boltzmann Cluster Oncology, Medical University of Vienna, Vienna, Austria

BJORN VAN ANROOIJ, BSc
Department of Allergology, Groningen Research Institute for Asthma and COPD, University Medical Center Groningen, University of Groningen, Groningen, The Netherlands

OMBRETTA VIAPIANA, MD
Rheumatology Section, Department of Medicine, University of Verona, Verona, Italy

CATHERINE R. WEILER, MD, PhD, FAAAAI
Assistant Professor of Medicine, Mayo Clinic College of Medicine; Cochair, Program of Excellence in Mast cell and Eosinophil Disorders, Division of Allergic Disease, Department of Internal Medicine, Rochester, Minnesota

PETER F. WELLER, MD
Chief, Division of Allergy and Inflammation; Chief, Division of Infectious Diseases, Professor of Medicine, Department of Medicine, Beth Israel Deaconess Medical Center, Harvard Medical School, Boston, Massachusetts

ROBERTA ZANOTTI, MD
Hematology Section, Department of Medicine, University of Verona, Verona, Italy

Contents

Cem Akin and Peter Valent

Mastocytosis is characterized by accumulation of pathologic mast cells in tissues. Most patients with mastocytosis experience mast cell activation symptoms in response to various triggers. The diagnosis of mastocytosis should be made from objective pathologic findings. Modern diagnostic criteria and classification of mastocytosis were proposed in 2000 by an international consensus group and formed the basis of the current World Health Organization (WHO) guidelines, which have been validated to correlate with prognosis and help selection of therapy. In this article, the WHO criteria for diagnosis and classification are summarized and practical aspects to avoid common pitfalls in diagnostic workup are discussed.

Glenn Cruse, Dean D. Metcalfe, and Ana Olivera

In this review, the authors discuss common gain-of-function mutations in the stem cell factor receptor KIT found in mast cell proliferation disorders and summarize the current understanding of the molecular mechanisms by which these transforming mutations may affect KIT structure and function leading to altered downstream signaling and cellular transformation. Drugs targeting KIT have shown mixed success in the treatment of mastocytosis and other hyperproliferative diseases. A brief overview of the most common KIT inhibitors currently used, the reasons for the varied clinical results of such inhibitors and a discussion of potential new strategies are provided.

Siham Bibi, Florent Langenfeld, Sylvie Jeanningros, Fabienne Brenet, Erinn Soucie, Olivier Hermine, Gandhi Damaj, Patrice Dubreuil, and Michel Arock

In all variants of mastocytosis, activating *KIT* mutations are frequently found. In adults, neoplastic mast cells (MCs) cells show the *KIT* mutation D816V, whereas in children, MCs invading the skin are frequently positive for non-*KIT* D816V mutations. The clinical course and prognosis of the disease vary among patients with systemic mastocytosis (SM). Additional *KIT*-independent molecular defects might cause progression. Additional oncogenic lesions have recently been identified in advanced SM. In advanced SM the presence of additional genetic lesions or altered signaling worsening the prognosis might lead to the use of alternative therapies such as combined antisignaling targeted treatments or stem cell transplantation.

Tetramer-forming tryptase (hTryptase-β) was recently discovered to have a prominent role in preventing the internal accumulation of life-threatening fibrin deposits and fibrin-platelet clots. The anticoagulant activity of hTryptase-β is an explanation for the presence of hemorrhagic disorders in some patients with anaphylaxis or mastocytosis. The fragments of hFibrinogen formed by the proteolysis of this prominent protein by hTryptase-β could be used as biomarkers in the blood and/or urine for the identification and monitoring of patients with mast cell–dependent disorders. Recombinant hTryptase-β has potential to be used in clinical settings where it is desirable to inhibit blood coagulation.

This article updates current knowledge about epidemiology, prognosis, and risk factors for major complications in mastocytosis. A prevalence of mastocytosis of 1 in 10000 inhabitants has been reported, but underdiagnosis is assumed. The prognosis for cutaneous and indolent systemic mastocytosis is excellent. For more advanced forms of disease, prognostic parameters have been identified. A high extent of skin involvement, increased basal serum tryptase values, and extensive blistering are risk factors for severe mast cell activation episodes in children, whereas these associations seem to be less strong or nonexistent for anaphylaxis and osteoporosis in adult patients with indolent systemic mastocytosis.

This article presents information for the identification and characterization of mast cells from bone marrow and other tissues using multiparametric flow cytometry. In addition, it provides guidelines for the application of this technique in the subclassification of systemic mastocytosis and assessment of the long-term prognosis of patients individually.

Mastocytosis is a disease of bone marrow origin histologically characterized by compact tissue infiltrates of atypical mast cells never seen in reactive states. Most patients with mastocytosis have transformed mast cells carrying an activating point mutation at codon 816 of *KIT* and also show an elevated serum tryptase level. In this article immunophenotypical features of mast cells are described. Based on these features, mast cells are not closely related to other myeloid cells. Using the knowledge on aberrantly expressed antigens by mast cells, the hematopathologist should be able to recognize the disease even in the presence of unusual morphologic findings or an associated hematologic non–mast cell lineage disease.

Mastocytosis encompasses a group of clinically and pathologically hetero-geneous disorders most commonly involving the skin, which typically takes the form of urticaria pigmentosa. Mastocytosis may also involve other organs, most often bone marrow, followed by gastrointestinal tract, liver, spleen, and lymph nodes. The presence of extracutaneous involvement by mastocytosis is a major diagnostic criterion for systemic disease. How-ever, mast cell infiltrates are often subtle in skin and extracutaneous organs, and the histologic features of mastocytosis at different anatomic sites may be variable. This article reviews the pathologic features and clinical corre-lates of mastocytosis involving skin and other extramedullary sites.

CD30 is a transmembrane receptor, normally not expressed by mast cells, which regulates proliferation/apoptosis and antibody responses. Aberrant expression of CD30 by mastocytosis mast cells and interaction with its ligand CD30L (CD153) appears to play an important role in the pathogenesis and clinical presentation of systemic mastocytosis. This article highlights the expression profile and role of CD30 and CD30L in physiologic and pathologic conditions, the applicability of CD30 as a marker for systemic mastocytosis, the consequences of mast cell–expressed CD30, and the possibility of future anti-CD30 based cytoreductive therapies.

Eosinophils and mast cells coexist in clonal and nonclonal disorders. The interplay between these cells is complex and not fully understood. Discussed are both allergic/nonclonal disorders in which both cell types are increased in number are likely to play a role in pathogenesis and clonal disorders in which both cell types are affected and play key roles in pathogenesis. Finally, some treatment options, keeping both disorders in mind, are discussed. Future directions in thinking about these disorders are also briefly explored.

Hymenoptera venom allergy is a typical IgE-mediated reaction caused by sensitization to 1 or more allergens of the venom, and accounts for 1.5% to

34% of all cases of anaphylaxis. Patients suffering from mastocytosis are more susceptible to the anaphylactic reactions to an insect sting. This article aims to answer the most important clinical questions raised by the diagnosis and treatment of insect venom allergy in mastocytosis patients. Total avoidance of Hymenoptera is not feasible, and there is no preventive pharmacologic treatment available, although venom immunotherapy reduces the risk of subsequent systemic reactions.

Bone involvement is frequent in patients with systemic mastocytosis. Osteoporosis is the most prevalent bone manifestation, but diffuse osteosclerosis or focal osteolytic or osteosclerotic lesions are not infrequent. The risk of osteoporotic fractures is high, especially at the spine and in men. Routine measurements of bone mineral density and vertebral morphometry are warranted. The bone turnover markers indicate the involvement of complex bone metabolism in mastocytosis-related manifestations. Bisphosphonates represent the first-line treatment for osteoporosis-related mastocytosis.

Drugs are known triggers of anaphylaxis in patients with mastocytosis even to the association between drug anaphylaxis and mastocytosis does not appear frequently appear. Nevertheless, mast cell disorders might be ruled out in cases of severe systemic reactions. Careful examination of the skin should accompany measurement of basal serum tryptase levels. The data published about drug anaphylaxis in patients with mast cell disorders are scarce, and it is not currently possible to provide clear recommendations. Most papers report cases of anaphylaxis during surgical procedures or radiocontrast media exposure. There are no specific recommendations to prevent severe reactions during such procedures, although some specialists suggest performing premedication with antihistamines and corticosteroids before anesthesia or radiocontrast media administration.

In approximately one-third of cases, patients with mastocytosis can display various disabling general and neuropsychological symptoms. General signs may have a major impact on quality of life. Neurologic symptoms are less frequent. In a majority of cases, the pathophysiology of these symptoms is not known but could be linked to tissular mast cell infiltration, mast cell mediator release, or both. Treatments aiming at reducing mast cell number and/or stabilizating mast cells may be useful. Preliminary results suggest that treatment with kinase inhibitors may improve symptoms of depression and cognitive impairment.

Mast Cell Sarcoma: Clinical Management **423**

Catherine R. Weiler and Joseph Butterfield

Mast cell sarcoma is a disorder that results in abnormal mast cells as identified by morphology, special stains, and in some publications, c-kit mutation analysis. It affects animal species such as canines more commonly than humans. In humans it is a very rare condition, with variable clinical presentation. There is no standard therapy for the disorder. It can affect any age group. It is occasionally associated with systemic mastocytosis and/or urticaria pigmentosa. The prognosis of mast cell sarcoma in published literature is very poor in humans.

Treatment Strategies in Mastocytosis **433**

Frank Siebenhaar, Cem Akin, Carsten Bindslev-Jensen, Marcus Maurer, and Sigurd Broesby-Olsen

Treatment recommendations for mastocytosis are based mostly on expert opinion rather than evidence obtained from controlled clinical trials. In this article, treatment options for mastocytosis are presented, with a focus on the control of mediator-related symptoms in patients with indolent disease.

Index **449**

IMMUNOLOGY AND ALLERGY CLINICS OF NORTH AMERICA

Foreword

The Amazing Mast Cell

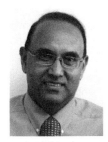

Rafeul Alam, MD, PhD
Consulting Editor

The mast cell represents one of the early innate immune cells that emerged before the adaptive immune cells. It expresses a variety of pathogen recognition receptors/sensors that explain its involvement in innate immune response.[1] The expression of the high-affinity IgE receptor made the mast cell an extraordinary effector cell of the adaptive immune system. Because of its secretion of histamine, leukotriene, and other vasoactive mediators, the mast cell is traditionally considered an effector cell of an immediate hypersensitivity reaction. However, the function of the mast cell goes beyond the immediate hypersensitivity reaction. The mast cell is involved in other types of hypersensitivity reactions including delayed hypersensitivity reaction and in innate immune response against bacteria and parasites.[1] In addition to allergic diseases and host defense, the mast cell has been implicated in the pathogenesis of such diverse diseases as rheumatoid arthritis, lupus, multiple sclerosis, pulmonary fibrosis, pain, atherosclerosis, and vascular diseases of the brain.[2] There is a growing body of evidence that suggests a close functional link between mast cells and neuronal cells.[3] This link might explain the CNS symptoms that many allergy sufferers experience during the allergy season. While under certain circumstances the mast cell promotes inflammation, in other situations it actually prevents inflammation and promotes healing. An example of the homeostatic function is its role in the inactivation of snake venom.[4]

Tremendous progress has been made in understanding the mechanism of mast cell activation and the various ligands that activate mast cells. Ligand (antigen)-independent activation of mast cells through the IgE receptor is a fascinating area. This might explain the beneficial effect of the anti-IgE antibody Omalizumab in chronic spontaneous urticaria. Mast cell activation syndrome is another condition that generates exciting basic science questions. It is unclear what activates mast cells in this condition. The various forms of mastocytosis remain a clinical challenge. I have invited Dr Cem Akin, a leader in the field, to update us on mast cells and mast cell disorders.

Supported by NIH Grants RO1 AI091614 and N01 HHSN272200700048C.

Immunol Allergy Clin N Am 34 (2014) xv–xvi
http://dx.doi.org/10.1016/j.iac.2014.02.002 **immunology.theclinics.com**

He has brought together an outstanding group of experts and topics for this issue. I hope you enjoy them.

Rafeul Alam, MD, PhD
Division of Allergy and Immunology
National Jewish Health
University of Colorado Denver
1400 Jackson Street
Denver, CO 80206, USA

E-mail address:
alamr@njhealth.org

REFERENCES

1. St John AL, Abraham SN. Innate immunity and its regulation by mast cells. J Immunol 2013;190:4458–63.
2. Voehringer D. Protective and pathological roles of mast cells and basophils. Nat Rev Immunol 2013;13:362–75.
3. Undem BJ, Taylor-Clark T. Mechanisms underlying the neuronal-based symptoms of allergy. J Allergy Clin Immunol 2014. pii:S0091-6749(13) 01847–2.
4. Metz M, Piliponsky AM, Chen CC, et al. Mast cells can enhance resistance to snake and honeybee venoms. Science 2006;313:526–30.

Preface

Mastocytosis

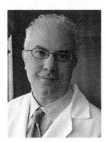

Cem Akin, MD, PhD
Editor

Mastocytosis is a rare disorder, or at least it has been considered rare, for a long time. A major breakthrough in the diagnosis of mastocytosis occurred in 2000 when a group of experts convened in Vienna and established diagnostic criteria based on objective pathologic findings. The recommendations of this consensus group were later adopted by the World Health Organization and formed the basis of our current diagnostic criteria. These guidelines introduced the concept of minor criteria that did not require the presence of large aggregates of mast cells in the bone marrow, which was the gold standard of diagnosis until that time. It suddenly became possible to diagnose mastocytosis in many new patients who did not have urticaria pigmentosa or large bone marrow aggregates of mast cells. Subsequent studies proved that mastocytosis was the underlying diagnosis in a considerable subset of patients with recurrent "idiopathic anaphylaxis" and anaphylactic reactions to hymenoptera venom. The increased awareness of mastocytosis along with expanded clinical availability of diagnostic testing such as D816V c-kit mutational analysis and serum tryptase levels resulted in increasing diagnoses. Today, referral centers for mastocytosis often evaluate patients in whom the diagnosis of mastocytosis was not recognized for many years as well as those with inappropriate diagnoses not meeting the World Health Organization criteria. Therefore, an educational gap still seems to remain in terms of when to suspect the diagnosis and how to order and interpret the correct diagnostic testing.

The authors of this issue were mainly chosen from an international group of experts who got together in Boston in 2011 to discuss and update the diagnostic criteria, classification, and recommendations on various other clinical aspects of disease. I would like to thank all of them for their valuable contributions of their expertise and time to this issue. I would also like to gratefully acknowledge the support of our individual patients and patient support groups in our quest to improve our understanding of the disease and ultimately to find better treatment options. Finally, I would like to thank Dr Rafeul Alam for his continued interest in mastocytosis and for inviting me to edit this issue. Patients with mastocytosis can present to a wide variety of medical specialists

Immunol Allergy Clin N Am 34 (2014) xvii–xviii
http://dx.doi.org/10.1016/j.iac.2014.02.005
0889-8561/14/$ – see front matter © 2014 Elsevier Inc. All rights reserved.

including allergists, internists, pediatricians, gastroenterologists, endocrinologists, hematologists, oncologists, orthopedic surgeons, dermatologists, and neurologists. I hope that this issue of the *Immunology and Allergy Clinics of North America* proves valuable in updating the current state of knowledge not only for allergists but also for all physicians and patients who would like to gain more information on mastocytosis.

Cem Akin, MD, PhD
Harvard Medical School
Mastocytosis Center
Brigham and Women's Hospital
Boston, MA 02115, USA

E-mail address:
cakin@partners.org

Erratum

An error was made in the February 2014 issue of *Immunology and Allergy Clinics,* Vol. 34, No. 1, on pages 73 and 141. One of the authors of "Physical Urticarias and Cholinergic Urticaria" and "Urticarial Vasculitis and Schnitzler Syndrome" was incorrectly listed as H.C. Torsten Zuberbier, MD. The author's correct name is Torsten Zuberbier, MD.

Immunol Allergy Clin N Am 34 (2014) xix
http://dx.doi.org/10.1016/j.iac.2014.01.007
0889-8561/14/$ – see front matter © 2014 Elsevier Inc. All rights reserved.

immunology.theclinics.com

Diagnostic Criteria and Classification of Mastocytosis in 2014

Cem Akin, MD, PhD[a],*, Peter Valent, MD[b]

KEYWORDS

- Mastocytosis • Diagnosis • Classification • World Health Organization • c-kit
- Tryptase

KEY POINTS

- The diagnosis of mastocytosis in skin is established by presence of characteristic maculopapular skin lesions and confirmed by skin biopsy.
- Systemic mastocytosis should be diagnosed based on World Health Organization (WHO) criteria. Presence of unexplained symptoms of mast cell activation should prompt the pathologic investigation; however, the diagnosis cannot be based on symptoms alone.
- According to WHO, mastocytosis is classified into 7 categories, with distinct clinicopathologic and prognostic features that guide the therapy.
- Tryptase level greater than 20 ng/mL is associated with systemic mastocytosis. However, lower tryptase levels can be seen in patients with cutaneous mastocytosis, monoclonal mast cell activation syndrome, and systemic mastocytosis with limited bone marrow involvement.
- More than 90% of adults and 80% of children with mastocytosis are detected to have somatic gain of function mutations in c-kit. In most patients with systemic mastocytosis, the c-kit mutation D816V is detectable.

DEFINITION AND OVERVIEW OF CATEGORIES

Mastocytosis is a disorder characterized by accumulation of pathologic mast cells in tissues, which is accompanied by symptoms of mast cell activation in most patients.[1–4] Most commonly affected tissues are skin, bone marrow, and gastrointestinal tract, followed by liver, spleen, and lymph nodes. Mastocytosis can affect both children and adults. In children, it commonly presents with skin lesions of urticaria

---

Conflict of Interest Disclosure: Dr C. Akin has a consultancy agreement with Novartis.
[a] Harvard Medical School, Director, Mastocytosis Center, Brigham and Women's Hospital, Harvard Medical School, 1 Jimmy Fund Way, Room 626B, Boston, MA 02115, USA; [b] Division of Hematology and Hemostaseology, Department of Internal Medicine I and Ludwig Boltzmann Cluster Oncology, Medical University of Vienna, Währinger Gürtel 18-20, A-1090, Vienna, Austria
* Corresponding author.
E-mail address: cakin@partners.org

Immunol Allergy Clin N Am 34 (2014) 207–218
http://dx.doi.org/10.1016/j.iac.2014.02.003
0889-8561/14/$ – see front matter © 2014 Elsevier Inc. All rights reserved.
immunology.theclinics.com

pigmentosa (UP) or mastocytomas within the first year of life.[5-7] Mastocytosis diagnosed in infancy has a good prognosis; there is no evidence of pathologic mast cell accumulation in tissues other than skin (cutaneous mastocytosis), and most patients experience resolution or fading of skin lesions by adolescence. In contrast, adult-onset mastocytosis is almost always associated with bone marrow involvement and has a persistent course. When mastocytosis is present in any extracutaneous tissue (proved by biopsy) and shows multifocal or diffuse organ infiltration, it is termed systemic mastocytosis (SM). SM is a heterogeneous group of disorders with variable prognosis.[8] Most patients have indolent SM (ISM), meaning that bone marrow examination shows abnormal mast cell collections but no other hematologic disease, and there is no evidence of end-organ damage attributable to mast cell infiltration. Patients with ISM have a comparable life expectancy with the general age-matched population.[9-11] Up to 20% of patients with SM may have a second bone marrow disease, usually with myeloproliferative or myelodysplastic features. These patients have SM associated with a hematologic non–mast cell clonal disease (SM-AHNMD). The prognosis in these patients depends on the course of the AHNMD.[10] A few patients (approximately 5%) have evidence of end-organ damage caused by mast cell infiltration (aggressive SM [ASM]), in whom the disease follows an accelerated course resembling a malignancy.[12,13] Mast cell leukemia (MCL) is a rare subset of SM, which is diagnosed when mast cells in bone marrow aspirate smears are greater than 20%.[14,15] In several of these cases, circulating mast cells are found. Mast cell sarcoma (MCS) and extracutaneous mastocytosis are extremely rare variants with solid mast cell tumors, bearing malignant and benign pathologic features, respectively.[16]

DIAGNOSIS

Mastocytosis commonly comes to clinical attention in one of the following clinical scenarios:

1. The patient (or parents if the patient is a child) notices the hyperpigmented skin lesions of UP (or mastocytoma in a child). Sometimes, these lesions may be noticed in dermatology evaluations for other purposes rather than by patients themselves, because they may resemble freckles earlier in the course.
2. The patient presents with symptoms of mast cell activation such as recurrent flushing, hypotension, near syncope or syncope, abdominal cramps, and diarrhea. Anaphylaxis is suspected, but an allergy evaluation often does not identify a culprit. A variation of this presentation involves patients who experience severe systemic reactions to Hymenoptera stings. Curiously, urticaria and angioedema are not commonly seen in mast cell activation episodes in mastocytosis.
3. The patient is detected to have hematologic abnormalities such as cytopenias or increased white blood or platelet counts, liver or spleen enlargement, fatigue, and weight loss, prompting a hematologic workup.
4. The patient may be detected to have sclerotic or lytic bone lesions in imaging studies, raising concern for metastatic disease.
5. A rare first presentation is osteoporosis and pathologic bone fractures (commonly vertebral compression fractures). This finding should raise suspicion in younger patients (especially males) who do not otherwise have any risk factors for osteoporosis.
6. The patient is referred because of nonspecific gastrointestinal symptoms suggestive of colitis and unexplained splenomegaly, and the hematologic evaluation shows mastocytosis.

7. The patient has been diagnosed with a myelodysplastic syndrome, acute myeloid leukemia (AML), or chronic myelomonocytic leukemia (CMML), and the molecular workup showed a c-kit mutation. In these cases, no histology was available or the pathologist had overlooked SM.

The first step in all patients who are suspected to have mastocytosis is a thorough skin examination to detect typical skin lesions (UP type). These lesions range in size from a few millimeters to a few centimeters and have a brownish hyperpigmentation along with a hyperemic component. The lesions are fixed and do not appear and disappear at different locations like classic urticarial wheals. They are usually nonpruritic at baseline but may be triggered to urticate with friction, temperature changes, fever, emotional or physical stress, exercise, alcohol, and spicy foods. Stroking of the lesion results in a wheal localized to the lesion (Darier sign); however, some patients may lack this sign if they are on H_1 antihistamines. Skin lesions in young children may not be hyperpigmented and may show blistering in the first 3 years of life. Although most experts can diagnose UP-like skin lesions on visual inspection, skin biopsy may confirm the diagnosis of mastocytosis (in the skin) in suspected cases. In these patients, skin biopsy shows a perivascular mast cell infiltrate in the upper dermis. Some scattered eosinophils may be mixed with the infiltrate, but other inflammatory cells are typically absent. Increased melanin deposition is noted in epidermis. Mastocytomas are typically solitary and larger lesions with histologic evidence of a solid mast cell tumor. Physical irritation of mastocytomas may cause systemic symptoms, such as hives. Teleangiectasia macularis eruptive perstans is a rare manifestation of cutaneous mastocytosis, in which the skin has flat teleangiactatic macules in a generalized distribution. Skin lesions in adults generally spare sun-exposed areas, such as face and hands, and tend to aggregate in areas prone to irritation, such as upper thighs and axillae. However, it is not uncommon to have lesions on scalp, face, and neck in young children.

After visualization of skin lesions, the patient is said to have mastocytosis in the skin, and a decision has to be made whether a bone marrow biopsy is necessary to look for evidence (criteria) of systemic mastocytosis or to classify the patient as having cutaneous mastocytosis if bone marrow histopathology is normal or criteria for SM are not fulfilled. A simple guide for this decision is the patient's age. Children in whom the skin lesions start in the first 2 years of life rarely have bone marrow involvement, and these children are presumed to have cutaneous mastocytosis. A bone marrow biopsy in children is not routinely recommended unless the child has a persistently high serum tryptase level (or shows an increasing trend in serial measurements) or has abnormal complete blood count or liver or spleen enlargement. In contrast, most patients with adult-onset disease have evidence of bone marrow involvement when skin lesions are detected, and therefore, a bone marrow biopsy is recommended to establish the diagnosis of SM, to assess bone marrow mast cell burden, and to rule out presence of other hematologic disease.

Therefore, a bone marrow biopsy is recommended in adult patients presenting with skin lesions of UP type as well as those presenting with clinical scenarios 2 to 5, outlined earlier. Biopsy of tissues other than bone marrow is not recommended to establish a diagnosis, because bone marrow is always involved, and the histopathologic aspects of mast cell disease are not well studied in other tissues. Gastrointestinal biopsies are sometimes needed to establish the cause of symptoms such as diarrhea and malabsorption, whether they are caused by mast cell infiltration or simply caused by systemic effects of mast cell mediator release, and a subset of patients were first diagnosed on gastrointestinal biopsies by astute pathologists.[17]

Diagnosis of SM is made according to the World Health Organization (WHO) criteria (**Box 1**). These criteria were established by an international group of experts in a consensus meeting in Vienna in 2000.[18–20] Until that time, the diagnosis was mainly made by visualization of large aggregates of mast cells in bone marrow and subjective assessment of increased mast cell numbers in tissues. The Vienna conference retained the mast cell aggregates as the major diagnostic criterion but also introduced the concept of minor criteria. Thus, the modern diagnostic criteria include 1 major and 4 minor criteria, as outlined in the following sections. The patient needs to have either the major and at least 1 minor, or 3 minor criteria, to diagnose SM.

Major Criterion

Multifocal dense aggregates of mast cells with more than 15 cells per aggregate in an extracutaneous tissue. The tissue of choice in diagnosis is bone marrow. Both a biopsy and an aspirate should be obtained. Biopsy should be of good quality without significant crush or bleeding artifact. Formalin-fixed, paraffin-embedded bone marrow biopsy sections should be stained for tryptase, CD117 and CD25 in addition to routine hematoxylin-eosin stains. In normal bone marrow, mast cells are distributed interstitially and singly, with a predominantly round shape. Although even a small clustering of mast cells should raise suspicion for mastocytosis, to meet the major criterion, the clusters should contain at least 15 mast cells. Mast cell clusters in mastocytosis occur paratrabecularly, perivascularly, or interstitially. Sometimes, a spindle-shaped infiltrate is observed to line the bone trabeculae. Eosinophils are frequently found in increased numbers around the infiltrate. Some samples may have a polytypic lymphocytic infiltrate around or within the lesions.[21,22] Patients with smoldering or ASM or MCL often have a high degree of involvement in bone marrow biopsy (>30%), with associated marked fibrosis. The cells have spindle shapes, oval and eccentric nuclei with pale cytoplasm in hematoxylin-eosin staining. Tryptase stain confirms the nature of the infiltrate as mast cells.

Minor Criteria

1. More than 25% of the cells have morphologic abnormalities such as spindle shapes, hypogranulation, eccentric nuclei, cytoplasmic projections, and multilobed

---

Box 1
Diagnostic criteria of SM

Major

Multifocal dense aggregates of mast cells with more than 15 cells per aggregate in an extracutaneous tissue

Minor

1. Greater than 25% of mast cells have morphologic abnormalities such as spindle shapes, cytoplasmic projections, hypogranulation (see text)

2. Expression of CD25 with or without CD2 by mast cells

3. Detection of a codon 816 c-kit mutation by a sensitive technique in lesional tissue or peripheral blood

4. Serum baseline tryptase greater than 20 ng/mL[a]

  [a] Not valid if there is AHNMD.
Data from Refs.[18–20]; see text for more detailed discussion; major +1 minor, or 3 minor, criteria are required.

or clefted nuclei.[23,24] Normal bone marrow mast cells have round cytoplasm, with a centrally located nucleus and dense granulation. In bone marrow aspirate smears, mast cells are usually located in or near bone spicules. The percentage of mast cells in bone marrow aspirate smears has been shown to correlate with advanced mastocytosis and prognosis. If mast cell percentage is greater than 20% in an aspicular area, the diagnosis is MCL. Mast cells of less than 5% are generally seen in ISM, whereas mast cells between 5% and 19% signify an intermediate prognosis,[23] which is often the case in ASM, and termed ASM in transformation (ASM-t), because these cases often progress to MCL.[15]

2. Mast cells aberrantly express CD25 and CD2.[25,26] Normal or reactive mast cells usually do not express these markers. CD25 is more sensitive and specific than CD2.[27,28] Expression of these markers can be detected by immunohistochemistry (IHC) or flow cytometry. IHC has the advantage of being applicable to archived paraffin-embedded samples.[29] Serial sections should be stained for tryptase to detect coexpression of CD25 in mast cells. CD2 staining does not always yield positive results, especially in advanced disease. Flow cytometry is also a sensitive and reliable method of detecting aberrant mast cell marker expression, if it is performed in reference centers with expertise on this technique. Because the mast cell percentage of the marrow aspirate is usually low (in many cases <1%), special gating techniques and acquisition of many events (at least 500,000 or preferably higher) are required for an accurate analysis.[26,30]

3. Using a sensitive technique, c-kit point mutation at codon 816 is detectable in peripheral blood or lesional tissue.[31–34] Detailed accounts of c-kit mutations in mastocytosis in pathogenesis of mastocytosis and their roles in altered signal transduction are discussed in other articles by Cruse and colleagues, Arock and colleagues in this issue. D816V c-kit mutation is detectable in more than 80% of patients with SM in bone marrow mast cells[34,35] and in approximately 40% of children with cutaneous mastocytosis in lesional skin.[36] Analysis of peripheral blood may yield false-negative results in most commercially available tests, because of the somatic nature of the mutation, although recently introduced polymerase chain reaction–based sensitive tests approach the sensitivity in bone marrow sorted mast cells.[33] Mutation may be confined to mast cells in patients with indolent disease, whereas it may involve multiple other myeloid and even lymphoid lineages in patients with advanced disease.[35,37,38] Patients with multilineage involvement were shown to have a higher risk of progression to aggressive mastocytosis and carry a poorer prognosis. c-kit D816V mutation renders the mast cells resistant to the currently available tyrosine kinase inhibitors, including matinib.[39–41]

4. Serum tryptase greater than 20 ng/mL.[42–46] Normal median tryptase level in the healthy population is 5 ng/mL. Mast cells are the major source of the neutral protease tryptase. Basophils and myeloid progenitors also produce smaller amounts of this enzyme. Therefore, tryptase levels may be increased in other myeloid neoplastic processes and do not count as a minor criterion in SM-AHNMD.[47] Commercially available tryptase assay uses an enzyme-linked immunosorbent assay method to measure a combination of mature tryptases and protryptases. Mature tryptase (β tryptase) is stored in mast cell granules and is released after a mast cell degranulation or anaphylactic event, with peak levels found in approximately 1 hour after the degranulation. β Tryptase levels are undetectable in sera from healthy individuals. In contrast, protryptases (mainly encoded by α tryptase) are targeted to cell membrane and constitutively secreted out of the mast cells. Therefore, the total tryptase level at baseline reflects α (pro) tryptase and correlates with total body mast cell burden. A basal tryptase level less than 20 ng/mL does not

rule out mastocytosis, whereas slight tryptase increases greater than 20 ng/mL can be seen in individuals other than those with mastocytosis (including those with renal disease, myeloid neoplasms, and idiopathic) and even in apparently healthy controls. Therefore, tryptase levels alone should not be used as the sole criterion to diagnose mastocytosis.

Some patients with mast cell activation symptoms and lower tryptase levels may not meet the full WHO criteria for the diagnosis of mastocytosis but may have CD25+ mast cells in bone marrow biopsies or have the c-kit D816V mutation detectable.[48–50] These patients meeting only 1 or 2 minor criteria are termed to have monoclonal mast cell activation syndrome (MMAS). It is not clear whether patients with MMAS progress to full-blown mastocytosis with time.

A rare histopathologic variant of SM termed well-differentiated SM (WDSM) is characterized by aggregates of mast cells with round shapes and fully granulated morphology with no CD25 expression.[51] Aberrant CD30 expression may be a useful marker for these patients, who generally have childhood-onset mastocytosis with skin lesions and progress to have adult-onset systemic disease.[52,53] Most patients with WDSM do not carry the D816V c-kit mutation and thus may respond to imatinib.[54] The WDSM morphology may be found in patients with ISM but can sometimes also be found in patients with advanced SM requiring therapy. Therefore also, the term WDSM should be used as a descriptive appendix to the final diagnosis, for example, ISM-WDSM, ASM-WDSM, or ASM with WDSM morphology. Sometimes, it is nearly impossible to differentiate between WDSM and reactive mast cell hyperplasia.

CLASSIFICATION

The WHO classification divides mastocytosis into 7 categories (**Box 2**). A major checkpoint in classification of mastocytosis is to determine whether the patient has cutaneous mastocytosis or SM. This determination correlates with the age of onset of disease and is defined by histopathologic criteria, as discussed earlier. If a diagnosis of SM is made, the next step is to classify the disease into 1 of 4 categories of SM.

1. ISM. Most patients with adult-onset disease fall into this category. Patients with ISM satisfy the WHO diagnostic criteria for SM but do not have other hematologic

---

Box 2
Classification of mastocytosis

- Cutaneous mastocytosis
- ISM
- Smoldering SM[a]
- SM-AHNMD
- ASM
- MCL
- MCS
- Extracutaneous mastocytoma

[a] The smoldering subtype of SM has recently been accepted as a separate category by the consensus group, but was not implemented as such in the WHO classification of 2008.

disorders or evidence of tissue dysfunction caused by mast cell infiltration. Prognosis of ISM is good, with chance of progression to one of the more advanced categories being less than 5%. Patients with ISM often have chronic symptoms of mast cell degranulation, such as flushing, pruritus, abdominal cramps, and diarrhea, and usually require symptomatic management with antimediator therapy. The risks of hypotensive anaphylaxis[55–57] and osteoporosis[58] are increased. A substantial subset of patients who experience systemic allergic reactions to Hymenoptera stings have been described as having ISM or MMAS.[59,60]

A WHO subvariant of ISM called smoldering SM is characterized by increased mast cell burden (>30% infiltration in bone marrow biopsy and tryptase levels >200 ng/mL) and may have splenomegaly or hepatomegaly without significant organ impairment and subtle dysplastic changes not meeting the full criteria of another hematologic disease or ASM (B findings).[61–63] These patients may be at a higher risk of progression to a more advanced category. WHO has included this variant as a subcategory of ISM. However, more recently, the smoldering type of SM has been recognized as a major defined category of SM, with unique clinical and molecular features. The key molecular feature is the clonal multilineage involvement, which can be shown by the presence of KIT D816V in various hematopoietic lineages.

2. SM-AHNMD. These patients meet the criteria for SM as well as a second hematologic disorder. The associated hematologic disorder is usually myeloid: myelodysplastic syndromes, CMML, myeloproliferative disorders (including those associated with JAK2 V617F mutation), and AML have all been described.[10,64] Lymphoproliferative disorders such as non-Hodgkin lymphoma and myeloma have also been occasionally described.[65,66] The SM component in SM-AHNMD may be indolent or aggressive, and each component should be diagnosed and treated according to its own treatment guidelines.

3. ASM. This category of mastocytosis has a clinical course similar to other malignancies leading to organ damage and is associated with poor prognosis. The symptoms are caused by extensive mast cell infiltration, causing tissue dysfunction (C findings).[18–20] Tissues involved in ASM include hematopoietic, gastrointestinal, and skeletal systems.[12] Pulmonary, renal, and central nervous system involvement is rare. C findings include cytopenias (absolute neutrophil count <1000/μL, hemoglobin <10 g/dL, platelets <100,00/μL) with a high degree of bone marrow involvement (usually >30%) or splenomegaly, increased levels in liver function tests with evidence of portal hypertension or ascites, extensive gastrointestinal infiltration documented by biopsy accompanied by malabsorption, hypoalbuminemia, weight loss and chronic diarrhea, or large osteolytic lesions with pathologic bone fractures. The last finding should not be confused by osteoporosis and resulting vertebral compression fractures, which are common in indolent mastocytosis. The local mast cell infiltration should be documented whenever possible. Tryptase levels in ASM are usually higher than 100 ng/mL and often increase rapidly over time.[67] In some of these patients, progression to MCL is seen within a few months. These cases may suffer from ASM-t, a condition defined by a mast cell count of 5% to 19% in bone marrow smears. Patients with ASM are candidates for mast cell cytoreductive or investigational therapies. In this regard, many patients with ASM have concomitant AHNMD (ASM-AHNMD). In these cases, the overall treatment plan has to be adapted to both conditions.

4. MCL. Mast cells are not components of normal peripheral blood. MCL is defined by a mast cell count of 20% or greater in bone marrow smears.[15] Although some mast cells in circulation can be detected in ASM, presence of 10% or more mast cells in

peripheral blood is highly suspicious (diagnostic) for MCL. In aleukemic variants of MCL, bone marrow aspirate smears contain 20% or more mast cells in aspicular areas, but circulating mast cells are less than 10%. Mast cells in MCL have high-grade morphology, with significant degranulation, multilobular or clefted nuclei, and may even show mitotic figures. Serum tryptase is often significantly increased and may be found greater than 500 or even greater than 1000 ng/mL. MCL may occur de novo or occasionally develop secondary to other mast cell disease categories, such as ASM. MCL has a poor prognosis, and patients often have C findings at diagnosis or develop them shortly thereafter, although a chronic form with a relatively stable course over several years has been recognized.[14] Similar to ASM, patients with MCL require cytoreductive and investigational therapies. In many cases, polychemotherapy is recommended, and in those who show a good response, stem cell transplantation has to be considered.

MCS is a rare malignant form of solid mast cell tumor with destructive infiltration and metastatic potential.[16] This issue contains an excellent review article by Weiler and Butterfield on all cases of this tumor published in the literature. MCS may progress to MCL within a short period. Skin involvement has also been described and was reported to develop in the background of UP. Extracutaneous mastocytoma is an exceedingly rare benign mast cell tumor, and the clinical experience is limited to a few case reports.[68]

SUMMARY

The current diagnostic criteria and classification of mastocytosis are well validated by clinical studies and have been shown to correlate with prognosis and to guide in the selection of therapy. As new knowledge is gained regarding clinical course, molecular pathogenesis and therapy for disease, evidence-based revisions to improve the current criteria should be considered by international consensus. Using the guidelines in this article, it should be straightforward to establish a diagnosis of mastocytosis in most cases. Cases with low mast cell burden or uncertain diagnostic interpretation should be referred to centers of expertise. In Europe, centers of excellence have been organized under the umbrella of the European Competence Network on Mastocytosis (http://www.ecnm.net). Although no similar organization exists in the United States, there are several centers of excellence, including the Brigham and Women's Hospital, Stanford, Mayo Clinic, MD Anderson, and National Institutes of Health. It is the hope for the future that these centers will develop and merge as a robust collaborative competence network in the United States. The patient support groups, such as the Mastocytosis Society, also provide valuable education and organize yearly meetings (http://www.tmsforacure.org/) and should thereby support academic studies and networking in this emerging field of science.

REFERENCES

1. Akin C, Metcalfe DD. Systemic mastocytosis. Annu Rev Med 2004;55:419.
2. Metcalfe DD. Mast cells and mastocytosis. Blood 2008;112:946.
3. Valent P, Akin C, Sperr WR, et al. Mastocytosis: pathology, genetics, and current options for therapy. Leuk Lymphoma 2005;46:35.
4. Arock M, Valent P. Pathogenesis, classification and treatment of mastocytosis: state of the art in 2010 and future perspectives. Expert Rev Hematol 2010;3:497.
5. Fried AJ, Akin C. Primary mast cell disorders in children. Curr Allergy Asthma Rep 2013;13:693.

6. Castells M, Metcalfe DD, Escribano L. Diagnosis and treatment of cutaneous mastocytosis in children: practical recommendations. Am J Clin Dermatol 2011;12:259.
7. Carter MC, Metcalfe DD. Paediatric mastocytosis. Arch Dis Child 2002;86:315.
8. Pardanani A, Tefferi A. Systemic mastocytosis in adults: a review on prognosis and treatment based on 342 Mayo Clinic patients and current literature. Curr Opin Hematol 2010;17:125.
9. Pardanani A, Lim KH, Lasho TL, et al. WHO subvariants of indolent mastocytosis: clinical details and prognostic evaluation in 159 consecutive adults. Blood 2010;115:150.
10. Pardanani A, Lim KH, Lasho TL, et al. Prognostically relevant breakdown of 123 patients with systemic mastocytosis associated with other myeloid malignancies. Blood 2009;114:3769.
11. Escribano L, Alvarez-Twose I, Sanchez-Munoz L, et al. Prognosis in adult indolent systemic mastocytosis: a long-term study of the Spanish Network on Mastocytosis in a series of 145 patients. J Allergy Clin Immunol 2009;124:514.
12. Valent P, Akin C, Sperr WR, et al. Aggressive systemic mastocytosis and related mast cell disorders: current treatment options and proposed response criteria. Leuk Res 2003;27:635.
13. Valent P, Sperr WR, Akin C. How I treat patients with advanced systemic mastocytosis. Blood 2010;116:5812.
14. Georgin-Lavialle S, Lhermitte L, Dubreuil P, et al. Mast cell leukemia. Blood 2013;121:1285.
15. Valent P, Sotlar K, Sperr WR, et al. Refined diagnostic criteria and classification of mast cell leukemia (MCL) and myelomastocytic leukemia (MML): a consensus proposal. Ann Oncol, in press.
16. Ryan RJ, Akin C, Castells M, et al. Mast cell sarcoma: a rare and potentially under-recognized diagnostic entity with specific therapeutic implications. Mod Pathol 2013;26:533.
17. Hahn HP, Hornick JL. Immunoreactivity for CD25 in gastrointestinal mucosal mast cells is specific for systemic mastocytosis. Am J Surg Pathol 2007;31:1669.
18. Valent P, Horny HP, Escribano L, et al. Diagnostic criteria and classification of mastocytosis: a consensus proposal. Leuk Res 2001;25:603.
19. Valent P, Horny HP, Li CY, et al. Mastocytosis. In: Jaffe ES, Harris NL, Stein H, et al, editors. World Health Organization (WHO) classification of tumours. Pathology and genetics. Tumours of haematopoietic and lymphoid tissues. Lyon (France): IARC Press; 2001. p. 291.
20. Horny HP, Metcalfe DD, Bennett JM, et al. Mastocytosis. In: Swerdlow SH, Campo E, Harris NL, et al, editors. WHO classification of tumours of haematopoietic and lymphoid tissues, vol. 2, 4th edition. Lyon (France): IARC Press; 2008. p. 54.
21. Akin C, Jaffe ES, Raffeld M, et al. An immunohistochemical study of the bone marrow lesions of systemic mastocytosis: expression of stem cell factor by lesional mast cells. Am J Clin Pathol 2002;118:242.
22. Horny HP, Lange K, Sotlar K, et al. Increase of bone marrow lymphocytes in systemic mastocytosis: reactive lymphocytosis or malignant lymphoma? Immunohistochemical and molecular findings on routinely processed bone marrow biopsy specimens. J Clin Pathol 2003;56:575.
23. Sperr WR, Escribano L, Jordan JH, et al. Morphologic properties of neoplastic mast cells: delineation of stages of maturation and implication for cytological grading of mastocytosis. Leuk Res 2001;25:529.

24. Horny HP, Valent P. Diagnosis of mastocytosis: general histopathological aspects, morphological criteria, and immunohistochemical findings. Leuk Res 2001;25:543.

25. Escribano L, Orfao A, Diaz-Agustin B, et al. Indolent systemic mast cell disease in adults: immunophenotypic characterization of bone marrow mast cells and its diagnostic implications. Blood 1998;91:2731.

26. Escribano L, Diaz-Agustin B, Lopez A, et al. Immunophenotypic analysis of mast cells in mastocytosis: when and how to do it. Proposals of the Spanish Network on Mastocytosis (REMA). Cytometry B Clin Cytom 2004;58:1.

27. Morgado JM, Sanchez-Munoz L, Teodosio CG, et al. Immunophenotyping in systemic mastocytosis diagnosis: 'CD25 positive' alone is more informative than the 'CD25 and/or CD2' WHO criterion. Mod Pathol 2012;25:516.

28. Pardanani A, Kimlinger TK, Reeder TL, et al. Differential expression of CD2 on neoplastic mast cells in patients with systemic mast cell disease with and without an associated clonal haematological disorder. Br J Haematol 2003; 120:691.

29. Sotlar K, Horny HP, Simonitsch I, et al. CD25 indicates the neoplastic phenotype of mast cells: a novel immunohistochemical marker for the diagnosis of systemic mastocytosis (SM) in routinely processed bone marrow biopsy specimens. Am J Surg Pathol 2004;28:1319.

30. Akin C, Valent P, Escribano L. Urticaria pigmentosa and mastocytosis: the role of immunophenotyping in diagnosis and determining response to treatment. Curr Allergy Asthma Rep 2006;6:282.

31. Nagata H, Worobec AS, Oh CK, et al. Identification of a point mutation in the catalytic domain of the protooncogene c-kit in peripheral blood mononuclear cells of patients who have mastocytosis with an associated hematologic disorder. Proc Natl Acad Sci U S A 1995;92:10560.

32. Longley BJ, Tyrrell L, Lu SZ, et al. Somatic c-KIT activating mutation in urticaria pigmentosa and aggressive mastocytosis: establishment of clonality in a human mast cell neoplasm. Nat Genet 1996;12:312.

33. Kristensen T, Vestergaard H, Bindslev-Jensen C, et al. Sensitive KIT D816V mutation analysis of blood as a diagnostic test in mastocytosis. Am J Hematol 2014 Jan 20. [Epub ahead of print]. http://dx.doi.org/10.1002/ajh.23672.

34. Akin C. Molecular diagnosis of mast cell disorders: a paper from the 2005 William Beaumont Hospital Symposium on Molecular Pathology. J Mol Diagn 2006;8:412.

35. Teodosio C, Garcia-Montero AC, Jara-Acevedo M, et al. An immature immunophenotype of bone marrow mast cells predicts for multilineage D816V KIT mutation in systemic mastocytosis. Leukemia 2012;26:951.

36. Bodemer C, Hermine O, Palmerini F, et al. Pediatric mastocytosis is a clonal disease associated with D816V and other activating c-KIT mutations. J Invest Dermatol 2010;130:804.

37. Akin C, Kirshenbaum AS, Semere T, et al. Analysis of the surface expression of c-kit and occurrence of the c-kit Asp816Val activating mutation in T cells, B cells, and myelomonocytic cells in patients with mastocytosis. Exp Hematol 2000;28:140.

38. Akin C. Multilineage hematopoietic involvement in systemic mastocytosis. Leuk Res 2003;27:877.

39. Akin C, Metcalfe DD. The biology of Kit in disease and the application of pharmacogenetics. J Allergy Clin Immunol 2004;114:13.

40. Ma Y, Zeng S, Metcalfe DD, et al. The c-KIT mutation causing human mastocytosis is resistant to STI571 and other KIT kinase inhibitors; kinases with enzymatic site

mutations show different inhibitor sensitivity profiles than wild-type kinases and those with regulatory-type mutations. Blood 2002;99:1741.

41. Akin C, Brockow K, D'Ambrosio C, et al. Effects of tyrosine kinase inhibitor STI571 on human mast cells bearing wild-type or mutated c-kit. Exp Hematol 2003;31:686.

42. Schwartz LB. Clinical utility of tryptase levels in systemic mastocytosis and associated hematologic disorders. Leuk Res 2001;25:553.

43. Schwartz LB. Diagnostic value of tryptase in anaphylaxis and mastocytosis. Immunol Allergy Clin North Am 2006;26:451.

44. Schwartz LB, Irani AM. Serum tryptase and the laboratory diagnosis of systemic mastocytosis. Hematol Oncol Clin North Am 2000;14:641.

45. Schwartz LB, Metcalfe DD, Miller JS, et al. Tryptase levels as an indicator of mast-cell activation in systemic anaphylaxis and mastocytosis. N Engl J Med 1987;316:1622.

46. Schwartz LB, Sakai K, Bradford TR, et al. The alpha form of human tryptase is the predominant type present in blood at baseline in normal subjects and is elevated in those with systemic mastocytosis. J Clin Invest 1995;96:2702.

47. Sperr WR, El-Samahi A, Kundi M, et al. Elevated tryptase levels selectively cluster in myeloid neoplasms: a novel diagnostic approach and screen marker in clinical haematology. Eur J Clin Invest 2009;39:914.

48. Akin C, Scott LM, Kocabas CN, et al. Demonstration of an aberrant mast-cell population with clonal markers in a subset of patients with "idiopathic" anaphylaxis. Blood 2007;110:2331.

49. Akin C, Valent P, Metcalfe DD. Mast cell activation syndrome: proposed diagnostic criteria. J Allergy Clin Immunol 2010;126:1099.

50. Valent P, Akin C, Escribano L, et al. Standards and standardization in mastocytosis: consensus statements on diagnostics, treatment recommendations and response criteria. Eur J Clin Invest 2007;37:435.

51. Akin C, Fumo G, Yavuz AS, et al. A novel form of mastocytosis associated with a transmembrane c-kit mutation and response to imatinib. Blood 2004; 103:3222.

52. Morgado JM, Perbellini O, Johnson RC, et al. CD30 expression by bone marrow mast cells from different diagnostic variants of systemic mastocytosis. Histopathology 2013;63:780.

53. Teodosio C, Garcia-Montero AC, Jara-Acevedo M, et al. Mast cells from different molecular and prognostic subtypes of systemic mastocytosis display distinct immunophenotypes. J Allergy Clin Immunol 2010;125:719.

54. Alvarez-Twose I, Gonzalez P, Morgado JM, et al. Complete response after imatinib mesylate therapy in a patient with well-differentiated systemic mastocytosis. J Clin Oncol 2012;30:e126.

55. Akin C. Anaphylaxis and mast cell disease: what is the risk? Curr Allergy Asthma Rep 2010;10:34.

56. Brockow K, Jofer C, Behrendt H, et al. Anaphylaxis in patients with mastocytosis: a study on history, clinical features and risk factors in 120 patients. Allergy 2008;63:226.

57. Gulen T, Hagglund H, Dahlen B, et al. High prevalence of anaphylaxis in patients with systemic mastocytosis–a single-centre experience. Clin Exp Allergy 2014;44:121.

58. van der Veer E, van der Goot W, de Monchy JG, et al. High prevalence of fractures and osteoporosis in patients with indolent systemic mastocytosis. Allergy 2012;67:431.

59. Bonadonna P, Perbellini O, Passalacqua G, et al. Clonal mast cell disorders in patients with systemic reactions to Hymenoptera stings and increased serum tryptase levels. J Allergy Clin Immunol 2009;123:680.

60. Alvarez-Twose I, Bonadonna P, Matito A, et al. Systemic mastocytosis as a risk factor for severe Hymenoptera sting-induced anaphylaxis. J Allergy Clin Immunol 2013;131:614.

61. Akin C, Scott LM, Metcalfe DD. Slowly progressive systemic mastocytosis with high mast-cell burden and no evidence of a non-mast-cell hematologic disorder: an example of a smoldering case? Leuk Res 2001;25:635.

62. Jordan JH, Fritsche-Polanz R, Sperr WR, et al. A case of 'smouldering' mastocytosis with high mast cell burden, monoclonal myeloid cells, and C-KIT mutation Asp-816-Val. Leuk Res 2001;25:627.

63. Valent P, Akin C, Sperr WR, et al. Smouldering mastocytosis: a novel subtype of systemic mastocytosis with slow progression. Int Arch Allergy Immunol 2002; 127:137.

64. Sperr WR, Horny HP, Valent P. Spectrum of associated clonal hematologic non-mast cell lineage disorders occurring in patients with systemic mastocytosis. Int Arch Allergy Immunol 2002;127:140.

65. Kluin-Nelemans HC, Ferenc V, van Doormaal JJ, et al. Lenalidomide therapy in systemic mastocytosis. Leuk Res 2009;33:e19.

66. Du S, Rashidi HH, Le DT, et al. Systemic mastocytosis in association with chronic lymphocytic leukemia and plasma cell myeloma. Int J Clin Exp Pathol 2010;3:448.

67. Sperr WR, Jordan JH, Fiegl M, et al. Serum tryptase levels in patients with mastocytosis: correlation with mast cell burden and implication for defining the category of disease. Int Arch Allergy Immunol 2002;128:136.

68. Castells MC. Extracutaneous mastocytoma. J Allergy Clin Immunol 2006;117:1513.

Functional Deregulation of KIT

Link to Mast Cell Proliferative Diseases and Other Neoplasms

Glenn Cruse, PhD, Dean D. Metcalfe, MD, Ana Olivera, PhD*

KEYWORDS

- Mastocytosis • KIT mutations • KIT signaling • KIT trafficking • KIT inhibitors

KEY POINTS

- KIT, the tyrosine kinase receptor for stem cell factor, is critical for the proliferation, survival, differentiation, and homing of hematopoietic bone marrow stem cells, particularly mast cells, which retain KIT expression and are dependent on KIT activity during their lifespan.
- Gain-of-function mutations in c-Kit resulting in ligand-independent receptor activity associate with hyperproliferative diseases, especially mast cell proliferation disorders (mastocytosis), gastrointestinal stromal tumors (GISTs) and other hematological neoplasms.
- Despite the large number of individual somatic oncogenic mutations identified, most are grouped within mutational hotspots in exon 11 (more frequent in GISTs), encoding for the regulatory juxtamembrane domain, and exon 17 (more frequent in mastocytosis and other germ line malignancies), encoding for the catalytic kinase domain of KIT.
- Structural changes in the receptor induced by these mutations affect the intracellular trafficking of KIT and quantitatively and qualitatively alter normal KIT signaling leading to enhanced proliferation.
- Challenges in the treatment of these diseases include the differential sensitivity to known KIT inhibitors depending on the type of mutation and their relatively low selectivity to KIT, the development of drug resistance, and the presence of other complementing co-oncogenic events or epigenetic modifications contributing to the pathology.

INTRODUCTION

The c-Kit proto-oncogene is the cellular, untruncated counterpart of the gene in the Hardy-Zuckerman feline sarcoma virus genome (v-Kit) responsible for its transforming activity.[1] Gain-of-function mutations in c-Kit promoting tumor formation and

Financial support was provided by the Division of Intramural Research of NIAID within the National Institutes of Health.

Disclaimers: None.

Mast Cell Biology Section, Laboratory of Allergic Diseases, National Institute of Allergy and Infectious Diseases (NIAID), National Institutes of Health, 10 Center Drive, Building 10, Room 11C207, MSC 1881, Bethesda, MD 20892, USA

* Corresponding author.

E-mail address: Ana.Olivera@nih.gov

Immunol Allergy Clin N Am 34 (2014) 219–237
http://dx.doi.org/10.1016/j.iac.2014.01.002   **immunology.theclinics.com**
0889-8561/14/$ – see front matter Published by Elsevier Inc.

progression have been identified in certain human cancers, a knowledge that has boosted an interest in targeting the activity of this receptor.

c-Kit encodes for a protein, KIT (CD117), belonging to a family of transmembrane growth factor receptors with intrinsic tyrosine kinase activity.[2] Its specific ligand is stem cell factor (SCF), also known as KIT ligand, mast cell growth factor, or steel factor.[3,4] SCF is primarily, but not exclusively, produced by stromal cells, such as fibroblasts, in 2 major forms, a soluble form and a membrane-bound form, which are present at varying ratios in different tissues.[3,5,6] Both forms activate KIT but may mediate qualitatively and quantitatively different types of responses,[7,8] although the specific mechanisms remain largely unknown.

KIT is highly expressed in hematopoietic stem cells from the bone marrow, and its activity is critical for constitutive hematopoiesis and for the proliferation, survival, differentiation, and homing of these cells.[8–10] Expression of KIT is generally lost during the differentiation process of most hematopoietic cells, with the exception of mast cells, which retain KIT through their lifespan. KIT, thus, plays an important role in mast cell proliferation, survival, and function.[11–15] KIT expression can be upregulated during an immune response in eosinophils[16] and dendritic cells,[17] whereas in both human basophils and eosinophils, KIT expression is generally found at low levels.[18,19] The expression of KIT is, however, not restricted to hematopoietic cells: it is expressed in melanocytes, interstitial cells of Cajal in the gastrointestinal tract,[20] and other cell types.[21–24] Accumulated evidence in rodent models with KIT alterations has provided insights on the cell populations that are most critically KIT dependent. Thus, mice carrying mutations that impair KIT structure or expression (such as WBB6F$_1$- Kit$^{W/W-v}$ and C57BL/6-Kit$^{W-sh/W-sh}$ mice) exhibit specific phenotypic abnormalities in their adulthood, including profound mast cell and melanocyte deficiency, macrocytic anemia, reduced fertility, and a lack of gut interstitial cells of Cajal resulting in reduced pacemaker activity in the small intestine.[4,20,24] The absence of KIT or its ligand in mice is embryonically or perinatally lethal, suggesting a critical, broader biologic role of SCF/KIT signaling during embryogenesis.[4] In humans, loss-of-function mutations in c-Kit associate with piebaldism, a rare, autosomal dominant disorder characterized by congenital white patches in the skin and hair caused by improper migration of melanoblasts in the embryo,[25] whereas acquired gain-of-function mutations in c-Kit result in particular neoplastic diseases.

In this review, the authors provide a general overview of the consequences of gain-of-function mutations in c-Kit, the structure and molecular mechanisms governing KIT signaling, and describe how gain-of-function mutations in c-Kit result in its overactive function and lead to cellular transformation, with particular focus on mast cells and disorders of pathologic mast cell proliferation.

C-KIT MUTATIONS AND LINK TO MALIGNANCIES

Human malignancies associated with activating c-Kit mutations include mast cell proliferative disorders; gastrointestinal stromal tumors (GISTs); and, less commonly, melanoma and acute myeloid leukemia. Increased expression of normal c-Kit may also contribute to tumorigenesis in solid lung cancers from small lung cells that do not normally express KIT and are exposed to environments rich in SCF. Activating mutations in small lung cancer cells, nonetheless, have rarely been found; their involvement in tumor progression is still unclear.[26–28] Dysregulation of KIT activity plays a central role, however, in the pathogenesis of those malignancies originated from cells dependent on SCF for differentiation/survival, such as mast cells and interstitial cells of Cajal.[29–33] GISTs are thought to derive from interstitial cells of Cajal; in up to 80% of sporadic GISTs, at least 17 different activating mutations involving exons 8, 11, 13, or 17 of c-Kit have been reported.[29,34] Similarly, approximately 90% of adults with diseases of abnormal mast cell proliferation (mastocytosis) have at least a point mutation consisting of a substitution of aspartic acid to valine in the catalytic domain of c-Kit (D816V), rendering it constitutively active.[35–37]

Although KIT is also critical for melanocyte physiology, transforming mutations in c-Kit appear only in about 3% of all melanomas, particularly in metastatic melanoma (reviewed in Ref.[38]). This finding is consistent with the observation that an activating c-Kit point mutation in genetically modified mouse melanocytes predominantly increased melanocyte migration over any effect in proliferation or pigment production.[39] Because maturation of hematopoietic cells other than mast cells results in downregulation of c-Kit expression, transforming mutations of this receptor rarely affect most hematopoietic lineages.[31] However, mutations or internal tandem duplications in c-Kit that contribute to pathogenesis have been observed in approximately 17% of acute myeloid leukemias (AML).[31,40,41] These mutations are acquired somatic mutations present in a clonal lineage population, and it is thought that the ultimate phenotype of malignant hemopoietic cells of a specific lineage expressing mutant KIT is influenced by additional complementing co-oncogenic events or epigenetic modifications that affect their differentiation process, proliferation, and survival.[31,42]

As it is discussed later, therapies blocking KIT activity have been somewhat successful in the treatment of some of these malignancies alone or in combination but not in others when complete remissions or improved survival time is rare. The success of therapy is linked to the type of mutation and/or the presence of additional mutations in c-Kit or other proto-oncogenes.

c-Kit and Neoplastic Growth of Mast Cells

Mast cells are derived from CD34[+] bone marrow hematopoietic pluripotent progenitors[43] but fully differentiate in tissues, where they establish residency (for review see Ref.[44]). Mast cells are usually located around blood vessels and nerves within the connective tissue, where SCF is abundant. The role of mast cells in the regulation of adaptive responses occurs primarily through cell surface receptors that bind immunoglobulin antibodies (Fc receptors), particularly FcεRI, the high receptor for immunoglobulin E (IgE) (reviewed in Ref.[45]). On encountering a multivalent allergen (antigen [Ag]), IgE receptors in the mast cell surface bound to Ag-specific IgE are aggregated and the proinflammatory mediators contained in mast cell granules are secreted by degranulation or are synthesized de novo, causing an immediate hypersensitivity allergic reaction. Mast cells also respond to a variety of stimuli in the tissue environment that can alter mast cell function and, thus, the allergic response. Among those, SCF can synergistically enhance mast cell degranulation, cytokine production, and chemotactic migration induced by other stimulants, particularly IgE/Ag (reviewed in Ref.[46]). Thus, changes in SCF concentrations in the tissue environment or dysregulated KIT activity may not only affect mast cell numbers and homeostasis[11] but also mast cell responsiveness.

Mast cells are found in excessive numbers in tissues in a heterogeneous group of disorders collectively known as *mastocytosis*. Diseases of pathologic mast cell proliferation are classified into disease variants based on clinical presentation, pathologic findings, and prognosis. There are excellent reviews covering the criteria and symptoms of these variants and, thus, they are not detailed here.[33,37,47] In general, mastocytosis is classified under cutaneous (the most benign form and best prognosis with mostly skin involvement) and systemic mastocytosis (with mast cell infiltrates and effects in the bone marrow and extracutaneous organs, such as liver, spleen, or lymph nodes). The occurrence of somatic activating mutations in the c-Kit gene in a hematopoietic progenitor cell is considered an important early event in the progression of mastocytosis. Particularly, a mutation in position 816 of KIT from aspartate to valine that results in constitutive ligand-independent tyrosine phosphorylation of KIT and tumorigenicity in mice[48] is highly associated with mastocytosis in adult patients but is less frequently found in cases of children with mastocytosis, which is usually cutaneous and often resolves before puberty.[37,49–51] Although this is suggestive of a different basis for the children's form of this disease, a recent study in a larger cohort of pediatric mastocytosis found that indeed 86% of these patients had activating mutations in c-Kit, with the D816V mutation present in 35% of cases.[52] The reasons for the frequent recession rate in children are, however, still unclear. It seems that the presence of gain-of-function mutations of KIT is a necessary prerequisite for mastocytosis in most cases, but the phenotypic diversity in mastocytosis may arise from a combination of additional acquired mutations or other inherited genetic polymorphisms. For example, recent studies in the authors' laboratory identified activating mutations in Neuroblastoma-RAt Sarcoma oncogen (N-RAS) in 2 out of 8 patients with advanced mastocytosis that seemed to precede the D816V c-Kit mutation because they were present in the CD34[+] progenitors, whereas the D816V mutation was not.[53] In addition to N-RAS mutations that may further promote the clonal expansion of mast cells and disease severity in some patients, other epigenetic changes or alterations in RNA splicing can also influence the pathogenesis of mastocytosis. Along these lines, a splice variant of KIT missing 4 amino acids (glycine-asparagine-asparagine-lysine [GNNK]) in the extracellular domain (GNNK−)[8] (**Fig. 1**) is preferentially

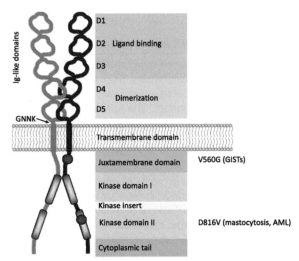

Fig. 1. Structure of KIT. KIT comprises 5 extracellular immunoglobulinlike domains, a membrane spanning domain, and 2 catalytic kinase domains. The first 3 immunoglobulinlike domains are responsible for binding to the KIT ligand, SCF. The 2 immunoglobulinlike domains proximal to the plasma membrane interact and facilitate dimerization of KIT. A region of 4 amino acids (GNNK) lies adjacent to the plasma membrane region, and alternative splicing of KIT results in GNNK+ and GNNK− isoforms. The JM domain of KIT contains the Tyr residues Y568 and Y570, which become phosphorylated on activation releasing its autoinhibitory function. Point mutations in the JM domain change its conformation and prevent its regulatory function. The V560G mutation is an example of an activating mutation in the JM domain, particularly in association with GISTs. There are 2 catalytic kinase domains (KD) separated by a kinase insert domain. Several activating mutations have been reported in the KD of KIT. The D816V mutation is a common mutation and is associated with mastocytosis.

expressed in patients with severe mastocytosis with the D816V mutation as compared with normal individuals,[54,55] a finding that correlates with the ability of this isoform to enhance KIT signaling and the maturation of mast cells.[55] In agreement with a participation of splice variant expression in the overall disease severity, no differences in the relative expression of the GNNK− and GNNK+ isoforms were found in the pediatric, less severe form of the disease.[52] Other alterations in c-Kit gene transcripts in patients with systemic mast cell activation disorders have been described[54]; however, the significance of these alternative splice forms is unclear.

In addition to promoting mast cell proliferation and survival, persistent activation of KIT may reduce the threshold of mast cell activation to other stimuli. Thus, it is not unexpected that patients suffer recurrent spontaneous episodes of flushing, shortness of breath, palpitations, nausea, diarrhea, abdominal pain, hypotension, or a combination of these symptoms[37] as a consequence of increased mast cell mediator release. In fact, the prevalence of anaphylaxis in adults diagnosed with mastocytosis is considerably higher than expected in the general population.[56] Despite the progress in the understanding of KIT signaling in mast cells, the exact triggers and specific signaling mechanisms involved in these episodes remain poorly understood.[37,56]

In the next section, the authors describe the structural and mechanistic characteristics of KIT in normal conditions and how the structure/function interrelationship of the SCF receptor can be altered by mutations in neoplastic diseases, particularly in mastocytosis.

MECHANISMS OF KIT ACTIVATION
Structure of KIT

KIT is a type III receptor tyrosine kinase (RTK) that exists as multiple splice variants and in various states of glycosylation, which may represent the maturity of the receptor. Therefore, the molecular weight of KIT ranges between 120 and 150 kDa depending on posttranslational modifications. KIT and other type III RTKs contain 5 extracellular immunoglobulinlike domains (D1 distal to D5 juxtamembrane [JM]) (**Fig. 1**) that form an elongated serpentine shape.[57] The distal D1, D2, and D3 domains constitute the SCF binding portion of KIT with SCF and KIT forming a 2:2 stoichiometry,[57] supporting suggestions that KIT dimerization is a consequence of bivalent binding to SCF homodimers.[32,58] The intracellular JM domain of KIT, in the inactive state, interacts with the kinase domains (KD) preventing its catalytic function and providing a negative switch regulatory mechanism.[59,60] KIT signaling in response to SCF is triggered by the intrinsic kinase activity of the receptor by way of 2 catalytic KD separated by a kinase insert domain (see **Fig. 1**). Transphosphorylation of tyrosine residues in the JM, kinase insert domain, and cytoplasmic tail participate in recruitment of signaling molecules to the receptor complex, initiating signaling cascades through several divergent pathways (**Fig. 2**).

Signaling Pathways of KIT in Mast Cells

As the authors have discussed, signaling through KIT is critical for human mast cell survival, growth, differentiation, and proliferation. In addition, SCF affects secretion, adhesion, and migration and, therefore, regulates most normal mast cell functions. Although the signaling pathways that are activated downstream of KIT are well established, the mechanisms that regulate specific responses to SCF signals are not well understood. One potential mechanism for directing specific mast cell responses to SCF stimulation is differential phosphorylation of residues within the cytoplasmic domains of KIT. The activation of KIT by SCF induces KIT dimerization and initiation of

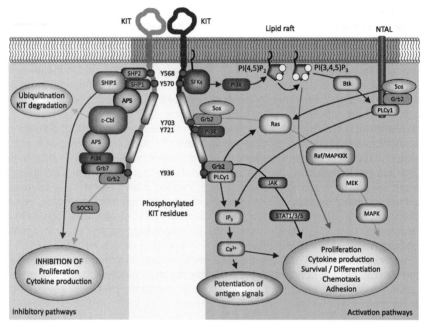

Fig. 2. KIT signaling pathways. KIT signaling occurs through several pathways. Phosphorylation of the JM Tyr residues recruits Src family kinases (SFKs), in particular Lyn, initiating PI3K signaling and the phosphorylation of other signaling and adaptor proteins. These events most likely occur within lipid rafts where the PI3K substrate, PI(4,5)P$_2$, is converted to PI(3,4,5)P$_3$, a signaling lipid that contributes to the activation of other enzymes. Adaptor proteins (non–T-cell activation linker [NTAL] and growth factor receptor–bound protein 2 [Grb2]) are phosphorylated by the receptor or by Src kinases and recruit other signaling proteins, forming signaling complexes. PLCγ1, for example, is recruited by the adaptor protein NTAL to lipid rafts, activated by phosphorylation and by PI(3,4,5)P$_3$, cleaving PI(3,4)P$_2$ to form IP$_3$, which induces the release of Ca^{2+} from intracellular stores; diacylglycerol, together with Ca^{2+}, activates PKC. Tyr residues within the kinase insert domain of KIT interact with PI3K and Grb2, leading to the activation of the Ras/Raf/mitogen-activated protein kinase (MAPK) pathway. Another pathway critical for KIT-mediated proliferation, particularly in gain-of-function KIT mutants, is the activation of the transcription factors signal transducer and activator of transcription (STAT)1/3/5. Janus kinase (JAK) is phosphorylated after KIT activation, and in turn phosphorylates STAT allowing its translocation to the nucleus, where it exerts its function. Inhibitory pathways of KIT also regulate responsiveness to SCF. The JM Tyr residues of KIT can recruit the phosphatases, SHP1, SHP2, and SHIP1, which may contribute to negative regulation of KIT signaling. In addition, recruitment of the ubiquitin E3 ligase, c-Cbl, via the dimeric adaptor protein containing PH and SH2 domains (APS), may be a critical determinant for ubiquitination and degradation of KIT. Both Tyr 936 and Tyr 570 seem to regulate the recruitment of c-Cbl and binding of APS. APS exists as a dimer and, thus, may require 2 simultaneously phosphorylated KIT residues to recruit c-Cbl. For simplification, only one extracellular domain of KIT is represented and bound ligand is not depicted. Btk, Bruton tyrosine kinase; Sos, son-of sevenless.

intrinsic tyrosine kinase activity, resulting in autophosphorylation of tyrosine residues that act as docking sites for signaling proteins containing either Src homology 2 (SH2) or phosphotyrosine-binding domains.[61–63] Thus, phosphorylation of specific KIT tyrosine residues triggers signal transduction through divergent pathways that may drive distinct mast cell responses.

One of the early signaling events after the activation of KIT is recruitment of Src family kinases (SFKs) to phosphorylated tyrosines (Y568 and Y570) in the JM domain of KIT.[64,65] SFK signaling may regulate several critical SCF-dependent mast cell functions. For example, transfection of a dominant negative form of the SFK, Lyn, inhibits mast cell proliferation and chemotaxis in response to SCF.[66] SFKs, such as Lyn, contain N-terminal myristoylation sites and, in some cases, a palmitoylation site, which are critical for anchoring the kinases, respectively, to the plasma membrane and to specialized membrane microdomains (lipid rafts).[67] Therefore, SFK signaling most likely occurs at the plasma membrane where the JM domain of KIT is easily accessible for binding membrane–anchored SFKs. Indeed, SFK signaling may actually be required for KIT internalization as well as migration.[68] Further indication that plasma membrane localization is key for KIT signaling through SFKs comes from the observation that KIT associates with lipid rafts after stimulation with SCF and that lipid rafts are essential for the activation of SFKs in response to SCF.[69,70]

Lipid rafts may also be important for signal transduction through the phosphatidylinositol-3-kinase (PI3K) pathway because disruption of lipid rafts specifically diminishes phosphorylation of the PI3K surrogate, protein kinase B AKT, in response to SCF stimulation.[69,70] PI3K phosphorylates the plasma membrane–associated phosphatidylinositol-4,5-biphosphate $(PI(4,5)P_2)$ to form phosphatidylinositol-3,4,5,-triphosphate $(PI(3,4,5)P_3)$, which in turn recruits pleckstrin homology (PH) domain–containing signaling proteins to the plasma membrane (reviewed by Ref.[71]). The classic class I PI3K complex consists of a regulatory p85 subunit and a catalytic p110 subunit. Bone marrow–derived mast cells (BMMCs) from mice with targeted deletion of PI3K exhibit reduced survival and proliferate less than wild-type BMMC in response to SCF, which is associated with a reduction in the phosphorylation status of the mitogen-activated protein kinase (MAPK) Jun-amino-terminal kinase (JNK).[72] In addition, PI3K also seems to play an important role in mast cell chemotaxis,[73] suggesting that PI3K and SFKs regulate similar functional responses to SCF.

The activation of KIT by SCF also triggers the activation of the MAPKs, extracellular-signal-regulated kinase 1 and 2 (ERK1 and ERK2), JNK, and p38. Phosphorylated tyrosine residues in activated KIT (see **Fig. 2**) are recognized by the SH2 domain of the adaptor protein growth factor receptor–bound protein 2 (Grb2), which then forms a complex with the guanine exchange factor (GEF) son-of sevenless (Sos). Sos activates the G protein Ras by promoting the exchange of GDP by GTP (see **Fig. 2**).[74] GTP-bound, active Ras initiates a cascade of serine/threonine kinases (Raf, MEK) that lead to the activation of the ERK1 and ERK2.[75] The pathway leading to p38 and JNK activation by KIT in mast cells is not well established.[46] The Ras-Raf-MEK-ERK pathway regulates many cellular processes, particularly survival, proliferation, and cytokine production in mast cells. Therefore, targeting this pathway is attractive for cancer treatment[76] and potentially mastocytosis.

Gain-of-Function c-Kit Mutations and Mechanisms for Constitutive Activation

The oncogenic c-Kit mutations found in neoplasms are gain-of-function mutations that result in ligand-independent tyrosine kinase activity and lead to ligand-independent proliferation, differentiation and/or survival of the affected cells.[31,32,77] Despite the large number of individual oncogenic mutations identified, most are grouped within mutational hot spots in exons 11 encoding for the JM domain and 17 encoding for the second KD of KIT. JM mutations appear more frequently in GISTs, while 90% of patients with systemic mastocytosis, most cases of AML and other germ cell cancers have the D816V c-Kit point mutation in the KD. The reasons for the preference for exon

17 mutations in hematologic malignancies as compared with exon 11 in GISTs are not known. Other exons, such as 8, 9, and 10, coding for the extracellular domain (8 and 9) and transmembrane domain of the receptor have been described in AML,[40] GISTs,[30,32] and in patients with childhood mastocytosis,[52] but the incidence of these mutations is much lower.[32] The authors refer the reader to other reviews or reports for more detailed listings of the specific oncogenic mutations.[33,37,47,52,78,79] In this section, the authors briefly review the current understanding on how these hot-spot point mutations mechanistically affect receptor function.

Activating mutations in JM domains mainly relieve the suppressive effect of the JM region on the activity of the receptor and are mechanistically regarded as regulatory, whereas those in the KD are catalytic in nature.[77,80] Less common mutations in the extracellular and transmembrane domains (ectodomains) may also lead to KIT hyperactivity, probably by stabilizing receptor dimers and facilitating the activation of the RTK.[57,81] Despite the distinct nature of the mechanisms by which different mutations lead to KIT hyperactivation, they are not completely dissociated because of the interconnected nature of the secondary-tertiary structures of KIT. The JM domain in resting conditions forms a hairpin loop that inserts into the active site of KIT, maintaining the activation loop (A-loop) inactive.[59,82] On binding to SCF and consequent dimerization, the primary sites in the JM domain (Y568 and Y570) are transphosphorylated, lifting the auto-inhibition and allowing further activation.[83] This activation process also involves a large rearrangement of the A-loop (from folded to extended) that facilitates access to Mg^{2+}-ATP and protein substrates to the kinase catalytic site.[83] Mutations in the JM region lead to the release of this regulatory suppression, permitting the extended, active conformation[83] and promoting ligand-independent dimerization,[77,84] favoring further signaling. Mutations in the KD, particularly the D816V mutation, not only cause a local structural unfolding in the A-loop (directly affecting the enzymatic site configuration)[60,85–87] but also a long-range structural rearrangement of the JM region that in turn weakens its interaction with the KD, relieving the regulatory inhibition. The greater freedom of movement of the JM domain in D816V mutants also allows for interactions with another KIT receptor and promotes dimerization.[80,82,84,86] Moreover, because of the increased catalytic activity in KD mutants, tyrosines Y568 and Y570 in the JM domain are phosphorylated; thus, their inhibition of the kinase is further disrupted.[32,80,88] Thus, the negative switch mechanism by the JM region may be suppressed not only by direct mutations in this region but also indirectly by mutations in the catalytic domain; furthermore, increased dimerization may occur in all mutated receptors. Structure-function studies on KIT have been instrumental in understanding why, in some instances, differences in the type of mutation lead to similar disease phenotypes and why drug sensitivity differs depending on the mutation site, as discussed later.

The structural changes in the receptor induced by these mutations also quantitatively and qualitatively affect normal KIT signaling and cell function. For example, p38-MAPK pathways are preferentially activated over ERK-MAPK pathways in JM deletion mutants.[87] Similarly, other important mitogenic pathways, such as AKT- and signal transducer and activator of transcription (STAT)-dependent pathways are also constitutively activated in JM and D816V mutants.[87,89,90] Mutations in the extracellular domain of the receptor, like those found in some pediatric mastocytosis patients, when introduced in rodent cells resulted in preferential AKT activation as compared with D816V mutations.[91] On the other hand, the interaction of JM docking sites with phosphatases, such as SH2-domain containing phosphatase (SHP) SHP1, SHP2, and SH2 domain-containing inositol-5-phosphatase (SHIP), are disrupted in JM KIT mutants. These phosphatases normally dephosphorylate the receptor, tyrosine kinases associated with the receptor, or, in the case of SHIP, cleave signaling lipids, such as phosphatidylinositol (3,4,5) triphosphate (PIP$_3$), thus downregulating KIT activity (see **Fig. 2**).[87,92] Disruption of their suppression results in enhanced KIT activity. Overall, the altered signaling in KIT mutants may be a consequence of preferential phosphorylation of certain tyrosine sites and/or alterations in the trafficking of the receptor (as discussed in the next section).

Trafficking of KIT and Its Impact on Signaling

There is growing evidence that trafficking and localization of RTKs modulate signal transduction and alter functional outcomes in response to ligand (for reviews see Refs.[93,94]). RTKs, including KIT, are activated by ligand binding at the plasma membrane where rapid signaling is initiated. Signaling at the plasma membrane is a key process for many receptors where interactions with plasma membrane-associated adaptor proteins, such as linker of activated T cells (LAT) and non–T-cell activation linker (NTAL), are critical for propagation of signaling (reviewed by Ref.[46]). In addition, signaling through both phospholipase C (PLC)γ1 and PI3K most likely require plasma membrane localization because their lipid substrate, PI(4,5)P$_2$, is plasma membrane–associated and access to PI(4,5)P$_2$ is limited in endosomes.[95] Therefore, receptor internalization and degradation attenuates the strength and duration of plasma membrane–associated signaling and, thus, has been considered as a negative regulator of receptor signal transduction. However, for some receptors, such as the RTK epidermal growth factor receptor (EGFR), internalization into endosomal compartments is required for full activation of MAPK.[96,97] Receptor endocytosis may, therefore, alter signal transduction pathways, and signaling at the plasma membrane may result in distinct responses compared with signaling within the endosomal compartments.

Much of the work performed on the effects of RTK trafficking on signal transduction thus far has been carried out with the EGFR. It has been demonstrated that the EGFR and downstream signaling pathways, such as MAPKs, signal in early endosomes[98–100] and that EGFR can continue to signal in late endosomes and multivesicular bodies until passage into the intraluminal vesicles of late endosomes and lysosomes halts signaling.[96,97,101] One reason for the requirement of internalization for RTK signal transduction seems to be the composition of signaling scaffold complexes within distinct endocytic compartments that facilitate certain signal transduction pathways (**Fig. 3**).[102–104] For example, signal transduction from EGFR to the ERK pathway in late endosomes depends on the localization of MEK1 kinase partner protein (MP1) and the adaptor protein p14, which are specific to late endosomes,[103] and disruption of p14-MP1-MEK1 endosomal signaling complex inhibits proliferation.[105]

These observations suggest that signaling in the endocytic system and the formation of signaling complexes specific to late endosomes could be critical for determining a proliferative response to growth factors. RTKs with activating mutations that drive hematopoietic cell transformation exhibit abnormal cellular localization, localizing mainly within the ER and Golgi instead of in the plasma membrane; this intracellular localization seems critical for the proliferative response (reviewed by Ref.[106]). Specifically, intracellular perinuclear signaling of KIT with the activating D816V mutation is sufficient to drive neoplasia, whereas plasma membrane signaling is dispensable in a mouse model of myelomonocytic neoplasia.[107] Prolonged endosomal signaling may, thus, be important for neoplastic transformation; factors that reduce receptor degradation pathways could promote this response. For example, altered trafficking of KIT in BMMC by targeting small ARF GTPase-activating protein 1 led to intracellular retention of KIT and hyperphosphorylation of ERK by reducing KIT

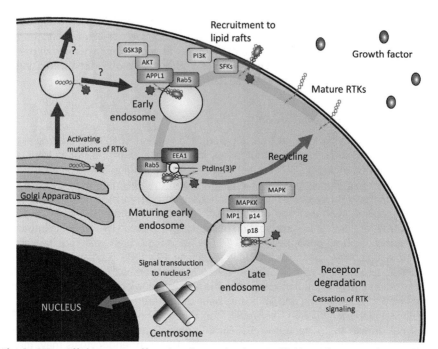

Fig. 3. RTK trafficking may affect signal transduction. Trafficking of RTKs, such as KIT, may regulate signal transduction pathways by binding to adaptor proteins specific to endosomal compartments and altering the type of signaling complexes recruited. Initiation of RTK signaling triggers recruitment to lipid rafts where interactions with plasma membrane–anchored signaling molecules is facilitated. In particular, lipid rafts may be critical for signaling through the SFKs, PI3K and PLCγ1. Internalization of RTKs can induce the activation of additional signaling pathways by recruitment of adaptor proteins, such as adaptor protein, phosphotyrosine interaction, PH domain, and leucine zipper containing 1 (APPL1), in very early endosomes, which can bind AKT and direct signaling through GSK3β. As the early endosome matures, it becomes positive for PtdIns(3)P, which recruits the early endosomal antigen 1 (EEA1) protein. At this point, the early endosome may sort receptors for recycling back to the plasma membrane. Receptors that are not recycled remain in the endosome as it matures to a late endosome and control switches from Rab5 to Rab7. Signaling still occurs within the limiting membrane of late endosomes where adaptor protein complexes of p14, p18, and MEK1 kinase partner protein (MP1), which are specific to the late endosomal compartments, may promote unique signaling to the MAPK pathway. The localization of late endosomes may also promote signal transduction to the nucleus because their close proximity to the centrosome allows weak signals to travel shorter distances and reach the nucleus. Eventually, receptors passage into intraluminal vesicles of multivesicular bodies and lysosomes, which results in cessation of signaling and receptor degradation. The schematic is an oversimplification, as multiple signaling pathways may well occur at all stages of receptor trafficking; but enrichment of particular adaptor proteins may promote a particular pathway by facilitating specific interactions. Activating mutations in RTKs favor their intracellular localization and trigger signaling from intracellular compartments in the absence of ligand. Further studies are needed to determine how the constitutively active RTKs traffic and signal in cells. Normal RTKs are depicted in green and mutated RTKs in red.

trafficking to lysosomes and, thus, degradation, which may predispose mice to myelodysplasia and acute myeloid leukemia.[108]

The regulation of KIT and RTK trafficking and signal transduction seems complex. However, understanding the interplay between these processes may prove critical for our understanding of how KIT regulates many distinct cellular functions, which could aid in the design of more effective inhibitors of KIT-mediated proliferative diseases.

KIT INHIBITORS AND TREATMENT OF MUTATED KIT-DRIVEN PROLIFERATIVE DISEASES

Pharmacologic targeting of KIT catalytic activity has been a major strategy for blocking KIT-mediated responses. This strategy is used because KIT with oncogenic c-Kit mutations is mostly expressed inside organelles, precluding the potential use of neutralizing antibodies. Another limiting factor in the treatment of KIT-related malignancies has been that inhibitors targeting the inactive ATP-binding site conformation of KIT, such as imatinib mesylate (imatinib, STI571, Gleevec or Glivec) and its derivatives (nilotinib [AMN107] and PD180970) are unsuccessful in inhibiting the active, extended conformation of KIT. Therefore, mutations that stabilize the active conformation (mostly KD mutations, including the common D816V mutation), as those found in most aggressive mastocytosis patients, are resistant to this drug. Nevertheless, imatinib has been an efficient drug with relatively few side effects[109] for the treatment of patients with GIST who harbor c-Kit mutations in exon 11 (corresponding to the JM domain) and some patients with mastocytosis with a V560G mutation in the JM domain, a novel mutation in the transmembrane region (F522C) and other mutations.[33] An additional drawback of imatinib has been the incidence in some of these patients of secondary resistance to the drug, apparently caused in part by the acquisition (or enrichment) of other mutations in the KD of the receptor that are insensitive to imatinib.[32,41]

Other compounds, including dasatinib (BMS-354825), have been found to target the catalytic activity associated with D816V and other KD mutations. Dasatinib was reported to inhibit KIT autophosphorylation and the growth of both human mast cell line (HMC)-1.1 and HMC-1.2 human mast cell lines, which express the V560G mutation or the V560G and D816V mutations, respectively.[12] Dasatinib was approved in 2010 as a first-line treatment of chronic myeloid leukemia (CML) in chronic phase and for the treatment of any-phase CML resistant or intolerant to a previous treatment.[110] The current data on early response to treatment to dasatinib are predictive of improved long-term outcomes in CML.[110] Dasatinib and derivatives, however, have wider specificity and affect multiple kinases, such as Src kinases, Tec kinases, Bruton tyrosine kinase, MAPKs, and AKT, as well as other receptor kinases[12] that are important for growth and other functions in mast cells and other cell types. Thus, although being potentially more effective by acting on various pathways, their distinct side effects should also be taken into consideration depending on the patient.[110–112] Another second-generation tyrosine kinase inhibitor is midostaurin (PKC412), an N-benzoyl derivative of staurosporine that inhibits protein kinase C (PKC) as well as KIT, Fms-like tyrosine kinase 3 (FLT-3), and platelet-derived growth factor receptor (PDGFR). Midostaurin has activity in vitro against the D816 KIT mutants by itself and shows synergistic effects in combination with other KIT inhibitors (reviewed in Ref.[79]). In a phase-2 study, midostaurin was orally administered to patients with various forms of advanced mastocytosis and showed a major response rate of 38%, which included improvement of hemoglobin and platelet counts, improvement of liver function abnormalities, and improvement of ascites.[113] The observation of a major response rate (as compared with any other type of clinical response) was significantly associated with the presence of a D816V mutation. Side effects were also present in these patients, and treatment was discontinued in 69% of the patients. Additional studies are needed to clarify the advantage of midostaurin versus other treatments.

The better understanding of the KIT structure, domains, and mechanisms of activation has allowed for rational drug design approaches to intercept the activity of KIT mutants, although this is at its early stages and there is need for further testing and clinical development. An example is the development of compounds (DP-2976 and DP-4851) designed to target access to the KIT switch pocket. The switch pocket can bind either the JM region maintaining the inactive conformation or the KD activation loop maintaining the active conformation. Both inhibitors potently and selectively inhibit the activity of normal KIT and KIT harboring the D816V mutation, proliferation of neoplastic and non-neoplastic mast cells, as well as the ability of KIT to enhance mast cell activation.[114]

CONCLUDING REMARKS AND FUTURE DIRECTIONS

Transforming point mutations in KIT, which are critical for the manifestation of neoplastic diseases, such as mastocytosis and GISTs, appear primarily in regions of the receptor involved in maintaining the normal structural, regulatory, and activation dynamics of KIT, thus rendering a constitutively active receptor. Despite the progress in identifying specific transforming mutations, the increased understanding of how these mutations affect KIT signaling and function, and the boosted interest in targeting KIT, important challenges in the treatment of these diseases still lie ahead. Both the heterogeneity in the phenotype of mastocytosis and the success of therapy may be in part related to the presence of a combination of KIT mutations and mutations in other proto-oncogenes. Even though joint drug treatments targeting KIT and other oncogenes could be successful, this will entail tailoring the type of therapy, if available, to the genotype of each patient.[41] Despite the interest and benefits of individualized treatments, more general pharmacologic approaches should not be overlooked. Studies on gene expression profiling in bone marrow mast cells[115] and whole peripheral blood[116] from cohorts of patients with mastocytosis suggest that several general biologic processes and pathways are commonly altered in these patients. For example, not surprisingly, metabolic pathways and pathways involved in proliferation and apoptosis are significantly changed in patients with mastocytosis.[115,116] One could speculate that drugs that reprogram metabolic pathways and restore normal energy and growth homeostasis of transformed cells, such as metformin (a drug approved for treatment of patients with type II diabetes that has shown promising effects in treating human cancers[117,118]), may help control the hyperproliferation of mast cells and the pathology associated with mastocytosis. Although the importance of metabolic pathways in the development or symptoms of mastocytosis is presently unknown, a further understanding may provide the grounds for novel therapeutic approaches for mastocytosis treatment in combination with specific KIT inhibitors. Other novel therapeutic approaches of increasing appeal and promise for cancer treatment include miRNA therapies, although adjustments in this technology are still needed to achieve the full potential.[119] The increased interest in miRNA technology is in part based on the finding that miRNA profiles can accurately predict the origin of the cancer tissue[120] and that manipulation of these molecules may affect the behavior of neoplastic cells.[119,121] No miRNA profiling has been so far strongly linked to specific patient populations with mastocytosis; however, the evidence of specific miRNAs involved in the regulation of the cell cycle in mast cells,[122] degranulation, cytokine production, migration of mast cells,[123] and in the expression of transcription factors mediating proliferation of primary and KIT-transformed mast cells[124] makes this approach one of promising potential.[125]

In summary, although complete remission for some of the proliferative diseases harboring KIT mutations has not yet been fully achieved, new drug designs of KIT inhibitors, together with the advances in individual genotyping and in identifying the molecular mechanisms that underlie these diseases, may afford new possibilities and potential breakthroughs in treatment.

REFERENCES

1. Yarden Y, Kuang WJ, Yang-Feng T, et al. Human proto-oncogene c-kit: a new cell surface receptor tyrosine kinase for an unidentified ligand. EMBO J 1987; 6:3341–51.
2. Qiu FH, Ray P, Brown K, et al. Primary structure of c-kit: relationship with the CSF-1/PDGF receptor kinase family–oncogenic activation of v-kit involves deletion of extracellular domain and C terminus. EMBO J 1988;7:1003–11.
3. Flanagan JG, Leder P. The kit ligand: a cell surface molecule altered in steel mutant fibroblasts. Cell 1990;63:185–94.
4. Broudy VC. Stem cell factor and hematopoiesis. Blood 1997;90:1345–64.
5. Toksoz D, Zsebo KM, Smith KA, et al. Support of human hematopoiesis in long-term bone marrow cultures by murine stromal cells selectively expressing the membrane-bound and secreted forms of the human homolog of the steel gene product, stem cell factor. Proc Natl Acad Sci U S A 1992;89:7350–4.
6. Reber L, Da Silva CA, Frossard N. Stem cell factor and its receptor c-Kit as targets for inflammatory diseases. Eur J Pharmacol 2006;533:327–40.
7. Miyazawa K, Williams DA, Gotoh A, et al. Membrane-bound Steel factor induces more persistent tyrosine kinase activation and longer life span of c-kit gene-encoded protein than its soluble form. Blood 1995;85:641–9.
8. Ashman LK. The biology of stem cell factor and its receptor C-kit. Int J Biochem Cell Biol 1999;31:1037–51.
9. Ogawa M, Matsuzaki Y, Nishikawa S, et al. Expression and function of c-kit in hemopoietic progenitor cells. J Exp Med 1991;174:63–71.
10. Bowie MB, Kent DG, Copley MR, et al. Steel factor responsiveness regulates the high self-renewal phenotype of fetal hematopoietic stem cells. Blood 2007;109: 5043–8.
11. Kitamura Y, Oboki K, Ito A. Molecular mechanisms of mast cell development. Immunol Allergy Clin North Am 2006;26:387–405.
12. Jensen BM, Akin C, Gilfillan AM. Pharmacological targeting of the KIT growth factor receptor: a therapeutic consideration for mast cell disorders. Br J Pharmacol 2008;154:1572–82.
13. Lennartsson J, Jelacic T, Linnekin D, et al. Normal and oncogenic forms of the receptor tyrosine kinase kit. Stem Cells 2005;23:16–43.
14. Linnekin D. Early signaling pathways activated by c-Kit in hematopoietic cells. Int J Biochem Cell Biol 1999;31:1053–74.
15. Galli SJ, Tsai M, Wershil BK, et al. Regulation of mouse and human mast cell development, survival and function by stem cell factor, the ligand for the c-kit receptor. Int Arch Allergy Immunol 1995;107:51–3.
16. Oliveira SH, Taub DD, Nagel J, et al. Stem cell factor induces eosinophil activation and degranulation: mediator release and gene array analysis. Blood 2002; 100:4291–7.

17. Krishnamoorthy N, Oriss TB, Paglia M, et al. Activation of c-Kit in dendritic cells regulates T helper cell differentiation and allergic asthma. Nat Med 2008;14: 565–73.
18. Yuan Q, Austen KF, Friend DS, et al. Human peripheral blood eosinophils express a functional c-kit receptor for stem cell factor that stimulates very late antigen 4 (VLA-4)-mediated cell adhesion to fibronectin and vascular cell adhesion molecule 1 (VCAM-1). J Exp Med 1997;186:313–23.
19. Heinemann A, Sturm GJ, Ofner M, et al. Stem cell factor stimulates the chemotaxis, integrin upregulation, and survival of human basophils. J Allergy Clin Immunol 2005;116:820–6.
20. Huizinga JD, Thuneberg L, Kluppel M, et al. W/kit gene required for interstitial cells of Cajal and for intestinal pacemaker activity. Nature 1995;373:347–9.
21. Al-Muhsen SZ, Shablovsky G, Olivenstein R, et al. The expression of stem cell factor and c-kit receptor in human asthmatic airways. Clin Exp Allergy 2004; 34:911–6.
22. Hollenbeck ST, Sakakibara K, Faries PL, et al. Stem cell factor and c-kit are expressed by and may affect vascular SMCs through an autocrine pathway. J Surg Res 2004;120:288–94.
23. Hirata T, Kasugai T, Morii E, et al. Characterization of c-kit-positive neurons in the dorsal root ganglion of mouse. Brain Res Dev Brain Res 1995;85:201–11.
24. Reber LL, Marichal T, Galli SJ. New models for analyzing mast cell functions in vivo. Trends Immunol 2012;33:613–25.
25. Oiso N, Fukai K, Kawada A, et al. Piebaldism. J Dermatol 2013;40:330–5.
26. Sekido Y, Takahashi T, Ueda R, et al. Recombinant human stem cell factor mediates chemotaxis of small-cell lung cancer cell lines aberrantly expressing the c-kit protooncogene. Cancer Res 1993;53:1709–14.
27. Sihto H, Sarlomo-Rikala M, Tynninen O, et al. KIT and platelet-derived growth factor receptor alpha tyrosine kinase gene mutations and KIT amplifications in human solid tumors. J Clin Oncol 2005;23:49–57.
28. Lu HY, Zhang G, Cheng QY, et al. Expression and mutation of the c-kit gene and correlation with prognosis of small cell lung cancer. Oncol Lett 2012;4:89–93.
29. Bachet JB, Landi B, Laurent-Puig P, et al. Diagnosis, prognosis and treatment of patients with gastrointestinal stromal tumour (GIST) and germline mutation of KIT exon 13. Eur J Cancer 2013;49:2531–41.
30. Hirota S, Isozaki K, Moriyama Y, et al. Gain-of-function mutations of c-kit in human gastrointestinal stromal tumors. Science 1998;279:577–80.
31. Ashman LK, Ferrao P, Cole SR, et al. Effects of mutant c-Kit in early myeloid cells. Leuk Lymphoma 1999;34:451–61.
32. Lennartsson J, Ronnstrand L. Stem cell factor receptor/c-Kit: from basic science to clinical implications. Physiol Rev 2012;92:1619–49.
33. Metcalfe DD. Mast cells and mastocytosis. Blood 2008;112:946–56.
34. Rammohan A, Sathyanesan J, Rajendran K, et al. A gist of gastrointestinal stromal tumors: a review. World J Gastrointest Oncol 2013;5:102–12.
35. Nagata H, Worobec AS, Oh CK, et al. Identification of a point mutation in the catalytic domain of the protooncogene c-kit in peripheral blood mononuclear cells of patients who have mastocytosis with an associated hematologic disorder. Proc Natl Acad Sci U S A 1995;92:10560–4.
36. Garcia-Montero AC, Jara-Acevedo M, Teodosio C, et al. KIT mutation in mast cells and other bone marrow hematopoietic cell lineages in systemic mast cell disorders: a prospective study of the Spanish Network on Mastocytosis (REMA) in a series of 113 patients. Blood 2006;108:2366–72.

37. Brockow K, Metcalfe DD. Mastocytosis. Chem Immunol Allergy 2010;95:110–24.
38. Tran A, Tawbi HA. A potential role for nilotinib in KIT-mutated melanoma. Expert Opin Investig Drugs 2012;21:861–9.
39. Alexeev V, Yoon K. Distinctive role of the cKit receptor tyrosine kinase signaling in mammalian melanocytes. J Invest Dermatol 2006;126:1102–10.
40. Malaise M, Steinbach D, Corbacioglu S. Clinical implications of c-Kit mutations in acute myelogenous leukemia. Curr Hematol Malig Rep 2009;4:77–82.
41. Ashman LK, Griffith R. Therapeutic targeting of c-KIT in cancer. Expert Opin Investig Drugs 2013;22:103–15.
42. Odenike O, Thirman MJ, Artz AS, et al. Gene mutations, epigenetic dysregulation, and personalized therapy in myeloid neoplasia: are we there yet? Semin Oncol 2011;38:196–214.
43. Kirshenbaum AS, Kessler SW, Goff JP, et al. Demonstration of the origin of human mast cells from CD34+ bone marrow progenitor cells. J Immunol 1991;146:1410–5.
44. Gurish MF, Austen KF. Developmental origin and functional specialization of mast cell subsets. Immunity 2012;37:25–33.
45. Rivera J, Gilfillan AM. Molecular regulation of mast cell activation. J Allergy Clin Immunol 2006;117:1214–25 [quiz: 1226].
46. Gilfillan AM, Tkaczyk C. Integrated signalling pathways for mast-cell activation. Nat Rev Immunol 2006;6:218–30.
47. Verstovsek S. Advanced systemic mastocytosis: the impact of KIT mutations in diagnosis, treatment, and progression. Eur J Haematol 2013;90:89–98.
48. Piao X, Bernstein A. A point mutation in the catalytic domain of c-kit induces growth factor independence, tumorigenicity, and differentiation of mast cells. Blood 1996;87:3117–23.
49. Nagata H, Okada T, Worobec AS, et al. c-kit mutation in a population of patients with mastocytosis. Int Arch Allergy Immunol 1997;113:184–6.
50. Longley BJ, Tyrrell L, Lu SZ, et al. Somatic c-KIT activating mutation in urticaria pigmentosa and aggressive mastocytosis: establishment of clonality in a human mast cell neoplasm. Nat Genet 1996;12:312–4.
51. Buttner C, Henz BM, Welker P, et al. Identification of activating c-kit mutations in adult-, but not in childhood-onset indolent mastocytosis: a possible explanation for divergent clinical behavior. J Invest Dermatol 1998;111:1227–31.
52. Bodemer C, Hermine O, Palmerini F, et al. Pediatric mastocytosis is a clonal disease associated with D816V and other activating c-KIT mutations. J Invest Dermatol 2010;130:804–15.
53. Wilson TM, Maric I, Simakova O, et al. Clonal analysis of NRAS activating mutations in KIT-D816V systemic mastocytosis. Haematologica 2011;96:459–63.
54. Molderings GJ, Kolck UW, Scheurlen C, et al. Multiple novel alterations in Kit tyrosine kinase in patients with gastrointestinally pronounced systemic mast cell activation disorder. Scand J Gastroenterol 2007;42:1045–53.
55. Chan EC, Bai Y, Bandara G, et al. KIT GNNK splice variants: expression in systemic mastocytosis and influence on the activating potential of the D816V mutation in mast cells. Exp Hematol 2013;41:870–81.e2.
56. Brockow K, Jofer C, Behrendt H, et al. Anaphylaxis in patients with mastocytosis: a study on history, clinical features and risk factors in 120 patients. Allergy 2008;63:226–32.
57. Yuzawa S, Opatowsky Y, Zhang Z, et al. Structural basis for activation of the receptor tyrosine kinase KIT by stem cell factor. Cell 2007;130:323–34.

58. Lemmon MA, Pinchasi D, Zhou M, et al. Kit receptor dimerization is driven by bivalent binding of stem cell factor. J Biol Chem 1997;272:6311–7.
59. Mol CD, Dougan DR, Schneider TR, et al. Structural basis for the autoinhibition and STI-571 inhibition of c-Kit tyrosine kinase. J Biol Chem 2004;279:31655–63.
60. Mol CD, Lim KB, Sridhar V, et al. Structure of a c-kit product complex reveals the basis for kinase transactivation. J Biol Chem 2003;278:31461–4.
61. Blume-Jensen P, Claesson-Welsh L, Siegbahn A, et al. Activation of the human c-kit product by ligand-induced dimerization mediates circular actin reorganization and chemotaxis. EMBO J 1991;10:4121–8.
62. Pawson T. Specificity in signal transduction: from phosphotyrosine-SH2 domain interactions to complex cellular systems. Cell 2004;116:191–203.
63. Ronnstrand L. Signal transduction via the stem cell factor receptor/c-Kit. Cell Mol Life Sci 2004;61:2535–48.
64. Linnekin D, DeBerry CS, Mou S. Lyn associates with the juxtamembrane region of c-Kit and is activated by stem cell factor in hematopoietic cell lines and normal progenitor cells. J Biol Chem 1997;272:27450–5.
65. Abram CL, Courtneidge SA. Src family tyrosine kinases and growth factor signaling. Exp Cell Res 2000;254:1–13.
66. O'Laughlin-Bunner B, Radosevic N, Taylor ML, et al. Lyn is required for normal stem cell factor-induced proliferation and chemotaxis of primary hematopoietic cells. Blood 2001;98:343–50.
67. Kovarova M, Tolar P, Arudchandran R, et al. Structure-function analysis of Lyn kinase association with lipid rafts and initiation of early signaling events after Fcepsilon receptor I aggregation. Mol Cell Biol 2001;21:8318–28.
68. Broudy VC, Lin NL, Liles WC, et al. Signaling via Src family kinases is required for normal internalization of the receptor c-Kit. Blood 1999;94:1979–86.
69. Jahn T, Leifheit E, Gooch S, et al. Lipid rafts are required for Kit survival and proliferation signals. Blood 2007;110:1739–47.
70. Arcaro A, Aubert M, Espinosa del Hierro ME, et al. Critical role for lipid raft-associated Src kinases in activation of PI3K-Akt signalling. Cell Signal 2007; 19:1081–92.
71. Foster FM, Traer CJ, Abraham SM, et al. The phosphoinositide (PI) 3-kinase family. J Cell Sci 2003;116:3037–40.
72. Fukao T, Yamada T, Tanabe M, et al. Selective loss of gastrointestinal mast cells and impaired immunity in PI3K-deficient mice. Nat Immunol 2002;3: 295–304.
73. Tan BL, Yazicioglu MN, Ingram D, et al. Genetic evidence for convergence of c-Kit- and alpha4 integrin-mediated signals on class IA PI-3kinase and the Rac pathway in regulating integrin-directed migration in mast cells. Blood 2003; 101:4725–32.
74. Chardin P, Camonis JH, Gale NW, et al. Human Sos1: a guanine nucleotide exchange factor for Ras that binds to GRB2. Science 1993;260:1338–43.
75. Roskoski R Jr. ERK1/2 MAP kinases: structure, function, and regulation. Pharmacol Res 2012;66:105–43.
76. Montagut C, Settleman J. Targeting the RAF-MEK-ERK pathway in cancer therapy. Cancer Lett 2009;283:125–34.
77. Kitayama H, Kanakura Y, Furitsu T, et al. Constitutively activating mutations of c-kit receptor tyrosine kinase confer factor-independent growth and tumorigenicity of factor-dependent hematopoietic cell lines. Blood 1995;85:790–8.
78. Boissan M, Feger F, Guillosson JJ, et al. c-Kit and c-kit mutations in mastocytosis and other hematological diseases. J Leukoc Biol 2000;67:135–48.

79. Ustun C, DeRemer DL, Akin C. Tyrosine kinase inhibitors in the treatment of systemic mastocytosis. Leuk Res 2011;35:1143–52.

80. Laine E, Chauvot de Beauchene I, Perahia D, et al. Mutation D816V alters the internal structure and dynamics of c-KIT receptor cytoplasmic region: implications for dimerization and activation mechanisms. PLoS Comput Biol 2011;7: e1002068.

81. Kohl TM, Schnittger S, Ellwart JW, et al. KIT exon 8 mutations associated with core-binding factor (CBF)-acute myeloid leukemia (AML) cause hyperactivation of the receptor in response to stem cell factor. Blood 2005;105:3319–21.

82. Laine E, Auclair C, Tchertanov L. Allosteric communication across the native and mutated KIT receptor tyrosine kinase. PLoS Comput Biol 2012;8:e1002661.

83. Zou J, Wang YD, Ma FX, et al. Detailed conformational dynamics of juxtamembrane region and activation loop in c-Kit kinase activation process. Proteins 2008;72:323–32.

84. Tsujimura T, Hashimoto K, Kitayama H, et al. Activating mutation in the catalytic domain of c-kit elicits hematopoietic transformation by receptor self-association not at the ligand-induced dimerization site. Blood 1999;93:1319–29.

85. Vendome J, Letard S, Martin F, et al. Molecular modeling of wild-type and D816V c-Kit inhibition based on ATP-competitive binding of ellipticine derivatives to tyrosine kinases. J Med Chem 2005;48:6194–201.

86. Lam LP, Chow RY, Berger SA. A transforming mutation enhances the activity of the c-Kit soluble tyrosine kinase domain. Biochem J 1999;338(Pt 1):131–8.

87. Casteran N, De Sepulveda P, Beslu N, et al. Signal transduction by several KIT juxtamembrane domain mutations. Oncogene 2003;22:4710–22.

88. Blume-Jensen P, Hunter T. Oncogenic kinase signalling. Nature 2001;411: 355–65.

89. Chian R, Young S, Danilkovitch-Miagkova A, et al. Phosphatidylinositol 3 kinase contributes to the transformation of hematopoietic cells by the D816V c-Kit mutant. Blood 2001;98:1365–73.

90. Ning ZQ, Li J, Arceci RJ. Signal transducer and activator of transcription 3 activation is required for Asp(816) mutant c-Kit-mediated cytokine-independent survival and proliferation in human leukemia cells. Blood 2001;97:3559–67.

91. Yang Y, Letard S, Borge L, et al. Pediatric mastocytosis-associated KIT extracellular domain mutations exhibit different functional and signaling properties compared with KIT-phosphotransferase domain mutations. Blood 2010;116: 1114–23.

92. Kozlowski M, Larose L, Lee F, et al. SHP-1 binds and negatively modulates the c-Kit receptor by interaction with tyrosine 569 in the c-Kit juxtamembrane domain. Mol Cell Biol 1998;18:2089–99.

93. Teis D, Huber LA. The odd couple: signal transduction and endocytosis. Cell Mol Life Sci 2003;60:2020–33.

94. Sorkin A, von Zastrow M. Endocytosis and signalling: intertwining molecular networks. Nat Rev Mol Cell Biol 2009;10:609–22.

95. Haugh JM, Meyer T. Active EGF receptors have limited access to PtdIns(4,5) P(2) in endosomes: implications for phospholipase C and PI 3-kinase signaling. J Cell Sci 2002;115:303–10.

96. Kranenburg O, Verlaan I, Moolenaar WH. Dynamin is required for the activation of mitogen-activated protein (MAP) kinase by MAP kinase kinase. J Biol Chem 1999;274:35301–4.

97. Vieira AV, Lamaze C, Schmid SL. Control of EGF receptor signaling by clathrin-mediated endocytosis. Science 1996;274:2086–9.

98. Wu P, Wee P, Jiang J, et al. Differential regulation of transcription factors by location-specific EGF receptor signaling via a spatio-temporal interplay of ERK activation. PLoS One 2012;7:e41354.

99. Hu J, Troglio F, Mukhopadhyay A, et al. F-BAR-containing adaptor CIP4 localizes to early endosomes and regulates epidermal growth factor receptor trafficking and downregulation. Cell Signal 2009;21:1686–97.

100. Brankatschk B, Wichert SP, Johnson SD, et al. Regulation of the EGF transcriptional response by endocytic sorting. Sci Signal 2012;5:ra21.

101. Burke P, Schooler K, Wiley HS. Regulation of epidermal growth factor receptor signaling by endocytosis and intracellular trafficking. Mol Biol Cell 2001;12:1897–910.

102. Kolch W. Meaningful relationships: the regulation of the Ras/Raf/MEK/ERK pathway by protein interactions. Biochem J 2000;351(Pt 2):289–305.

103. Teis D, Wunderlich W, Huber LA. Localization of the MP1-MAPK scaffold complex to endosomes is mediated by p14 and required for signal transduction. Dev Cell 2002;3:803–14.

104. Taub N, Teis D, Ebner HL, et al. Late endosomal traffic of the epidermal growth factor receptor ensures spatial and temporal fidelity of mitogen-activated protein kinase signaling. Mol Biol Cell 2007;18:4698–710.

105. Teis D, Taub N, Kurzbauer R, et al. p14-MP1-MEK1 signaling regulates endosomal traffic and cellular proliferation during tissue homeostasis. J Cell Biol 2006;175:861–8.

106. Toffalini F, Demoulin JB. New insights into the mechanisms of hematopoietic cell transformation by activated receptor tyrosine kinases. Blood 2010;116:2429–37.

107. Xiang Z, Kreisel F, Cain J, et al. Neoplasia driven by mutant c-KIT is mediated by intracellular, not plasma membrane, receptor signaling. Mol Cell Biol 2007;27:267–82.

108. Kon S, Minegishi N, Tanabe K, et al. Smap1 deficiency perturbs receptor trafficking and predisposes mice to myelodysplasia. J Clin Invest 2013;123:1123–37.

109. Levitzki A, Mishani E. Tyrphostins and other tyrosine kinase inhibitors. Annu Rev Biochem 2006;75:93–109.

110. Jabbour E, Lipton JH. A critical review of trials of first-line BCR-ABL inhibitor treatment in patients with newly diagnosed chronic myeloid leukemia in chronic phase. Clin Lymphoma Myeloma Leuk 2013;13(6):646–56.

111. Delgado L, Giraudier S, Ortonne N, et al. Adverse cutaneous reactions to the new second-generation tyrosine kinase inhibitors (dasatinib, nilotinib) in chronic myeloid leukemia. J Am Acad Dermatol 2013;69:839–40.

112. Saglio G, Baccarani M. First-line therapy for chronic myeloid leukemia: new horizons and an update. Clin Lymphoma Myeloma Leuk 2010;10:169–76.

113. Gotlib J, DeAngelo DJ, George TI, et al. KIT inhibitor midostaurin exhibits a high rate of clinically meaningful and durable responses in advanced systemic mastocytosis: report of a fully accrued phase II trial. Blood (ASH Annual Meeting Abstracts) 2010;116:316.

114. Bai Y, Bandara G, Ching Chan E, et al. Targeting the KIT activating switch control pocket: a novel mechanism to inhibit neoplastic mast cell proliferation and mast cell activation. Leukemia 2013;27:278–85.

115. Teodosio C, Garcia-Montero AC, Jara-Acevedo M, et al. Gene expression profile of highly purified bone marrow mast cells in systemic mastocytosis. J Allergy Clin Immunol 2013;131:1213–24, 1224.e1–4.

116. Niedoszytko M, Oude Elberink JN, Bruinenberg M, et al. Gene expression profile, pathways, and transcriptional system regulation in indolent systemic mastocytosis. Allergy 2011;66:229–37.
117. Ben Sahra I, Le Marchand-Brustel Y, Tanti JF, et al. Metformin in cancer therapy: a new perspective for an old antidiabetic drug? Mol Cancer Ther 2010;9: 1092–9.
118. O'Neill LA, Hardie DG. Metabolism of inflammation limited by AMPK and pseudo-starvation. Nature 2013;493:346–55.
119. Burnett JC, Rossi JJ. RNA-based therapeutics: current progress and future prospects. Chem Biol 2012;19:60–71.
120. Rosenfeld N, Aharonov R, Meiri E, et al. MicroRNAs accurately identify cancer tissue origin. Nat Biotechnol 2008;26:462–9.
121. Sethi A, Sholl LM. Emerging evidence for MicroRNAs as regulators of cancer stem cells. Cancers (Basel) 2011;3:3957–71.
122. Mayoral RJ, Pipkin ME, Pachkov M, et al. MicroRNA-221-222 regulate the cell cycle in mast cells. J Immunol 2009;182:433–45.
123. Mayoral RJ, Deho L, Rusca N, et al. MiR-221 influences effector functions and actin cytoskeleton in mast cells. PLoS One 2011;6:e26133.
124. Lee YN, Brandal S, Noel P, et al. KIT signaling regulates MITF expression through miRNAs in normal and malignant mast cell proliferation. Blood 2011; 117:3629–40.
125. Deho L, Monticelli S. Human mast cells and mastocytosis: harnessing microRNA expression as a new approach to therapy? Arch Immunol Ther Exp (Warsz) 2010;58:279–86.

Molecular Defects in Mastocytosis
KIT and Beyond KIT

Siham Bibi, PhD[a], Florent Langenfeld, PhD[a],
Sylvie Jeanningros, MSc[a], Fabienne Brenet, PhD[b,c,d,e],
Erinn Soucie, PhD[b,c,d,e], Olivier Hermine, MD, PhD[f,g],
Gandhi Damaj, MD[g,h], Patrice Dubreuil, PhD[b,c,d,e,g],
Michel Arock, PharmD, PhD[a,*]

KEYWORDS

- Systemic mastocytosis • KIT • Mutation • Signaling • TET2 • ASXL1 • Spliceosome
- Targeted therapy

KEY POINTS

- The KIT D816V mutation is found in almost all the adult patients presenting with different subvariants of systemic mastocytosis (SM).
- The clinical course and prognosis of the different subvariants vary greatly among patients with SM.
- Additional genetic lesions and aberrant overexpression of signaling pathways are found in aggressive SM and SM with associated hematologic non–mast cell-lineage disease.
- These additional genetic aberrations or overexpression of signaling pathways are associated with progression of the disease and worsen significantly the prognosis of patients with SM.

Disclosure: O. Hermine and P. Dubreuil receive research funding and honorarium from AB Science. Other authors declare no competing financial interests.
M. Arock is supported by Fondation de France; F. Langenfeld is supported by a fellowship from Ligue Nationale Contre le Cancer; P. Dubreuil is supported by La Ligue Nationale Contre le Cancer (équipe labellisée) and INCa; F. Brenet is supported by a fellowship from Fondation pour la Recherche Médicale and E. Soucie by a fellowship from Fondation de France.

[a] Molecular Oncology and Pharmacology, LBPA CNRS UMR8113, Ecole Normale Supérieure de Cachan, 61, Avenue du Président Wilson, Cachan 94235, France; [b] Signaling, Hematopoiesis and Mechanism of Oncogenesis, Inserm U1068, CRCM, 27, Bd Leï Roure BP 30059, Marseille 13009, France; [c] Institut Paoli-Calmettes, 232, Bd Sainte-Marguerite BP 156, Marseille 13009, France; [d] Aix-Marseille University, UM 105, 27, Bd Leï Roure BP 30059, Marseille 13284, France; [e] CNRS, UMR7258, CRCM, 27, Bd Leï Roure BP 30059, Marseille 13009, France; [f] Clinical Hematology Department, Faculty of Medicine and AP-HP Necker-Enfants Malades, Paris Descartes University, 12, Rue de l'École de Médecine, 75006, Paris, France; [g] Faculty of Medicine et AP-HP Necker-Enfants Malades, Mastocytosis Reference Center, 149, Rue de Sèvres, 75015 Paris, Paris Cedex 15 75743, France; [h] Clinical Hematology Department, Hôpital Sud, CHU Amiens, Ave René Laënnec - Salouël, Amiens 80054, France
* Corresponding author.
E-mail address: arock@ens-cachan.fr

INTRODUCTION

Mast cells (MCs) are multifunctional immune cells derived from hematopoietic stem cell (HSC) in the bone marrow (BM). Committed BM MC progenitors (MCPs) are released into the bloodstream, where they have been identified in humans as CD34+/KIT+/CD13+/FcεRI– cells.[1] Human MCPs migrate into the peripheral tissues, where they differentiate terminally into 2 major subtypes: $MC_{tryptase}$ (MC_T) and $MC_{tryptase-chymase}$ (MC_{TC}). MC_T are found preferentially in mucosal tissues, whereas MC_{TC} are prominent in serosal tissues.[2,3] For both MC subtypes, the major growth and differentiation factor is stem cell factor (SCF), which binds KIT (CD117), a transmembrane receptor with intrinsic tyrosine kinase (TK) activity.[4]

Mastocytosis comprises a heterogeneous group of rare diseases characterized by abnormal accumulation of more or less atypical MCs in 1 or more organs.[5] Although mastocytosis can affect either children or adults, the behavior of the disease appears different not only in children (disease frequently restricted to the skin and attenuating at puberty) versus adults (disease constantly systemic and chronic) but also between adults with systemic involvement.[5] Adult patients may suffer from an indolent form of the disease or may show aggressive or even leukemic variants.[6] However, in most adults, a recurrent abnormality in the *KIT* gene (mainly *KIT* D816V) is found in neoplastic MCs.[7] This discrepancy between the recurrent genotype and the variable severity of the disease has led several teams to investigate for, then to find, the presence of associated non-*KIT* molecular defects, particularly in advanced systemic mastocytosis (advSM).[8–10]

In the first part of this review, an overview of the implications of *KIT* in MC development and functions is provided. The mechanisms involved in the transforming potential of *KIT* mutants found in the various subcategories of mastocytosis and their consequences for treatment are then discussed. The additional genetic defects found in several cohorts of patients and their impact in terms of severity and progression of the disease are described, as well as their possible implications for future therapeutic considerations.

CRITICAL ROLES OF SCF AND *KIT* IN THE DEVELOPMENT AND BIOLOGY OF MCs

Mice with loss-of-function mutations affecting either synthesis of SCF (Sl/Sld mice) or *Kit* (W/Wv mice) are virtually devoid of MCs, showing the importance of the SCF/Kit axis in MCs.[11] In contrast, gain-of-function mutations in the *KIT* proto-oncogene are associated with enhanced survival and autonomous growth of MCs and their progenitors.[12] In addition, the injection of SCF increases the number of MCs by more than 100 times near the site of injection.[13] MCs are the only terminally differentiated hematopoietic cells expressing KIT, and SCF promotes not only differentiation of MCs from their MCPs but also adhesion, migration, and survival, as well as mediator release from mature MCs.[2]

Structure of SCF

SCF is encoded by a gene on chromosome 12q22-12q24 in humans.[14] The gene is alternatively spliced, leading to 2 SCF isoforms, which differ in the absence or presence of a particular proteolytic cleavage site. The isoform containing the cleavage site undergoes proteolysis and becomes soluble (sSCF of 18 kDa), as a 165 amino acid protein, with the first 141 residues necessary for its receptor-binding activity.[15] The isoform lacking the cleavage site remains cell associated as a 31-kDa membrane-bound form (mSCF).[15]

Normal Structure of KIT

The proto-oncogene *KIT*, located on chromosome 4q12 in humans,[16] contains 21 exons transcribed/translated into a transmembrane receptor TK (RTK) of 145 kDa and 976 amino acids.[17] KIT structure is characterized by 5 immunoglobulin (Ig)-like subunits in the extracellular domain (ECD), which contains the binding site for SCF, and is linked to a cytoplasmic region by a single transmembrane helix (**Fig. 1**).[18]

The cytoplasmic region of KIT consists of an autoinhibitory juxtamembrane domain (JMD) and a kinase domain (KD) arranged in a proximal (N-) and a distal (C-) lobe linked by a hinge region (see **Fig. 1**). The C-lobe of KIT includes a large kinase insert domain of 77 residues.

Binding of SCF to the ECD induces KIT dimerization, initiating the transphosphorylation of specific tyrosine residues.[18] The intracellular portion of KIT shows 21 tyrosine residues, from which at least 10 are phosphorylated after activation of the receptor.[18] They serve as binding sites to recruit downstream signaling

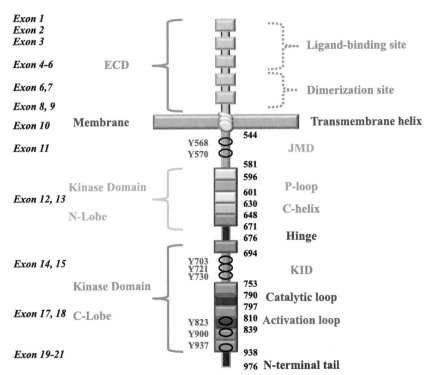

Fig. 1. Structure of normal KIT (KIT wild type). The *KIT* gene contains 21 exons transcribed/translated into a transmembrane RTK of 145 kDa and 976 amino acids. KIT structure is characterized by 5 Ig-like subunits in the extracellular domain (ECD), which contains the binding site for SCF and a dimerization site and is linked to a cytoplasmic region by a single transmembrane helix. The cytoplasmic region of KIT consists of an autoinhibitory juxtamembrane domain (JMD) of 35 residues and of a kinase domain (KD) arranged in a proximal (N-) and a distal (C-) lobe linked by a hinge region. The C-lobe includes a large kinase insert domain (KID) of 77 residues. In human KIT, the KID and the JMD contain 3 and 2 tyrosine residues, respectively. The receptor is presented under its monomeric form, and a dimer results from stem cell factor (SCF) ligation.

proteins, crucial for the control of cellular activities such as proliferation or apoptosis.[19]

Two crucial regulatory segments, the activation loop (A-loop, residues 810–835) and the JMD (residues 547–581), undergo extensive conformational rearrangements during the activation/deactivation process. In the inactive autoinhibited state of the receptor, the A-loop is adjacent to the active site, and the highly conserved catalytic D810-F811-G812 (DFG) motif adopts an out conformation: the phenylalanine is flipped into the adenosine triphosphate (ATP)-binding site, impairing ATP and Mg^{2+} cofactor binding.[20] This conformation is stabilized by the JMD that inserts itself directly into the active site and prevents the A-loop from adopting an active conformation.[21] On activation, the JMD moves from its autoinhibitory position to a completely solvent-exposed emplacement.[22] This intermediate conformation presenting an inactive, but not autoinhibited, state of the KD is followed by a conformational swap of the A-loop from an inactive packed arrangement to an active extended conformation.[22] This transition, together with a switch of the DFG motif to an "in" conformation, favors the stabilization of the active state, allowing ATP entrance and binding in the catalytic site.[22]

Physiologic Signaling by Normal KIT in MCs

Binding of SCF to KIT leads to the recruitment of several downstream signaling pathways, which account for MC survival, proliferation, activation or migration. KIT wild type (WT) recruits the PI3-kinases (PI3-K)/AKT/mechanistic target of rapamycin (mTOR) pathway,[23,24] the Janus Kinase 2 (JAK2)-Signal Transducer and Activator of Transcription (STAT)1/5 signaling,[25] the Src family kinases (SFK) pathway,[26,27] the mitogen-activated protein kinase pathway,[28–30] and phospholipases (particularly phospholipase C-γ).[31] A more detailed survey on normal KIT signaling is provided in the article by Olivera and colleagues elsewhere in this issue.

CLASSIFICATION OF MASTOCYTOSIS

Mastocytosis is schematically divided into cutaneous mastocytosis (CM) and systemic mastocytosis (SM).[6] Localized MC tumors (ie, mastocytomas and MC sarcoma [MCS]) are rare.[32] CM is usually diagnosed in childhood.[33] However, in most adult patients, the disease is systemic (SM), although the skin is often also affected.[34]

In patients with SM, the diagnosis is usually established by BM investigation using classic staining and specific tryptase stains.[35] Besides, apart from the BM, other organs, such as the liver or the gastrointestinal tract, may also be involved.[36] In addition, a high incidence of associated hematologic non-MC lineage diseases (AHNMD) is found in patients with SM.[37]

The 2008 World Health Organization (WHO) classification defined the following categories of SM: indolent SM (ISM), SM-AHNMD, aggressive SM (ASM), and MC leukemia (MCL).[38] In addition, the WHO classification included CM and the rare, localized, MC tumors, namely mast cell sarcoma (MCS) and extracutaneous mastocytomas (**Table 1**).[38]

The diagnosis of SM is based on 1 major and 4 minor criteria.[39] The major criterion of SM is the multifocal infiltration of MCs in the BM or other extracutaneous organs.[40] Minor SM criteria relate to the morphology of MCs by histology and on BM smears, aberrant expression of CD2 or CD25 by neoplastic MCs, an increased serum tryptase level (>20 ng/mL), and the presence of an activating *KIT* mutation at codon 816.[40] If at least 1 major and 1 minor criterion, or at least 3 minor criteria, are fulfilled, the final diagnosis is SM.

Table 1
WHO 2008 classification of mastocytosis

Category of Mastocytosis	Abbreviation	Subvariants
Cutaneous mastocytosis	CM	Urticaria pigmentosa (UP) Maculopapular CM (MPCM) Diffuse CM Mastocytoma of skin
Indolent systemic mastocytosis	ISM	Smoldering SM (SSM) Isolated bone marrow mastocytosis Well-differentiated SM
Systemic mastocytosis with an associated clonal hematologic non–mast cell disease	SM-AHNMD	SM-acute myeloid leukemia (AML) SM-myelodysplastic syndrome (MDS) SM-MPN SM-chronic myelomonocytic leukemia (CMML) SM-chronic eosinophilic leukemia (CEL) SM-non-Hodgkin lymphoma (NHL) SM-myeloma
Aggressive systemic mastocytosis	ASM	Lymphadenopathic SM with eosinophilia
Mast cell leukemia	MCL	Aleukemic MCL
Mast cell sarcoma	MCS	
Extracutaneous mastocytoma	ECM	

Adapted from Horny HP, Metcalfe DD, Bennett JM, et al. Mastocytosis. In: Swerdlow SH, Campo E, Harris NL, et al, editors. WHO classification of tumours of haematopoietic and lymphoid tissues. Lyon (France): IARC Press; 2008. p. 54–63.

KIT D816V is detectable not only in ISM but also in advSM.[41] From this observation, it must be concluded that, apart from *KIT* mutations, other factors might trigger the growth and survival of neoplastic MCs and that *KIT*-independent pathways may account for disease progression. Several of these additional *KIT*-independent oncogenic pathways may relate to the activation of LYN or BTK,[42] or additional genetic defects.[43] There is also a special subvariant of SM, termed smoldering SM (SSM), which presents with high MC burden, B-findings (borderline benign), such as hypercellular BM, dysplasia, organomegaly without organ failure, and high serum tryptase levels, but has a clinical course stable over years. However, some of these patients progress to ASM, SM-AHNMD, or even MCL over time, whereas others remain in the smoldering state for decades.[44] Thus, SSM is by some aspects an advSM. In SSM, the *KIT* D816V mutation is usually found in MCs, as well as in non-MC-lineage cells, which often are dysplastic or even mimic a myeloproliferative or myelodysplastic disease.[45]

INVOLVEMENT OF *KIT* DEFECTS IN MASTOCYTOSIS

Since SCF was identified as the major cytokine responsible for MC proliferation, various teams have investigated whether increased secretion of SCF could be involved in the pathophysiology of mastocytosis. No convincing data appeared, and investigations were thereafter conducted on its receptor KIT, which was reported to be responsible for autonomous growth of cell lines harboring *KIT* mutations, by constitutively activating downstream pathways in the absence of SCF.[46,47] Neoplastic MCs of patients with SM[48] and then of children with CM[49] were more recently found to present similar recurrent anomalies of the *KIT* gene structure (mainly *KIT* D816V in adults). An additional proof of the involvement of *KIT* defects in the pathophysiology of SM was provided by a model of animals transgenic for human *KIT* D816V, in which MC hyperplasia was observed, along with the expression of the transgene in MCs.[50]

Although additional genetic defects apart from *KIT* mutations have recently been found in neoplastic cells of patients with advSM,[8–10,43] *KIT* mutations are the only genetic alteration found in most mastocytosis cases (CM in children and ISM in adults) (**Fig. 2**). The following section emphasizes similarities and differences of the *KIT* defects found in mastocytosis variants as well as how the nature of the *KIT* mutant may affect the treatment of patients.

Pediatric CM

Unlike in adult patients, the frequency and the role of *KIT* mutations in childhood-onset mastocytosis, and whether it is a clonal disease, have long remained unclear. Longley and colleagues[49] found that 6 pediatric patients lacked mutations in codon 816, but 3 had a dominant inactivating mutation, K839E. Similarly, Buttner and colleagues[51] reported that none of 11 pediatric patients had codon 816 mutations, suggesting that childhood mastocytosis may be a reactive rather than a clonal disease. Conversely, Yanagihori and colleagues[52] found mutations in codon 816 in 10 of 12 children with mastocytosis, and Verzijl and colleagues[53] found that 25% of children with urticaria pigmentosa had the D816V mutation.

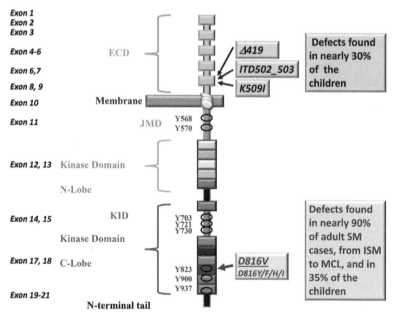

Fig. 2. KIT structure, showing localization of the more frequently observed mutations in the *KIT* sequence in pediatric or adult patients with mastocytosis. The receptor is presented under its monomeric form, whereas its wild type counterpart dimerizes on ligation with SCF before being activated in normal cells. The *KIT* D816V PTD mutant is found in up to 90% of the adult patients with SM, whereas ECD mutants are found in nearly 40% of affected children. Only the major mutations found in pediatric patients are represented here; see **Table 2** for a complete list of *KIT* mutants retrieved in children. Δ, deletion; ITD, internal tandem duplication; JMD, juxtamembrane domain; KI, kinase insert; PTD, phosphotransferase domain; TMD, transmembrane domain.

In a recent study conducted on a large cohort of pediatric patients (50 patients younger than 16 years), we examined the presence of *KIT* mutations.[54] We found 18 children (36%) with the D816V point mutation and 3 additional patients with other mutations in codon 816: D816Y (n = 2) and D816I (n = 1). Other new *KIT* mutations were identified in our cohort, mainly located in exons 8 and 9 (Δ417-418, D419Y, C443Y, S476I, ITD502-503, K509I) and exon 11 (D572A). All these new mutations were mutually exclusive of mutations in codon 816 and caused constitutive activation of KIT.[54] Further study of 60 additional pediatric cases provided similar results compared with our first set of patients (**Table 2**, Dubreuil and colleagues, unpublished data, 2014). From our studies, 76% of the pediatric patients have alterations in *KIT*, supporting the hypothesis that childhood mastocytosis is a clonal disease similar to SM in adults but with a less restricted spectrum of *KIT* mutations than in adults. However, how the pediatric form can spontaneously resolve remains to be elucidated.

ISM

KIT D816V mutant is the most frequent *KIT* abnormality, detected in virtually 100% of the ISM cases, when using a sensitive technique on purified BM MCs.[55,56] In a small fraction of patients with ISM, the disease progresses into an aggressive variant and the presence of *KIT* D816V mutation in non-MC lineages seems to be a predictor for risk of progression to ASM.[55] However, in a recent study conducted on 25 patients with ISM, the *KIT* D816V mutation was detected in both BM and peripheral blood (PB) cells in all cases using a very sensitive quantitative polymerase chain reaction,

Table 2
Analysis of *KIT* mutations in an extended pediatric cohort of 110 patients

Affected Exon	KIT Mutation (aa)	Number of Patients Affected	Frequency (%)
8	Del417-418-419 InsAsn-Ala	1	0.91
8	Del417-418-419 InsIle	1	0.91
8	Del417-418-419 InsTyr	1	0.91
8	Del419Asp	19	17.27
8	419ins6	1	0.91
8	C443Y	1	0.91
9	S451C	1	0.91
9	S476I	1	0.91
9	Ins6 501-502	2	1.82
9	Ins6 502-503	6	5.45
9	Ins6 504	1	0.91
9	Ins12 505-508	1	0.91
9	K509I	6	5.45
11	D572A	1	0.91
11	Del564-576	1	0.91
17	D816I	2	1.82
17	D816V	34	30.91
17	D816Y	3	2.73
NA	WT	27	24.55

meaning that circulating *KIT* D816V+ non-MCs in PB can be considered characteristic of ISM.[57]

Well-differentiated SM and SSM are subsets of ISM.[45] SSM has been described earlier. Well-differentiated SM is characterized by BM compact multifocal infiltrates, by round mature, CD25-negative MCs, and by a non-816 mutation of *KIT* or the absence of *KIT* mutation.[58]

ASM

ASM is a subvariant of SM with a progressive evolution and a poor prognosis (median survival of 41 months) compared with ISM.[59] C-findings (clinical findings) are found, corresponding to organ(s) failure, such as impaired BM function, hepatic failure and ascites, splenomegaly with hypersplenism, severe osteolysis and fractures, or malabsorption and weight loss.[60] In addition, ASM can transform into MCL.[61] Most patients with ASM present the *KIT* D816V mutation, but other *KIT* mutations (D820G or V559I) may also be found.[62,63] Neoplastic MCs in ASM typically show an immature phenotype with clonal involvement of all myeloid lineages by the *KIT* D816V mutation.[64]

Recently, reports, including ours, have proposed that additional genetic lesions apart from the *KIT* D816V mutation are present in ASM.[9,10,43] This feature may explain the aggressiveness of the disease, as well as the resistance of many *KIT* D816V+ patients with ASM to midostaurin, a drug active *in vitro* on this mutant.[65]

SM-AHNMD

SM-AHNMD is a complex subtype of advSM. The SM compartment can be ISM, ASM, or MCL (MCL is rarely associated with AHNMD),[66] whereas the AHNMD is of myeloid origin in most cases (see **Table 1**).[67] However, AHNMDs cover all major subtypes of hematologic malignancies, including lymphomas (see **Table 1**).[68] These various AHNMDs may present with their own recurrent genetic defects, such as t(8;21) in acute myeloid leukemia (AML) cells or *JAK2* V617F mutation in *BCR-ABL1*-negative myeloproliferative neoplasm (MPN).[37] However, the existence of a clonal relationship between the 2 disease components in SM-AHNMD has been largely unexplored. In a recent study, 48 patients with SM-AHNMD were tested for the presence of mutant *KIT* in the SM and AHNMD components of the disease.[69] The *KIT* D816V mutant was retrieved in the SM compartment of almost all the patients excepted those with an SM-chronic eosinophilic leukemia[69] and in AHNMD cells of most patients with SM–chronic myelomonocytic leukemia (CMML), suggesting that the *KIT* D816V mutant appears in a common MC/monocytic precursor, unlike patients with SM-MPN (20%) or SM-AML (30%), in whom *KIT* D816V was less frequently detectable in the non-MC malignant compartment. None of the patients in whom AHNMDs were lymphoproliferations showed the *KIT* 816 mutation.[69]

MCL

In a recent review compiling all the published cases (n = 51) of MCL, *KIT* D816V mutation was detected only in 13 of 28 patients with MCL analyzed (46%).[61] In 2 patients without *KIT* D816V, *KIT* was WT, whereas in 6 other cases, mutations were found in exon 9 (n = 3), exon 10 (n = 1), exon 11 (n = 1), or exon 13 (n = 1).[61]

MCS

MCS is an extremely rare, aggressive neoplasm composed of atypical malignant MCs presenting as a solitary mass.[32] *KIT* mutational status has been investigated in a few cases and showed either the absence of mutations or mutations in non-816 locations, such as *KIT* Δ419 or *KIT* N822K.[70]

Familial Forms of Mastocytosis

Familial occurrence of mastocytosis has been reported in more than 50 families since the mid-1880s. Most of the cases were pediatric CM without *KIT* mutations or with uncommon mutations (ie, K509I, A533D, N822I, M835K, S849I or deletion of amino acids 419 or 559–560).[71–73] Most of these *KIT* defects have been found activating and some were sensitive to imatinib, at least *in vitro*. In most cases, the *KIT* mutation found was of a germline nature, but we recently reported a family (mother and son) with adult-onset SM associated with a somatic *KIT* D816V mutation.[74]

ABNORMAL SIGNALING EVOKED BY THE *KIT* D816V ONCOGENIC MUTANT

This section focuses on the signaling pathways evoked by the KIT D816V mutant receptor (**Fig. 3**), which is the most prominently KIT mutant found in all the variants of SM.

Although the mechanism behind the constitutive activation of the KIT D816V mutant receptor is still not fully understood, 1 possibility is that mutation within the phospho-transferase domain (PTD) results in a structural change that relieves autoinhibitory mechanisms. This hypothesis remains speculative, because no crystal structure of the KD of KIT with an activating mutation has been yet published.

Recently, an *in silico* analysis has suggested that D816 mutations cause a structural change in the A-loop but also weaken the binding of the JMD to the KD.[22] Consequently, the inhibitory effect of the JMD on kinase activity is suppressed.[22] In addition, it was proposed that the extended JMD could make contact with another KIT receptor, thereby promoting dimerization in the absence of ligand.[22] In support of this hypothesis, recombinant KD with the D816Y mutation, but not the WT KD, was found to form dimers in solution.[75]

Several groups have compared the ability of WT and oncogenic mutants of *KIT* to induce signal transduction and found that they differ not only quantitatively but also qualitatively. This finding is potentially important, because it suggests that there might be ways to selectively target oncogenic signaling with less impact on the normal situation. The reason for the different signaling abilities can stem from changes in intracellular localization of the mutant KIT, altered substrate specificity, or a combination of both.

Changes in Intracellular Localization

KIT with gain-of-function mutations in the KD shows reduced cell surface expression, and inhibition of kinase activity in KIT KD mutations restored cell surface expression of the mutant receptor.[76] Another study reported that KIT D816V was primarily localized to and could transmit oncogenic signals from the Golgi apparatus, whereas KIT trapped in the endoplasmic reticulum (ER) could not.[77] In an attempt to elucidate the role of localization on signaling, cells with activating mutations of *KIT* were treated with brefeldin A, which causes protein accumulation in the ER, and then various signaling pathways were analyzed. Certain proteins such as AKT and Extracellular signal-Regulated Kinases (ERK)1/2 were not activated in brefeldin A–treated cells, whereas other proteins (eg, STAT5) were phosphorylated, suggesting that signals induced from different compartments can be qualitatively different.[78] Although KIT D816V has an increased intracellular localization, some is still surface exposed, and this has functional consequences. For instance, cells expressing *KIT* D816V still migrate toward soluble SCF.[79] Furthermore, even in cells expressing *KIT* D816V, SCF is still required to promote activation of AKT and ERK1/2.[80] In contrast, other pathways such as c-Jun N-terminal Kinases (JNKs), Casitas B-lineage Lymphoma (c-CBL), and Src Homology 2 domain-Containing (SHC) are constitutively activated in cells

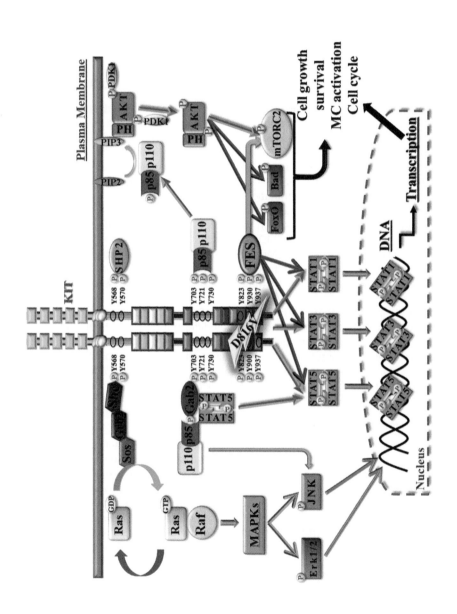

expressing *KIT* D816V. The reason for the dependence of intracellular localization for signaling is unclear but may relate to which downstream substrates are available at different locations. Alternatively, it could be the result of modifications in the receptors (eg, phosphorylation or selectively dephosphorylation) by other enzymes that are located only in certain compartments.

Altered Substrate Specificity

A recent study reported that KIT D816V showed a substrate specificity that resembled that of SRC and Abelson murine leukemia viral oncogene homolog (ABL) TKs.[81] Consequently, the mutant KIT could activate ERK1/2 independently of SRC, whereas KIT WT required SRC activity for these processes.[81] Several studies have tried to identify signaling pathways critical for the transforming abilities of mutant KIT. Particularly, we showed that the Feline Sarcoma Oncogene (FES) TK was important for negative regulation of STAT and positive regulation of mTOR phosphorylation downstream of KIT D816V.[82] More recently, the mTOR complex, composed by 2 molecules, mTORC1 and mTORC2, has been shown upregulated in neoplastic and developing immature MCs compared with their mature normal counterparts.[83] In addition, the use of selective inhibitors showed that, whereas mTORC1 may contribute to MC survival, mTORC2 was critical only for homeostasis of neoplastic and dividing immature MCs.[83] Because mTORC2 plays little role in the homeostasis of differentiated, nonproliferating, mature MCs, the investigators hypothesized that mTORC2 inhibition *via* a targeted approach might reduce the proliferation in MC disorders and leave normal differentiated MCs largely unaffected.[83]

The importance of the PI3-K/AKT pathway in mastocytosis has been reported recently. AKT activation has been identified as a key signaling molecule involved in KIT-dependent differentiation and growth of neoplastic MCs harboring oncogenic *KIT* mutants.[84] AKT was found phosphorylated in neoplastic MCs from patients suffering from *KIT* D816V+ SM and in the HMC-1.2 cell line, raising the hypothesis that AKT activation plays a critical role in the pathogenesis of mastocytosis.[74,84,85]

Because STAT5 is involved in growth and survival of normal MCs,[25] several teams studied the implication of STAT5 in neoplastic MC growth, survival, and transformation, and light was shed on its implication downstream of KIT D816V. A first study

---

Fig. 3. Aberrant signaling evoked by the KIT D816V mutant receptor. Although the receptor is presented under a dimeric form as a transmembrane protein, it has been postulated that the KIT D816V protein could activate substrates and be located in the cell cytoplasm. That KIT D816V dimerizes spontaneously with itself or with KIT WT, or is capable of transmitting oncogenic signals as a single molecule, remains largely unexplored. The *KIT* D816V oncogenic mutation alters the substrate specificity of the mutant protein, which shows a substrate specificity that resembled that of SRC and ABL TKs. In addition, FES TK is activated by mutant KIT protein and negatively regulates the STAT pathway, although it induced phosphorylation of mTOR. Furthermore, AKT activation has been identified as a key signaling molecule involved in KIT D816V-dependent differentiation and growth of neoplastic MCs. Also, STAT5 is believed to play a pivotal role in growth of *KIT* D816V+ neoplastic MCs and is constitutively phosphorylated in such cells, probably because KIT D816V can promote direct STAT5 activation, thus diverting the canonical JAK-STAT pathway. A noncanonical pSTAT5 cytoplasmic retention system is found in neoplastic MCs, namely pSTAT5 retention by docking to the p85 regulatory subunit of PI3K *via* the GAB2 scaffold protein that controls the AKT signaling. This cytoplasmic retention system might block nuclear accumulation of pSTAT5, keeping STAT5-mediated transcription at bay. Green arrows, activation; red arrows, inhibition; black arrows, induction of survival or functions.

showed that knockdown of STAT5 led to growth inhibition of neoplastic MC.[84] A second study has shown that neoplastic MCs express cytoplasmic and nuclear phospho-STAT5 (p-STAT5).[86] Furthermore, the same team showed that KIT D816V promotes direct STAT5-activation, and that p-STAT5 contributes to growth of neoplastic MCs.[86]

CONSEQUENCES OF THE VARIOUS DEFECTS IN *KIT* FOR TARGETED THERAPY

There are strong changes in the sensitivity of KIT mutants to TK inhibitors (TKIs) type II (eg, imatinib or masitinib) compared with KIT WT.[87] Thus, before using targeted therapies aiming to inhibit KIT TK activity for the treatment of patients with SM, it is mandatory to know exactly the *KIT* mutational status of each patient. However, even with adequate targeting of the KIT mutant, the results could be deceiving, and no complete remission should be obtained with SM, particularly in advSM. For this reason, combined therapies, or therapies targeting signaling downstream KIT could be a promising approach for the future.

PTD Mutants

The A-loop mutations D816V/H/Y/N induce high KIT resistance to imatinib *in vitro*, as well as *ex vivo* on patients' cells.[87] Given this resistance of *KIT* D816V toward imatinib, several other more or less targeted TKIs have been tested *in vitro* and in clinical studies for patients with advSM.

Dasatinib is also a potent inhibitor of SFKs, which are important mediators of KIT actions, and thus, this inhibitor potentially has dual targets of KIT kinase activity *per se* and SFK-mediated responses.[88] However, although dasatinib strongly inhibits KIT D816 mutants in cell lines, as well as in cells of patients with SM, only a few patients with ASM have been treated with dasatinib, with disappointing results.[89]

PKC412 (midostaurin) is an *N*-benzoylstaurosporine with potent inhibitory activity against protein kinase C, vascular endothelial growth factor receptor 2 (VEGFR-2), Alpha-type platelet-derived growth factor receptor (PDGFRa), Fms-related tyrosine kinase 3 (FLT3), kinase insert domain receptor (KDR), and KIT.[90] PKC412 decreased KIT phosphorylation in both HMC-1.1 cells and HMC-1.2 cells as well as in patients' cells at pharmacologic concentrations *in vitro*.[91] Several clinical trials are ongoing to examine the potential effects of this multikinase inhibitor in patients with SM.[65] In patients with ASM, midostaurin was shown to be well tolerated and there was a high rate of durable responses, accompanied by significant reductions in MC burden, including in MCL.[65]

JMD, Transmembrane Domain, and Extracellular Membrane Domain Mutants

By contrast to the PTD mutation D816V, the JMD mutation V560D/G increases the drug sensitivity of the receptor.[92] Imatinib inhibits at low concentrations the proliferation of the HMC-1.1 subclone with only *KIT* V560G mutation.[92] However, this mutant is rarely seen in SM, and thus, only limited data are available on the efficacy of imatinib in such patients. In addition, not all JMD mutations may be sensitive to imatinib (eg, V559I).[93]

A transmembrane domain mutation in *KIT* is a rare event in SM. Only 1 well-documented case has been reported. Akin and colleagues[94] described the case of a 25-year-old patient with SM with a germline *KIT* F522C mutation and a history of CM during childhood. Therapy with imatinib resulted in a dramatic improvement in MC burden and clinical symptoms in this patient.[94]

Most of the *KIT* mutants found in the ECD of the receptor, particularly those described in pediatric patients, were found highly sensitive to imatinib, at least *in vitro.*[74] Imatinib was even shown to be effective in a case of MCL with a defect in the ECD of KIT (p.A502_Y503dup).[95]

However, in rare cases of SM (or even MCL) with no defect in KIT (*KIT* WT), imatinib or masitinib have shown a significant activity *in vivo* in isolated cases.[96,97]

OTHER (ADDITIONAL) MOLECULAR DEFECTS FOUND IN VARIOUS FORMS OF MASTOCYTOSIS: BEYOND *KIT*

TET2 Mutations

TET2 functions and impact in hematologic malignancies

TET2 is a member of a family of 3 proteins (TET1, TET2, and TET3) that catalyze the conversion of 5-methylcytosine (5-mC) to 5-hydroxymethylcytosine (5-hmC) in the DNA.[98] 5-hmC may initiate DNA demethylation by actively excluding DNA methyltransferases from CpG islands. Thus, the TET family could be implied in epigenetic regulation *via* the induction of 5-hmC.

The *TET2* gene is located on chromosome 4q24, which is a breakpoint in various AML-associated translocations.[99] Mice knockout or heterozygous for *TET2* have abnormal hematopoiesis with, first, HSC expansion, then, the development of myeloid malignancies resembling CMML or myelodysplasia.[100] Recently, several investigators have identified *TET2* mutations, scattered across several of its 12 exons in 1 or both *TET2* alleles, as an early event during the development of various malignancies, including MPN, CMML, myelodysplastic syndrome (MDS), leukemia, and B- and T-cell lymphomas.[101] Patients with mutant *TET2*+ myeloid disorders show a decreased level of 5-hmC with hypomethylation or hypermethylation of DNA.[102] Altogether these data show that *TET2* plays a role in various hematologic malignancies.

TET2 and mastocytosis

The first report of an association between mastocytosis and alterations in *TET2* came from Tefferi and colleagues in 2009.[43] On a cohort of 48 patients with SM (comprising 6 patients with *FIP1L1-PDGFRA* fusion gene), these investigators found at the BM level that 29% of patients with SM, but no *FIP1L1-PDGFRA*+ patients, had *TET2* mutations. The presence of *TET2* defects was documented in 15% of 13 patients with ISM, 40% of 5 patients with ASM, and 35% of 23 patients with SM-AHNMD.[43] In addition, the investigators reported a significant association between monocytosis and the presence of *TET2* mutations. Furthermore, they showed a correlation between *TET2* lesions and presence of *KIT* D816V mutant. *KIT* D816V was found in 50% of patients with the *TET2* mutation, but in only 20% of patients without alteration in the *TET2* gene.[43] From these data, the investigators concluded that *TET2* mutations are frequent in SM, segregate with *KIT* D816V, and influence phenotype, without necessarily altering prognosis.

The presence of *TET2* mutations in mastocytosis was further confirmed by Traina and colleagues[8] on 26 patients (15 ISM, 8 SM-AHNMD, 2 ASM, and 1 MCS); these investigators found *TET2* mutations in 6 patients (23%), mostly in patients with SM-AHNMD (5 of the 6 patients with *TET2* mutations), whereas only 1 patient with ISM was found positive. Although the number of affected cases was low, the investigators claimed that the presence of *TET2* mutations conferred a poor prognosis regarding overall survival (OS).[8]

In a recent report, Schwaab and colleagues[10] have analyzed the complete coding regions of *TET2*, as well as of several other genes of interest, in a cohort of 39 patients with advSM. Regarding *TET2* defects, the investigators found 29 mutations identified in 15 patients. These 15 patients had an SM-AHNMD, with the SM compartment being indolent, aggressive, or even leukemic, whereas the AHNMD was frequently an MDS or a CMML.[10] In addition, the investigators compared the OS of the patients with KIT D816V mutation alone with one of the KIT D816V+ patients bearing TET2 mutations and found a shorter OS in the second group of patients.[10]

We have recently analyzed a cohort of 74 patients with mastocytosis, categorized according to the WHO classification into aggressive or nonaggressive disease.[9] Consistent with previous studies, most of our patients (82.5%) were positive for KIT mutation (78.4% KIT D816V+). TET2 mutations were detected in 20.3% of the patients and were distributed along the gene in a pattern similar to that reported in AML and CMML.[9] Two distinct mutations in the TET2 gene were detected in some patients, and in all cases, TET2 mutation occurred in conjunction with KIT mutation. TET2 mutation correlated significantly with aggressive forms of mastocytosis.[9] Both TET2 and KIT mutations were found in primary MCs sorted from patients, and clonal analysis from BM biopsies of 2 patients was also consistent with a model in which TET2 mutation is an early event preceding clonal disease onset of aggressive disease.[9]

To understand the mechanism underlying the impact of TET2 on the severity of the disease, we derived BM-derived MCs (BMMCs) from Tet2-/- mice and we transduced these BMMCs with KIT D816V, together with BMMCs obtained from Tet2 WT mice. We observed a significant and competitive growth advantage for KIT D816V+ Tet2-/- BMMCs compared with KIT D816V+ Tet2 WT cells.[9]

Taken together, these data provide evidence for the existence of an oncogenic cooperation between KIT and TET2 mutations in MCs and show TET2 mutation as a potential marker to diagnose and predict severe forms of mastocytosis. However, this observation does not apply to all the subtypes of advSM. In a recent study focused on 62 patients with SM-AHNMD, 27% of the patients were found to have a TET2 mutation.[103] However, in our hands, in univariate analysis as well as in multivariate analysis, the presence of TET2 mutation was not associated with an affected OS.[103]

Mutations in the Spliceosome Machinery

In humans, most protein-coding transcripts contain introns that are removed by messenger RNA splicing carried out by spliceosomes. Mutations in the spliceosome machinery, which include the splicing factor 3 subunit b1 (SF3b1), the U2 small nuclear RNA auxiliary factor 1 (U2AF1) and the serine arginine rich splicing factor 2 (SRSF2) have recently been identified using whole exome/genome technologies in MDS, CMML, and primary fibrosis.[104]

There is only 1 published report, by Schwaab and colleagues,[10] in which the structure of SF3B1 has been analyzed. Although the cohort comprised several patients with SM-CMML or SM-MDS, none of the 39 patients tested was found positive for hotspot mutations lying in the exon 15 of SF3B1.[10] More recently, we have analyzed the structure of SF3B1 on a cohort of 72 patients and found mutations in only 4 patients (5.6%), with 2 patients having mutations in codon 14 and 2 patients in codon 15.[105] We also analyzed the structure of U2AF1 and found only 2 patients with a mutation in codon 2. Mutations in SF3B1, U2AF1, and SRSF2 were found mutually exclusive in our cohort of patients.[105]

Schwaab and colleagues[10] also analyzed the occurrence of SRSF2 mutations in their cohort of 39 patients. These investigators found 14 patients (35%) presenting a mutation in the hotspot region of SRSF2.

We also tested a cohort of 72 patients for SRSF2-P95 mutation and found that after KIT mutations (81%), the SRSF2-P95 hotspot mutation was the most frequent defect found in our patients: 17 of 72 (23.6%) patients, whereas TET2 mutants were found in 21% of the patients.[105] We found that SRSF2-P95 hotspot mutation was highly correlated with the presence of an AHNMD (17 patients of 17 positive had an AHNMD). Nevertheless, we were able to show at the single-cell level that, in these cases of SRSF2-P95+ SM-AHNMD, the mutant was found in MCs as well as in monocytes, supporting a role for SRSF2-P95 mutation in MC transformation. In addition, we found TET2 and SRSF2-P95 mutations were statistically highly associated, suggesting a mechanistic link between these 2 factors. However, the presence of the SRSF2-P95 mutation in patients did not induce a shortening in OS.[105]

Regarding U2AF1 mutations in mastocytosis, Schwaab and colleagues[10] found only 2 patients of 39 with this defect. One of the 2 patients had an ISM and presented only with the U2AF1 mutation, whereas the other patient had an SM-MDS/MPN and presented several additional genetic defects.[10] Confirming this low frequency, we also analyzed the structure of U2AF1 in our cohort of 72 patients and found also only 2 patients affected by a mutation of this gene.[105]

ASXL1 Mutations

The gene ASXL1 (additional sex combs–like 1) is located in the chromosomal region 20q11 and encodes for a protein of the polycomb group and trithorax complex family ASXL1.[106] ASXL1 can interact with retinoic acid receptor and seems to be involved in chromatin remodeling, but its function remains unknown.[107] ASXL1 is expressed in most hematopoietic cell types, and a knockout mouse model showed mild defects in myelopoiesis but did not develop MDS or other hematologic malignancy.[108] Several studies have shown that ASXL1 mutations (particularly frequent in exon 12 and often heterozygous) occur frequently in MDS, AML, chronic myelogenous leukemia (CML), CMML, and MPN and worsen the prognosis.[109,110]

The first description of occurrence of ASXL1 defects in mastocytosis came in 2012 from the group of Traina and colleagues,[8] who sequenced ASXL1 gene in 26 patients with SM (15 ISM, 8 SM-AHNMD, 2 ASM, and 1 MCS) and found 3 different ASXL1 heterozygous mutations in 3 of the 26 (12%) patients with SM. ASXL1 mutations were found in 1 of 15 of the patients with ISM and 2 of 8 of the patients with SM-AHNMD.[8] An ASXL1 defect was the only genetic alteration (apart from a KIT D816V mutation) found in the patient with ISM, whereas the 2 patients with SM-AHNMD found positive for ASXL1 mutation were also positive for TET2 defects.

More recently, Schwaab and colleagues[10] found ASXL1 defects in 8 patients of 39. All 8 patients were found to have an SM-AHNMD, with the SM compartment being either indolent, aggressive, or even leukemic, whereas the AHNMD was found frequently to be CMML.[10] Four of 8 presented with an associated TET2 mutation, and 7 of 8 presented with 1 or several additional defects.[10] In addition, the investigators compared the OS of the patients with KIT D816V mutation alone with OS of the KIT D816V+ patients bearing at least 1 additional genetic defect. In all cases, including for ASXL1 mutations, OS was significantly shorter in the second group of patients.[10]

In our cohort of 62 French patients with SM-AHNMD (AHNMD being mostly myeloid, and comprising MDS, CMML, or MPN), we have analyzed the structure of KIT, TET2, ASXL1, and CBL genes (see earlier discussion). We found defects in ASXL1 in 14% of the patients.[103] In univariate analysis, we found that the presence of C-findings, the AHNMD subtypes (SM-MDS/CMML/AML vs SM-MPN/hypereosinophilia), neutropenia, high monocyte levels, and the presence of ASXL1 mutation had statistically significant detrimental effects on OS.[103] In our hands, with the use of multivariate analysis and a penalized Cox model, only the presence of the ASXL1 mutation remained an independent prognostic factor, which had a significant and negative effect on OS.[103]

The literature tends to show that *ASXL1* mutations are found at a frequency ranging between 12% and 20% of patients with SM, preferably in advSM, and in most cases in SM-AHNMD. In addition, it seems that the presence of *ASXL1* mutants could be detrimental for patients' outcome.

RAS Mutations

Acquired mutations in the *RAS* family are frequently implicated in malignant transformation and tumor maintenance.[111] RAS and proliferation of MCs were linked a long time ago by studying an interleukin 3–dependent mouse MC line (BP-3c) immortalized after introduction of the *v-HRas* oncogene producing mastocytoma.[112] More recently, another study confirmed that *NRASV12* expression induces the development of an ASM or even an MCL-like disease in mice.[113] Using an improved mouse BM transduction and transplantation model, a third study showed that an oncogenic form of *NRAS* induced rapidly and efficiently a CMML-like or AML-like disease and also an SM-like disease *in vivo*.[114] These last 2 studies indicated that oncogenic *NRAS* could be of importance in the pathogenesis of mastocytosis *in vivo*.

Wilson and colleagues[115] evaluated the coexistence of *NRAS*, *KRAS*, *HRAS*, or *MRAS* mutations on 44 *KIT* D816V+ patients (27 with ISM, 9 with SSM, 4 with SM-AHNMD, and 4 with ASM). These investigators found activating *NRAS* mutations in 2 patients (4.5%), one with ASM and the other with SM-CMML. In these 2 patients, BM CD34+ were positive for *NRAS* mutation but negative for *KIT* D816V mutant, whereas clonal MCs and circulating myeloid and lymphoid mature cells harbored both mutations, suggesting that *NRAS* mutations may have the potential to precede *KIT* D816V in clonal development.[115]

More recently, the Reiter group analyzed 39 *KIT* D816V+ patients with various subtype of ASM for the presence of *KRAS* and *NRAS* mutations.[10] These investigators found 4 patients (10.2%) with *KRAS* mutations (3 with an ASM and 1 MCL) and 2 other patients with ASM (5.1%) with *NRAS* mutant forms. No mutations in *RAS* were found in the 10 patients with ISM included in the cohort.[10]

We have recently analyzed the presence of *NRAS* mutations in our cohort of 72 patients with different subtypes of mastocytosis and found only 2 patients classified in the ASM-AHNMD group with mutant *NRAS* (2.8%).[105]

CBL, DNMT3A, ETV6, EZH2, RUNX1, and SETBP1 Mutations

These mutations are usually found at lower frequencies than *TET2*, *ASXL1*, or *SRSF2* mutations and are more frequently found in patients with SM-AHNMD. Because few data are available, it is difficult to determine whether they target both the MC and the non-MC components of the disease or only the non-MC part of the malignant cells, or to characterize their impact on prognosis, response to treatment, or OS of the patients. Here, we propose a rapid survey of their frequency, analyzing the few cohorts of patients published.

CBL mutants were found at a frequency ranging from 3.8% (1 of 26 patients)[8] to 20.5% (8 of 39)[10] patients in mastocytosis. In both reports, the mutants were exclusively found in patients with SM-AHNMD, except for 1 mutation in a patient with ISM.

The presence of *DNMT3A* mutations in mastocytosis has been analyzed by Traina and colleagues,[8] and 3 patients of 26 (11.5%) were found to have mutations in *DNMT3*: 2 patients with *KIT* D816V+ ISM and 1 patient with *KIT* WT SM-CMML.

The complete coding regions of the *ETV6* gene were analyzed in the cohort of 39 patients by Schwaab and colleagues[10] and 1 mutation was found in 1 patient with Unclassifiable myelodysplastic/myeloproliferative neoplasm (MDS/MPNu), who also presented mutations in *ASXL1*, *CBL*, and *U2AF1* genes.

The *EZH2* gene was analyzed by Traina and colleagues,[8] who found no alteration of the gene in a cohort of 26 patients, whereas the Reiter group found 2 of 39 patients with advSM (5.1%) with alterations in the structure of the gene, consisting of a missense mutation and 2 splice sites.[10] One patient was categorized as having an SM-MDS/MPNu, with associated defects in *TET2*, *ASXL1*, and *CBL*, whereas the other patient, categorized as ASM-MDS/MPNu, presented associated defects in *TET2* and *CBL*.[10]

In the same study, Schwaab and colleagues[10] analyzed additional genes known to be involved in hematologic malignancies, *SETBP1* and *RUNX1*. *SETBP1* gene codes for a nuclear localizing protein with mutations (mostly heterozygous missenses) that have been recently described in atypical CML, AML, MDS, and CMML with a low frequency.[116] Only 1 patient (2.5%) with *KIT* D816V+ ISM was found positive for *SETBP1* mutation. Runt-related transcription factor 1 (*RUNX1*), also known as AML1 protein or core-binding factor subunit α_2 (*CBFA2*) is a transcription factor regulating HSC differentiation. Mutations in *RUNX1* are implicated in MDS and AML and associated with a poor prognosis.[117] Such mutations (9 missense mutations, 1 frameshift) were also reported in 9 of the 39 *KIT* D816V+ patients with mastocytosis (23%) analyzed by the Reiter group.[10] All patients who tested positive for *RUNX1* mutations were patients with ASM, with or without AHNMD. Seven of these 9 patients presented with 1 or more additional genetic defects targeting *TET2*, *SRSF2*, or less frequently, *ASXL1*, and 3 of the 4 patients found positive for *KRAS* mutations in the whole cohort were also positive for *RUNX1* mutations.[10]

SUMMARY AND FUTURE CONSIDERATIONS

In SM, the *KIT* D816V mutant is detected in most (>90%) patients.[45] Although TKIs specific for KIT D816V have shown excellent activity toward KIT D816V *in vitro*,[91,118] these compounds have only modest activity *in vivo*. One possible explanation could be that the molecular pathogenesis of SM, particularly in advSM is more complex than the presence of a single gene defect in *KIT* and that additional genetic defects could

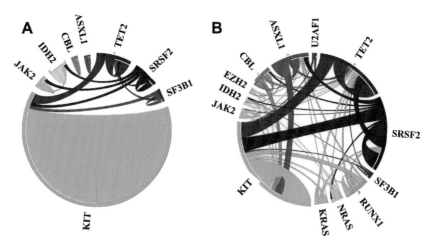

Fig. 4. Circos (circular genome data visualization) diagrams depicting the relative frequency and associations of the major mutations found in SM in nonaggressive (NA) forms (*A*) and in aggressive (A) forms (*B*) based on data from our work on 73 patients with SM (31 A, 42 NA)[105] and from the Reiter group study of 47 patients with SM (38 A, 9 NA).[10] (NA forms: SSM (±AHNMD), ISM (±AHNMD), CM, SM, MCL); (A forms: ASM (±AHNMD), MCS, MCL).

also influence the severity and progression of SM. This theory might explain the poor response to TKIs targeting KIT defects.

Data summarized here confirm that such genetic complexity exists in SM. Thus, in advSM (but not in ISM), there is increasing evidence that most patients present with 1 or several additional genetic defects, which might explain the aggressive evolution. Although some of these additional defects seem to be a rare event, encountered in only a few percent of patients with advSM tested, others are common and found in many of these patients. This finding is particularly the case for *TET2* mutants, which are found in up to 30% of patients with advSM.[9,10] Experiments conducted by our team showed that *KIT* D816V and *TET2* mutations cooperate *in vitro* and *in vivo* to induce a more aggressive cell phenotype when present together.[9] Also, mutations in *SRSF2* and in *ASXL1* are present in many of the patients tested and are related to a more aggressive disease.[10] In addition, a significant part of the patients may have 2 to more than 5 additional mutations, as shown by studies in which *KIT* D816V+ patients were found simultaneously positive for *TET2*, *SRSF2*, *ASXL1*, *CBL*, and *RUNX1* defects.[10] In line with the complexity of the associations of genetic defects found in SM by different teams, we present in **Fig. 4** Circos (circular genome data visualization) diagrams depicting the relative frequencies and associations of the major mutations in systemic SM in nonaggressive forms and in aggressive forms based on data from our work on 73 patients with SM (31 aggressive, 42 nonaggressive)[105] and from the Reiter group study on 47 patients with SM (38 aggressive, 9 nonaggressive).[10]

Data presented in this article suggest that ISM might be mainly a disease related to the sole presence of the *KIT* D816V mutant, whereas additional genetic defects (preexisting or acquired during disease evolution) might be responsible for progression to advanced phases of SM. However, in SM-AHNMD, these additional genetic defects could be related to the coexistence of 2 different diseases. This theory means that analysis of purified cell populations obtained by cell sorting or of single-cell derived clusters is mandatory to identify in which cell compartment one or the other of the mutations could be found. If these additional genetic defects are of obvious prognostic significance, their interest for future therapeutic in advSM remains to be explored.

REFERENCES

1. Kirshenbaum AS, Goff JP, Semere T, et al. Demonstration that human mast cells arise from a progenitor cell population that is CD34(+), c-kit(+), and expresses aminopeptidase N (CD13). Blood 1999;94:2333–42.
2. Metcalfe DD. Mast cells and mastocytosis. Blood 2008;112:946–56.
3. Li L, Meng XW, Krilis SA. Mast cells expressing chymase but not tryptase can be derived by culturing human progenitors in conditioned medium obtained from a human mastocytosis cell strain with c-kit ligand. J Immunol 1996;156:4839–44.
4. Valent P. The riddle of the mast cell: kit(CD117)-ligand as the missing link? Immunol Today 1994;15:111–4.
5. Valent P. Systemic mastocytosis. Cancer Treat Res 2008;142:399–419.
6. Arock M, Valent P. Pathogenesis, classification and treatment of mastocytosis: state of the art in 2010 and future perspectives. Expert Rev Hematol 2010;3: 497–516.
7. Feger F, Ribadeau Dumas A, Leriche L, et al. Kit and c-kit mutations in mastocytosis: a short overview with special reference to novel molecular and diagnostic concepts. Int Arch Allergy Immunol 2002;127:110–4.

8. Traina F, Visconte V, Jankowska AM, et al. Single nucleotide polymorphism array lesions, TET2, DNMT3A, ASXL1 and CBL mutations are present in systemic mastocytosis. PLoS One 2012;7:e43090.

9. Soucie E, Hanssens K, Mercher T, et al. In aggressive forms of mastocytosis, TET2 loss cooperates with c-KITD816V to transform mast cells. Blood 2012; 120:4846–9.

10. Schwaab J, Schnittger S, Sotlar K, et al. Comprehensive mutational profiling in advanced systemic mastocytosis. Blood 2013;122:2460–6.

11. Morii E. Development of mast cells: analysis with mutant mice. Int J Hematol 2007;86:22–6.

12. Piao X, Bernstein A. A point mutation in the catalytic domain of c-kit induces growth factor independence, tumorigenicity, and differentiation of mast cells. Blood 1996;87:3117–23.

13. Costa JJ, Demetri GD, Harrist TJ, et al. Recombinant human stem cell factor (kit ligand) promotes human mast cell and melanocyte hyperplasia and functional activation in vivo. J Exp Med 1996;183:2681–6.

14. Anderson DM, Williams DE, Tushinski R, et al. Alternate splicing of mRNAs encoding human mast cell growth factor and localization of the gene to chromosome 12q22-q24. Cell Growth Differ 1991;2:373–8.

15. Ashman LK. The biology of stem cell factor and its receptor C-kit. Int J Biochem Cell Biol 1999;31:1037–51.

16. Giebel LB, Strunk KM, Holmes SA, et al. Organization and nucleotide sequence of the human KIT (mast/stem cell growth factor receptor) proto-oncogene. Oncogene 1992;7:2207–17.

17. Chabot B, Stephenson DA, Chapman VM, et al. The proto-oncogene c-kit encoding a transmembrane tyrosine kinase receptor maps to the mouse W locus. Nature 1988;335:88–9.

18. Roskoski R Jr. Structure and regulation of Kit protein-tyrosine kinase–the stem cell factor receptor. Biochem Biophys Res Commun 2005;338:1307–15.

19. Roskoski R Jr. Signaling by Kit protein-tyrosine kinase–the stem cell factor receptor. Biochem Biophys Res Commun 2005;337:1–13.

20. Huse M, Kuriyan J. The conformational plasticity of protein kinases. Cell 2002; 109:275–82.

21. Chan PM, Ilangumaran S, La Rose J, et al. Autoinhibition of the kit receptor tyrosine kinase by the cytosolic juxtamembrane region. Mol Cell Biol 2003;23:3067–78.

22. Laine E, Chauvot de Beauchene I, Perahia D, et al. Mutation D816V alters the internal structure and dynamics of c-KIT receptor cytoplasmic region: implications for dimerization and activation mechanisms. PLoS Comput Biol 2011;7: e1002068.

23. Kim MS, Radinger M, Gilfillan AM. The multiple roles of phosphoinositide 3-kinase in mast cell biology. Trends Immunol 2008;29:493–501.

24. Vadlakonda L, Dash A, Pasupuleti M, et al. The paradox of Akt-mTOR interactions. Front Oncol 2013;3:165.

25. Morales JK, Falanga YT, Depcrynski A, et al. Mast cell homeostasis and the JAK-STAT pathway. Genes Immun 2010;11:599–608.

26. Timokhina I, Kissel H, Stella G, et al. Kit signaling through PI 3-kinase and Src kinase pathways: an essential role for Rac1 and JNK activation in mast cell proliferation. EMBO J 1998;17:6250–62.

27. O'Laughlin-Bunner B, Radosevic N, Taylor ML, et al. Lyn is required for normal stem cell factor-induced proliferation and chemotaxis of primary hematopoietic cells. Blood 2001;98:343–50.

28. Lennartsson J, Blume-Jensen P, Hermanson M, et al. Phosphorylation of Shc by Src family kinases is necessary for stem cell factor receptor/c-kit mediated activation of the Ras/MAP kinase pathway and c-fos induction. Oncogene 1999;18: 5546–53.

29. Nishida K, Wang L, Morii E, et al. Requirement of Gab2 for mast cell development and KitL/c-Kit signaling. Blood 2002;99:1866–9.

30. Samayawardhena LA, Hu J, Stein PL, et al. Fyn kinase acts upstream of Shp2 and p38 mitogen-activated protein kinase to promote chemotaxis of mast cells towards stem cell factor. Cell Signal 2006;18:1447–54.

31. Trieselmann NZ, Soboloff J, Berger SA. Mast cells stimulated by membrane-bound, but not soluble, steel factor are dependent on phospholipase C activation. Cell Mol Life Sci 2003;60:759–66.

32. Ryan RJ, Akin C, Castells M, et al. Mast cell sarcoma: a rare and potentially under-recognized diagnostic entity with specific therapeutic implications. Mod Pathol 2013;26:533–43.

33. Briley LD, Phillips CM. Cutaneous mastocytosis: a review focusing on the pediatric population. Clin Pediatr (Phila) 2008;47:757–61.

34. Pardanani A. Systemic mastocytosis: disease overview, pathogenesis, and treatment. Hematol Oncol Clin North Am 2012;26:1117–28.

35. Valent P, Aberer E, Beham-Schmid C, et al. Guidelines and diagnostic algorithm for patients with suspected systemic mastocytosis: a proposal of the Austrian competence network (AUCNM). Am J Blood Res 2013;3:174–80.

36. Sokol H, Georgin-Lavialle S, Canioni D, et al. Gastrointestinal manifestations in mastocytosis: a study of 83 patients. J Allergy Clin Immunol 2013;132: 866–73.e1–3.

37. Stoecker MM, Wang E. Systemic mastocytosis with associated clonal hematologic nonmast cell lineage disease: a clinicopathologic review. Arch Pathol Lab Med 2012;136:832–8.

38. Valent P, Horny H-P, Li CY, et al. Mastocytosis (mast cell disease). In: Jaffe ES, Harris NL, Stein H, et al, editors. World Health Organization (WHO) classification of tumours. Pathology & genetics. Tumours of haematopoietic and lymphoid tissues. Lyon (France): IARC Press; 2001. p. 291–302.

39. Valent P, Akin C, Escribano L, et al. Standards and standardization in mastocytosis: consensus statements on diagnostics, treatment recommendations and response criteria. Eur J Clin Invest 2007;37:435–53.

40. Valent P, Horny HP, Escribano L, et al. Diagnostic criteria and classification of mastocytosis: a consensus proposal. Leuk Res 2001;25:603–25.

41. Valent P, Akin C, Sperr WR, et al. Mastocytosis: pathology, genetics, and current options for therapy. Leuk Lymphoma 2005;46:35–48.

42. Gleixner KV, Mayerhofer M, Cerny-Reiterer S, et al. KIT-D816V-independent oncogenic signaling in neoplastic cells in systemic mastocytosis: role of Lyn and Btk activation and disruption by dasatinib and bosutinib. Blood 2011;118: 1885–98.

43. Tefferi A, Levine RL, Lim KH, et al. Frequent TET2 mutations in systemic mastocytosis: clinical, KITD816V and FIP1L1-PDGFRA correlates. Leukemia 2009;23: 900–4.

44. Jordan JH, Fritsche-Polanz R, Sperr WR, et al. A case of 'smouldering' mastocytosis with high mast cell burden, monoclonal myeloid cells, and C-KIT mutation Asp-816-Val. Leuk Res 2001;25:627–34.

45. Valent P. Mastocytosis: a paradigmatic example of a rare disease with complex biology and pathology. Am J Cancer Res 2013;3:159–72.

46. Furitsu T, Tsujimura T, Tono T, et al. Identification of mutations in the coding sequence of the proto-oncogene c-kit in a human mast cell leukemia cell line causing ligand-independent activation of c-kit product. J Clin Invest 1993;92: 1736–44.
47. Tsujimura T, Furitsu T, Morimoto M, et al. Ligand-independent activation of c-kit receptor tyrosine kinase in a murine mastocytoma cell line P-815 generated by a point mutation. Blood 1994;83:2619–26.
48. Longley BJ, Tyrrell L, Lu SZ, et al. Somatic c-KIT activating mutation in urticaria pigmentosa and aggressive mastocytosis: establishment of clonality in a human mast cell neoplasm. Nat Genet 1996;12:312–4.
49. Longley BJ Jr, Metcalfe DD, Tharp M, et al. Activating and dominant inactivating c-KIT catalytic domain mutations in distinct clinical forms of human mastocytosis. Proc Natl Acad Sci U S A 1999;96:1609–14.
50. Zappulla JP, Dubreuil P, Desbois S, et al. Mastocytosis in mice expressing human Kit receptor with the activating Asp816Val mutation. J Exp Med 2005;202:1635–41.
51. Buttner C, Henz BM, Welker P, et al. Identification of activating c-kit mutations in adult-, but not in childhood-onset indolent mastocytosis: a possible explanation for divergent clinical behavior. J Invest Dermatol 1998;111:1227–31.
52. Yanagihori H, Oyama N, Nakamura K, et al. c-kit Mutations in patients with childhood-onset mastocytosis and genotype-phenotype correlation. J Mol Diagn 2005;7:252–7.
53. Verzijl A, Heide R, Oranje AP, et al. C-kit Asp-816-Val mutation analysis in patients with mastocytosis. Dermatology 2007;214:15–20.
54. Bodemer C, Hermine O, Palmerini F, et al. Pediatric mastocytosis is a clonal disease associated with D816V and other activating c-KIT mutations. J Invest Dermatol 2010;130:804–15.
55. Garcia-Montero AC, Jara-Acevedo M, Teodosio C, et al. KIT mutation in mast cells and other bone marrow hematopoietic cell lineages in systemic mast cell disorders: a prospective study of the Spanish Network on Mastocytosis (REMA) in a series of 113 patients. Blood 2006;108:2366–72.
56. Kristensen T, Vestergaard H, Moller MB. Improved detection of the KIT D816V mutation in patients with systemic mastocytosis using a quantitative and highly sensitive real-time qPCR assay. J Mol Diagn 2011;13:180–8.
57. Kristensen T, Broesby-Olsen S, Vestergaard H, et al. Circulating KIT D816V mutation-positive non-mast cells in peripheral blood are characteristic of indolent systemic mastocytosis. Eur J Haematol 2012;89:42–6.
58. Teodosio C, Garcia-Montero AC, Jara-Acevedo M, et al. Mast cells from different molecular and prognostic subtypes of systemic mastocytosis display distinct immunophenotypes. J Allergy Clin Immunol 2010;125:719–26, 726.e1–4.
59. Gotlib J, Pardanani A, Akin C, et al. International Working Group-Myeloproliferative Neoplasms Research and Treatment (IWG-MRT) & European Competence Network on Mastocytosis (ECNM) consensus response criteria in advanced systemic mastocytosis. Blood 2013;121:2393–401.
60. Hauswirth AW, Simonitsch-Klupp I, Uffmann M, et al. Response to therapy with interferon alpha-2b and prednisolone in aggressive systemic mastocytosis: report of five cases and review of the literature. Leuk Res 2004;28: 249–57.
61. Georgin-Lavialle S, Lhermitte L, Dubreuil P, et al. Mast cell leukemia. Blood 2013;121:1285–95.
62. Pignon JM, Giraudier S, Duquesnoy P, et al. A new c-kit mutation in a case of aggressive mast cell disease. Br J Haematol 1997;96:374–6.

63. Nakagomi N, Hirota S. Juxtamembrane-type c-kit gene mutation found in aggressive systemic mastocytosis induces imatinib-resistant constitutive KIT activation. Lab Invest 2007;87:365–71.
64. Sperr WR, Valent P. Diagnosis, progression patterns and prognostication in mastocytosis. Expert Rev Hematol 2012;5:261–74.
65. Ustun C, DeRemer DL, Akin C. Tyrosine kinase inhibitors in the treatment of systemic mastocytosis. Leuk Res 2011;35:1143–52.
66. Valent P, Sperr WR, Akin C. How I treat patients with advanced systemic mastocytosis. Blood 2010;116:5812–7.
67. Sotlar K, Fridrich C, Mall A, et al. Detection of c-kit point mutation Asp-816 –> Val in microdissected pooled single mast cells and leukemic cells in a patient with systemic mastocytosis and concomitant chronic myelomonocytic leukemia. Leuk Res 2002;26:979–84.
68. Pardanani A, Lim KH, Lasho TL, et al. Prognostically relevant breakdown of 123 patients with systemic mastocytosis associated with other myeloid malignancies. Blood 2009;114:3769–72.
69. Sotlar K, Colak S, Bache A, et al. Variable presence of KITD816V in clonal haematological non-mast cell lineage diseases associated with systemic mastocytosis (SM-AHNMD). J Pathol 2010;220:586–95.
70. Georgin-Lavialle S, Aguilar C, Guieze R, et al. Mast cell sarcoma: a rare and aggressive entity–report of two cases and review of the literature. J Clin Oncol 2013;31:e90–7.
71. Zhang LY, Smith ML, Schultheis B, et al. A novel K509I mutation of KIT identified in familial mastocytosis–in vitro and in vivo responsiveness to imatinib therapy. Leuk Res 2006;30:373–8.
72. Wasag B, Niedoszytko M, Piskorz A, et al. Novel, activating KIT-N822I mutation in familial cutaneous mastocytosis. Exp Hematol 2011;39:859–65.e2.
73. Hoffmann KM, Moser A, Lohse P, et al. Successful treatment of progressive cutaneous mastocytosis with imatinib in a 2-year-old boy carrying a somatic KIT mutation. Blood 2008;112:1655–7.
74. Yang Y, Letard S, Borge L, et al. Pediatric mastocytosis-associated KIT extracellular domain mutations exhibit different functional and signaling properties compared with KIT-phosphotransferase domain mutations. Blood 2010;116: 1114–23.
75. Kim SY, Kang JJ, Lee HH, et al. Mechanism of activation of human c-KIT kinase by internal tandem duplications of the juxtamembrane domain and point mutations at aspartic acid 816. Biochem Biophys Res Commun 2011; 410:224–8.
76. Bougherara H, Georgin-Lavialle S, Damaj G, et al. Relocalization of KIT D816V to cell surface after dasatinib treatment: potential clinical implications. Clin Lymphoma Myeloma Leuk 2013;13:62–9.
77. Xiang Z, Kreisel F, Cain J, et al. Neoplasia driven by mutant c-KIT is mediated by intracellular, not plasma membrane, receptor signaling. Mol Cell Biol 2007;27: 267–82.
78. Choudhary C, Olsen JV, Brandts C, et al. Mislocalized activation of oncogenic RTKs switches downstream signaling outcomes. Mol Cell 2009;36:326–39.
79. Taylor ML, Dastych J, Sehgal D, et al. The Kit-activating mutation D816V enhances stem cell factor–dependent chemotaxis. Blood 2001;98:1195–9.
80. Chian R, Young S, Danilkovitch-Miagkova A, et al. Phosphatidylinositol 3 kinase contributes to the transformation of hematopoietic cells by the D816V c-Kit mutant. Blood 2001;98:1365–73.

81. Sun J, Pedersen M, Ronnstrand L. The D816V mutation of c-Kit circumvents a requirement for Src family kinases in c-Kit signal transduction. J Biol Chem 2009;284:11039–47.

82. Voisset E, Lopez S, Dubreuil P, et al. The tyrosine kinase FES is an essential effector of KITD816V proliferation signal. Blood 2007;110:2593–9.

83. Smrz D, Kim MS, Zhang S, et al. mTORC1 and mTORC2 differentially regulate homeostasis of neoplastic and non-neoplastic human mast cells. Blood 2011; 118:6803–13.

84. Harir N, Boudot C, Friedbichler K, et al. Oncogenic Kit controls neoplastic mast cell growth through a Stat5/PI3-kinase signaling cascade. Blood 2008;112: 2463–73.

85. Gabillot-Carre M, Lepelletier Y, Humbert M, et al. Rapamycin inhibits growth and survival of D816V-mutated c-kit mast cells. Blood 2006;108:1065–72.

86. Baumgartner C, Cerny-Reiterer S, Sonneck K, et al. Expression of activated STAT5 in neoplastic mast cells in systemic mastocytosis: subcellular distribution and role of the transforming oncoprotein KIT D816V. Am J Pathol 2009;175: 2416–29.

87. Gotlib J. KIT mutations in mastocytosis and their potential as therapeutic targets. Immunol Allergy Clin North Am 2006;26:575–92.

88. Lindauer M, Hochhaus A. Dasatinib. Recent Results Cancer Res 2010;184: 83–102.

89. Aichberger KJ, Sperr WR, Gleixner KV, et al. Treatment responses to cladribine and dasatinib in rapidly progressing aggressive mastocytosis. Eur J Clin Invest 2008;38:869–73.

90. Gani OA, Engh RA. Protein kinase inhibition of clinically important staurosporine analogues. Nat Prod Rep 2010;27:489–98.

91. Gleixner KV, Peter B, Blatt K, et al. Synergistic growth-inhibitory effects of ponatinib and midostaurin (PKC412) on neoplastic mast cells carrying KIT D816V. Haematologica 2013;98(9):1450–7.

92. Frost MJ, Ferrao PT, Hughes TP, et al. Juxtamembrane mutant V560GKit is more sensitive to imatinib (STI571) compared with wild-type c-kit whereas the kinase domain mutant D816VKit is resistant. Mol Cancer Ther 2002;1:1115–24.

93. Ashman LK, Griffith R. Therapeutic targeting of c-KIT in cancer. Expert Opin Investig Drugs 2013;22:103–15.

94. Akin C, Fumo G, Yavuz AS, et al. A novel form of mastocytosis associated with a transmembrane c-kit mutation and response to imatinib. Blood 2004;103: 3222–5.

95. Mital A, Piskorz A, Lewandowski K, et al. A case of mast cell leukaemia with exon 9 KIT mutation and good response to imatinib. Eur J Haematol 2011;86: 531–5.

96. Alvarez-Twose I, Gonzalez P, Morgado JM, et al. Complete response after imatinib mesylate therapy in a patient with well-differentiated systemic mastocytosis. J Clin Oncol 2012;30:e126–9.

97. Georgin-Lavialle S, Lhermitte L, Suarez F, et al. Mast cell leukemia: identification of a new c-Kit mutation, dup(501-502), and response to masitinib, a c-Kit tyrosine kinase inhibitor. Eur J Haematol 2012;89:47–52.

98. Tan L, Shi YG. Tet family proteins and 5-hydroxymethylcytosine in development and disease. Development 2012;139:1895–902.

99. Solary E, Bernard OA, Tefferi A, et al. Ten-eleven translocation-2 (TET2) gene in hematopoiesis and hematopoietic diseases. Leukemia 2013. [Epub ahead of print].

100. Li Z, Cai X, Cai CL, et al. Deletion of Tet2 in mice leads to dysregulated hemato-poietic stem cells and subsequent development of myeloid malignancies. Blood 2011;118:4509–18.
101. Holmfeldt L, Mullighan CG. The role of TET2 in hematologic neoplasms. Cancer Cell 2011;20:1–2.
102. Ko M, Huang Y, Jankowska AM, et al. Impaired hydroxylation of 5-methylcyto-sine in myeloid cancers with mutant TET2. Nature 2010;468:839–43.
103. Damaj G, Joris M, Chandesris O, et al. ASXL1 but not TET2 mutations adversely impact overall survival of patients suffering systemic mastocytosis with associ-ated clonal hematologic non-mast-cell diseases. PLoS One 2014;1:e85362.
104. Visconte V, Makishima H, Maciejewski JP, et al. Emerging roles of the spliceoso-mal machinery in myelodysplastic syndromes and other hematological disor-ders. Leukemia 2012;26:2447–54.
105. Hanssens K, Brenet F, Agopian J, et al. SRSF2-P95 hotspot mutation is highly associated with advanced forms of mastocytosis and mutations in epigenetic regulator genes. Haematologica 2014. [Epub ahead of print].
106. Cho YS, Kim EJ, Park UH, et al. Additional sex comb-like 1 (ASXL1), in cooper-ation with SRC-1, acts as a ligand-dependent coactivator for retinoic acid receptor. J Biol Chem 2006;281:17588–98.
107. Katoh M. Functional and cancer genomics of ASXL family members. Br J Cancer 2013;109:299–306.
108. Fisher CL, Pineault N, Brookes C, et al. Loss-of-function additional sex combs like 1 mutations disrupt hematopoiesis but do not cause severe myelodysplasia or leukemia. Blood 2010;115:38–46.
109. Delhommeau F, Jeziorowska D, Marzac C, et al. Molecular aspects of myelopro-liferative neoplasms. Int J Hematol 2010;91:165–73.
110. Abdel-Wahab O, Tefferi A, Levine RL. Role of TET2 and ASXL1 mutations in the pathogenesis of myeloproliferative neoplasms. Hematol Oncol Clin North Am 2012;26:1053–64.
111. Prior IA, Lewis PD, Mattos C. A comprehensive survey of Ras mutations in can-cer. Cancer Res 2012;72:2457–67.
112. Moroni C, Diamantis ID, Wodnar-Filipowicz A, et al. Multistage mastocytoma model characterized by autocrine IL-3 production. Haematol Blood Transfus 1989;32:407–10.
113. Wiesner SM, Jones JM, Hasz DE, et al. Repressible transgenic model of NRAS oncogene-driven mast cell disease in the mouse. Blood 2005;106:1054–62.
114. Parikh C, Subrahmanyam R, Ren R. Oncogenic NRAS rapidly and efficiently in-duces CMML- and AML-like diseases in mice. Blood 2006;108:2349–57.
115. Wilson TM, Maric I, Simakova O, et al. Clonal analysis of NRAS activating muta-tions in KIT-D816V systemic mastocytosis. Haematologica 2011;96:459–63.
116. Makishima H, Yoshida K, Nguyen N, et al. Somatic SETBP1 mutations in myeloid malignancies. Nat Genet 2013;45:942–6.
117. Osato M. Point mutations in the RUNX1/AML1 gene: another actor in RUNX leukemia. Oncogene 2004;23:4284–96.
118. Shah NP, Lee FY, Luo R, et al. Dasatinib (BMS-354825) inhibits KITD816V, an imatinib-resistant activating mutation that triggers neoplastic growth in most patients with systemic mastocytosis. Blood 2006;108:286–91.

Mast Cell–Restricted Tetramer-Forming Tryptases and Their Beneficial Roles in Hemostasis and Blood Coagulation

Alicia Prieto-García, MD, PhD[a],*, Mariana C. Castells, MD, PhD[b,1],
Philip M. Hansbro, PhD[c], Richard L. Stevens, PhD[b,1]

KEYWORDS

- Mast cell • hTryptase-β • mMCP-6 • mMCP-7 • Fibrinogen
- Fibrin thrombin-dependent coagulation • Anaphylaxis

KEY POINTS

- Tryptase-β–dependent proteolysis of the α chain of hFibrinogen impairs its ability to form thrombin-dependent fibrin.
- The antithrombotic activity of hTryptase-β hinders the internal accumulation of life-threatening fibrin deposits and fibrin-platelet clots in tissues when activated mast cells (MCs) exocytose histamine and other vasopermeability factors which, in turn, induce vasodilation and edema of tissues.
- The anticoagulant activity of MC-restricted tryptases explains why there are 2 genes in mice and humans that encode similar tetramer-forming tryptases that can proteolytically damage fibrinogen, and why there is no endogenous protease inhibitor in normal blood that can rapidly inactivate these enzymes.
- The anticoagulant activity of tetramer-forming tryptases also explains the presence of hemorrhagic disorders in some patients with anaphylaxis or mastocytosis.
- Recombinant hTryptase-β could be a more effective and safer anticoagulant in the clinic than porcine-derived heparin oligosaccharides.
- C-terminal fragments of the α chain of hFibrinogen in blood and/or urine potentially could be biomarkers for the identification of patients who have undergone systemic anaphylaxis, have mastocytosis, or have an MC activation disorder.

Funding Sources: NIH grant AI059746, and a grant from The Mastocytosis Society.
Disclosures: No conflicts of interest.
[a] Allergy Service, Hospital Universitario Gregorio Marañón, Instituto de Investigación Sanitaria Gregorio Marañón, Dr Esquerdo 46, Madrid 28007, Spain; [b] Division of Rheumatology, Immunology, and Allergy, Department of Medicine, Brigham and Women's Hospital, Harvard Medical School, 1 Jimmy Fund Way, Smith Building, Boston, MA 02115, USA; [c] Priority Research Centre for Asthma and Respiratory Disease, Hunter Medical Research Institute and University of Newcastle, 1 Kookaburra Circuit, Newcastle, NSW 2300, Australia
[1] Joint senior authors.
* Corresponding author.
E-mail address: aliprietog@gmail.com

Immunol Allergy Clin N Am 34 (2014) 263–281
http://dx.doi.org/10.1016/j.iac.2014.01.001
0889-8561/14/$ – see front matter © 2014 Elsevier Inc. All rights reserved.

immunology.theclinics.com

INTRODUCTION

Mast cells (MCs) are key effector cells in immediate hypersensitivity reactions because of their release of numerous proinflammatory mediators. The presence of too many MCs in tissues leads to mastocytosis (**Fig. 1**). However, the conservation of MCs in evolution and the failure to identify a human who lacks MCs suggests critical beneficial roles for these immune cells in our survival. In that regard, it has been demonstrated that the tetramer-forming tryptases exocytosed from activated MCs are needed for efficient host defense against certain bacterial, helminth, and virus infections.[1–6] Moreover, the loss of human immunodeficiency virus 1–infected hTryptase-β⁺ MCs and their progenitors in patients with AIDS is now believed to be a contributing factor in their inability to combat opportunistic infections.[7–9]

Tetramer-forming tryptases are stored in the MC's secretory granules ionically bound to serglycin proteoglycans (SGPGs), which usually have heparin chains. These serine proteases are useful clinical and experimental biomarkers for mastocytosis, anaphylaxis, and the MC activation syndrome. Such markers can be measured by enzyme-linked immunosorbent assays and can be detected in peripheral blood for longer periods of time than other mediators exocytosed from activated MCs (eg, histamine and arachidonic acid metabolites).[10–12] The expression of hTryptase-β is also highly restricted to MCs. Despite its diagnostic value, the biological function of the hTryptase-β in plasma and blood has largely remained unknown.

The ability to form fibrin when the skin and other connective tissues are wounded is essential for preventing blood loss and the entry of pathogens into the body. Nevertheless, the formation of intravascular fibrin deposits and fibrin-platelet clots can have dangerous consequences. When the MCs in skin and other connective tissue sites degranulate, these immune cells quickly release the contents of their secretory granules, which include histamine and tetramer-forming tryptases bound to SGPGs that usually contain heparin glycosaminoglycans (GAGs). Histamine is the major

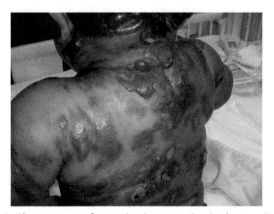

Fig. 1. Mastocytosis. The presence of an activating mutation in the tyrosine kinase receptor Kit/CD117 in the mast cell (MC)-committed progenitors of a mastocytosis patient eventually causes the accumulation of too many mature hTryptase-β⁺ MCs in the skin and other connective tissues. The activation of these MCs and the exocytosis of their granule mediators can lead to numerous clinical problems, as occurred in the skin of this patient with bullous mastocytosis. Because the C-terminus of the α chain of hFibrinogen is preferentially cleaved by hTryptase-β, the identification of peptides derived from the protein's α chain in the circulation via an enzyme-linked immunosorbent assay could be of therapeutic valuable in the early identification of mastocytosis patients, as well as monitoring their treatment.

vasopermeability factor that induces the substantial edema that occurs at tissue sites where MCs degranulate, owing to its ability to bind to the H1 receptors on surfaces of vascular endothelial cells. This signaling reaction causes the redistribution of adhesion proteins and the loss of tight junctions between adjacent endothelial cells, which then allows the influx of fibrinogen and other circulating proteins into the inflammatory site.[13] Despite the rapid accumulation of fibrinogen, fibrin deposits are rare in the edema sites that form when cutaneous MCs degranulate. Recently, the authors uncovered a beneficial role for mouse and human tetramer-forming tryptases in anaphylaxis, namely, by preventing the formation of fibrin clots when vasodilation and plasma extravasation into a connective tissue occur following MC activation.[14] This vital antithrombotic function is mainly due to the ability of hTryptase-β to proteolytically damage fibrinogen before thrombin can convert the latter precursor protein to fibrin. The anticoagulant activity of hTryptase-β is an explanation for the hemorrhagic disorders that can occur in patients with anaphylaxis or mastocytosis. To understand the function of MC-restricted tetramer-forming tryptases, it is necessary to know the structural and biological characteristics of this family of serine proteases as outlined herein.

HUMAN MC TRYPTASES

It is now apparent that the hTryptase-β[15,16] preparations purified from the MCs isolated from human skin and lung biopsies in the 1980s by numerous groups consisted of a complex mixture of serine proteases derived from the *TPSAB1* and *TPSB2* genes on chromosome 16p13.3.[17] Miller and colleagues[18] isolated the first cDNA that originated from the human *TPSAB1* gene. When expressed, it was discovered that recombinant hTryptase-α had very little, if any, enzymatic activity, owing to an Asp^{246}/Gly^{246} mutation in its catalytic domain (**Fig. 2**).[19–21] Because one of the amino acids in the enzyme's propeptide also differed from that in pro-hTryptase-β, it was concluded

A Human TPSAB1 (GenBank GeneID 7177; Accession # NP_003285)

```
  1 mlnllllalp vlasrayaap apgqalqrvg ivggqeaprs kwpwqvslrv hgpywmhfcg
 61 gslihpqwvl taahcvgpdv kdlaalrvql reqhlyyqdq llpvsriivh pqfytaqiga
121 dialleleep vvnsshvhtv tlppasetfp pgmpcwvtgw gdvdnderlp ppfplkqvkv
181 pimenhicda kyhlgaytgd dvrivrddml cagntrrdsc qgdsggplvc kvngtwlqag
241 vvswgegcaq pnrpgiytrv tyyldwihhy vpkkp
```

B Human TPSB2 (GenBank GeneID 64499; Accession # NP_077078)

```
  1 mlnllllalp vlasrayaap apgqalqrvg ivggqeaprs kwpwqvslrv rdrywmhfcg
 61 gslihpqwvl taahcvgpdv kdlaalrvql reqhlyyqdq llpvsriivh pqfytaqiga
121 dialleleep vnvsshvhtv tlppasetfp pgmpcwvtgw gdvdnderlp ppfplkqvkv
181 pimenhicda kyhlgaytgd dvrivrddml cagntrrdsc qgdsggplvc kvngtwlqag
241 vvswgegcaq pnrpgiytrv tyyldwihhy vpkkp
```

Fig. 2. Allelic variations of the human *TPSAB1* (*A*) and *TPSB2* (*B*) genes. Based on the information at GenBank's Single-Nucleotide Polymorphism database, the Human Genome Consortium identified numerous mutations in the 2 genes that change the amino acids highlighted in yellow in the translated zymogens. Frame-shift or premature translational-termination mutations that cause the expression of truncated proteins are highlighted in blue. In each instance, the first 30 amino acids of the 275-mer zymogen (*red*) correspond to the signal/propeptide. The amino acids that comprise the mature domain of each processed tryptase are in black type. The arrowhead (*green*) points to the location of the Asp mutation that blocks the substrate-binding cleft of hTryptase-α.

that MCs might be unable to remove the propeptide from the defective zymogen, thereby causing the nonprocessed zymogen to be constitutively secreted rather than be targeted to the cell's secretory granules.[22]

The following year, Miller, Vanderslice, and their colleagues[23,24] isolated the first cDNAs from the human *TPSAB1* and *TPSB2* genes that encoded enzymatically active serine proteases, which they initially designated as hTryptase-β1, -β2, and -β3. Except for residue 132 that dictated how many *N*-linked glycans were bound to these proteases, the amino acid sequences of hTryptase-β1 and -β2 were identical. It therefore was not surprising that the 2 recombinant enzymes had identical substrate specificities when combinational peptide libraries were scanned.[1,19,25] Chromosome 16p13.3 is a recombination hot spot,[26] and many point mutations in the human *TPSAB1* and *TPSB2* genes have been identified by the Human Genome Consortium in recent years. Some of these mutations result in the expression of truncated proteases. Additional isoforms have been identified that are caused by alternate splicing of the precursor transcript and by differential posttranslational modification of the translated protein.[26,27] Most of the allelic isoforms of the *TPSAB1* and *TPSB2* genes that encode proteins with different amino acid sequences (see **Fig. 2**) have not been evaluated experimentally. Thus, investigators generally refer to any enzymatically active product of the human *TPSAB1* and *TPSB2* genes as hTryptase-β.

hTryptase-α is encoded by one of the most studied mutated alleles of the *TPSAB1* gene. Whereas hTryptase-α lacks enzymatic activity because of mutations in its propeptide[28] and catalytic domain,[19–21] the neutrophil serine protease gene family member azurocidin/CAP37 has bactericidal bioactivity even though it also lacks enzymatic activity.[29–31] It therefore is possible that hTryptase-α and other enzymatically inactive proteins encoded by some of the mutated alleles of the human *TPSAB1* and *TPSB2* genes noted in **Fig. 2** have bioactivity even though they lack enzymatic activity. Tryptase-α is constitutively secreted by MCs instead of being stored in the cell's secretory granules.[22] Many humans have the α allele in their *TPSAB1* gene.[32–34] Although it is common for a human to have one defective allele in their *TPSAB1* and/or *TPSB2* genes, no hTryptase-β-null human has been identified.[33,34] These genome data support the mouse data, which led to the conclusion that enzymatically active tetramer-forming tryptases normally have beneficial roles in mammals.

Human MCs also express hTryptase-δ and hTryptase-γ/transmembrane tryptase/Prss31, which originate from the respective *TPSD1* and *TPSG1* genes also located on chromosome 16p13.3. hTryptase-γ differs from hTryptase-β in that it is preferentially retained on the outer leaflet of the plasma membrane when MCs degranulate, owing to its unique C-terminal membrane-spanning domain.[35] Because of this feature, hTryptase-γ can regulate those cell types physically contacted in tissues by activated MCs. The substrate preference of recombinant hTryptase-γ[35,36] overlaps that of recombinant hTryptase-β,[1,25] and transgenic mice that lack the orthologues of these human enzymes have reduced inflammation in experimental arthritis, colitis, and chronic obstructive pulmonary disease.[37–40] β-Tryptases are the major enzymatically active proteases stored in the secretory granules of human MCs, and these tetramer-forming enzymes can diffuse away somewhat from activated MCs in tissues, in contrast to membrane-retained hTryptase-γ. It therefore has been proposed that the latter enzyme is less important than the former in the pathogenesis of anaphylaxis.[41]

MOUSE MC TRYPTASES

Mouse chromosome 17A3.3 contains 13 genes that encode tryptic-like serine proteases.[42] MCs express 4 of these enzymes, namely, mouse MC protease (mMCP)-6/Tpsb2,[43] mMCP-7/Tpsab1,[44] mMCP-11/Prss34,[42] and transmembrane tryptase/tryptase γ/Prss31.[45] Like their human orthologues, mMCP-6/Tpsb2 and mMCP-7/Tpsab1 are tetramer-forming tryptases.[46] The amino acid sequences of BALB/c mMCP-6 and mMCP-7 are 75% identical, but mMCP-6 is more abundant in the constitutive MCs that reside in the peritoneal cavity than mMCP-7.[47] Mouse transmembrane tryptase/tryptase-γ/Prss31 also remains on the outer surface of activated MCs, like its human orthologue.[35,45,48] The connective-tissue MCs in every examined mouse strain express mMCP-6. By contrast, mMCP-7 and Prss31 are expressed in strain-dependent manners in wild-type (WT) mice.[45,49,50] For example, the MCs in BALB/c mice contain very little Prss31, presumably because of a defective promoter, whereas the MCs in C57BL/6 (B6) mice constitutively lack mMCP-7 owing to a splice-site mutation in its gene. However, the MCs in all examined WT mouse strains express at least 2 tryptases. Although mouse MCs and basophils express mMCP-11/Prss34, less is known about this soluble tryptase, as no human orthologue exists.[42,51]

SERGLYCIN PROTEOGLYCANS

The electron-dense secretory granules inside MCs contain protease-resistant SGPGs,[52–55] which contain highly sulfated heparin and/or chondroitin sulfate diB/E GAGs.[56–62] The GAG-attachment region of serglycin, with its Ser-Gly repeated amino acid sequence, cannot be cleaved by any known protease. This feature is biologically significant because the primary function of SGPGs in mammalian MCs is to package large amounts of enzymatically active neutral proteases in the cell's granules in such a way that does not result in appreciable autolysis of the bound proteases.[63–65] A positively charged surface is formed when each MC-restricted protease is properly folded. This face is recognized in the Golgi by the negatively charged GAGs attached to SGPGs.[66–70] The resulting zymogen-SGPG complex is then targeted to the secretory granule, where the removal of the propeptide takes place. SGPGs are therefore essential in the posttranslational processing and storage of histamine and varied peptidases in the secretory granules of MCs.

STRUCTURAL ANALYSIS OF MC TRYPTASES

The catalytic Ser-His-Asp triad of amino acids residing at the center of the active site of trypsin is also present in each MC tryptase. However, mice and human tetramer-forming tryptases have more restricted substrate preferences than trypsin and other serine proteases.[1,25,71,72] A comparison of the primary amino acid sequences of the mature domains of 223-mer trypsin and 245-mer mMCP-7 reveal 7 insertions and 2 deletions in the latter MC enzyme. Because of structural differences in the surface loops that form their active sites, the substrate-binding clefts of mMCP-7, mMCP-6, and hTryptase-β are more restricted than that in trypsin. The crystal structure of hTryptase-β2 also revealed that this serine protease has a unique doughnut-shaped structure.[70] The tetramer unit is formed by the interactions of specific Tyr and Pro residues in 6 loop segments of the monomers. A conserved Trp domain in the folded tryptase monomer is also essential in the formation of the tetramer unit.[46] The active site of each monomer faces toward the 50 Å × 30 Å central pore of the tetramer unit,[70] thereby sterically blocking the active site of each monomer. This structural feature explains why so few large-sized proteins are cleaved by hTryptase-β, mMCP-6, and mMCP-7. The presence of the associated SGPG provides stability to the 3-dimensional structure and also helps to restrict the enzyme's substrate specificity.[72,73] Although heparin-containing SGPGs are necessary to maintain the enzymatic activity of the hTryptase-β tetramer, homotypic tetramers of enzymatically active mMCP-7 free of SGPGs have been detected in the plasma of V3 mastocytosis mice following systemic anaphylaxis.[69] mMCP-7 is therefore an exception in that it is not dependent on SGPGs once it is exocytosed from activated MCs.[69,71]

BIOACTIVITY OF MC TRYPTASES

Mouse and human tryptases are stored in the cell's acidic secretory granules as mature enzymatically active enzymes. The proteolytic activities of mouse and human tryptases are optimal at neutral pH. The low pH of the secretory granules is another way that MCs hinder the intracellular autolysis of their tryptases. When exocytosed, MC tetramer-forming tryptases cannot be inhibited efficiently by any protease inhibitor present in the normal blood of humans and mice, including α1-antitrypsin and α2-macroglobulin.[69,74]

The BALB/c V3 mastocytosis mouse contains large numbers of mMCP-6+/mMCP-7+ MCs in its spleen and liver.[75] Studies performed on these mastocytosis mice reveal that mMCP-6 and mMCP-7 are packaged in the MC's granules ionically bound to SGPGs.[69] However, after inducing systemic anaphylaxis, much of exocytosed mMCP-7 quickly dissociates from its SGPG in the neutral pH environment. By contrast, exocytosed mMCP-6–SGPG complexes remain intact for hours in the extracellular matrix close to degranulated MCs.

mMCP-7 homotypic tetramers dissociate from SGPGs at neutral pH because the SGPG-binding domain of this tryptase preferentially contains His residues[68] instead of Arg/Lys residues, as occurs in mMCP-6 and in hTryptase-β.[69] The amino acid has a positive charge in the MC's acidic granules, thereby allowing mMCP-7 to ionically recognize negatively charged SGPGs. The loss of this positive charge when mMCP-7 is exocytosed into the neutral pH environment of the extracellular matrix is the structural feature that allows mMCP-7 homotypic tetramers to more easily diffuse away from the activated MCs in sites of inflammation. Thus, substantial amounts of mMCP-7 were found in the circulation 15 minutes after systemic anaphylaxis was induced in V3 mastocytosis mice. The discovery that circulating mMCP-7 was enzymatically active confirmed the in vitro data that showed the resistance of tetramer-forming tryptases to inactivation by circulating protease inhibitors.[69] The retention of exocytosed mMCP-6 in the extracellular matrix close to tissue activated MCs suggests a local action, whereas the rapid dissipation of mMCP-7 suggests a more distant action. Although small amounts of hTryptase-β have been found in human blood after MC activation in systemic anaphylaxis,[11,76] most of this exocytosed enzyme is held in tissues for hours like mMCP-6 ionically bound to heparin SGPGs. Most of these exocytosed tryptase-SGPG macromolecular complexes eventually are endocytosed and proteolytically destroyed in the primary lysosomes of macrophages and other nearby cells in the inflammatory site.[77]

SUBSTRATE PREFERENCES OF MC TRYPTASES

Recombinant BALB/c mMCP-6 and mMCP-7 had similar, but distinct, substrate preferences when tested against Lys/Arg-containing combinational peptide libraries.[71,72] The substrate specificities of recombinant hTryptase-β more closely resembled that of recombinant mMCP-6. Recombinant mMCP-7 preferentially cleaved peptides after an Arg residue in the amino acid sequence Ser-Leu-Ser-Ser-Arg-Gln-Ser.[71] The C-terminus of the α chain of hFibrinogen contains such a sequence. Owing to the inward location of the active sites of the 4 monomers in the tetramer unit, very few candidate proteins are susceptible to tetramer-forming tryptases. The C-terminus of the α chain of mouse and human fibrinogen are cleaved by mMCP-6, mMCP-7, and hTryptase-β because the exposed susceptible sequence extends out and away from the rest of the precursor plasma protein, thereby allowing it to pass through the central pore of the tetramer unit (**Fig. 3**).

The mMCP-6–susceptible peptides identified in the phage-display peptide library combinational studies revealed that this tryptase prefers substrates with more Pro, Lys, and/or Arg residues.[72] In contrast to mMCP-7, mMCP-6 and hTryptase-β remain ionically bound to SGPGs for hours after the macromolecular complexes are exocytosed from cutaneous MCs. This finding suggested that SGPGs and their covalently bound GAGs could influence the substrate specificities of their bound tryptases outside of the MC. A phage-display peptide library analysis using mMCP-6–heparin[72] and hTryptase-β–heparin[1,25] complexes showed that these complexes prefer substrates with the sequence Lys/Arg-Pro-X-Lys/Arg, where X may be up to 3 non-charged amino acids. The second Lys/Arg residue in the sequence is the P1 residue where the susceptible peptide is cleaved. Whether mMCP-6–chondroitin sulfate E and hTryptase-β–chondroitin sulfate E complexes have similar substrate preferences have not been evaluated.

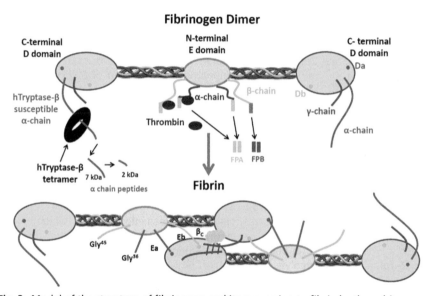

Fig. 3. Model of the structure of fibrinogen and its conversion to fibrin by thrombin, as well as its proteolytic damage by MC-restricted tetramer-forming tryptases. Native fibrinogen exists in blood and plasma as a head-to-head dimer that consists of 2 sets of 3 nonidentical polypeptide chains termed α (*blue*), β (*green*), and γ (*red*), which are joined together in the N-terminal E-domain by disulfide bridges. Each α chain in the dimer contains the inhibitory fibrinopeptide A (FPA, *light blue*) that is susceptible to thrombin (*brown*), which recognizes Arg-Gly sequences in the α and β chains. The proteolytic removal of FPA and then fibrinopeptide B (FPB, *dark green*) from the protein's β chain initiates fibrin assembly by exposing the Ea and Eb sequences in the N-terminal E-domain that recognize the respective Da and Db sequences in the C-terminal D-domain. Factor XIIIa cross-links Lys residues present in the γ chains of adjacent fibrin molecules to form stabilized fibrils. Less clear is the role of the C-terminus of the α chain in the conversion of fibrinogen to fibrin. However, this is the region of fibrinogen that is preferentially cleaved by tetramer-forming tryptases (*black doughnut*), resulting in the generation of a 7-kDa peptide that is further processed to a 2-kDa peptide.

Many in vitro studies have been carried out in attempts to identify those proteins that are preferentially cleaved by mouse and human tetramer-forming tryptases in the presence or absence of heparin. Although candidates have been identified, the data obtained in the in vitro studies carried out in the 1980s and 1990s are difficult to interpret today because the investigators at that time were unaware that their hTryptase-β preparations contained a complex mixture of functionally distinct enzymes (see **Fig. 2**). The possibility of heterotypic tetramers also was not considered, nor was the importance of the cofactor roles of chondroitin sulfate E–containing and heparin-containing SGPGs. Although the physiologic substrates of many of the identified hTryptase-β isoforms (see **Fig. 2**) remain to be determined, the in vitro data of pooled enzyme preparations identified several susceptible substrates, including high molecular weight kininogen, vasoactive intestinal peptide, pro-metalloproteinases, pro-urokinase, fibronectin, and complement factor C3.

THROMBIN-DEPENDENT CONVERSION OF FIBRINOGEN TO FIBRIN

Fibrinogen is the most important component of the coagulation system, and is a 340-kDa glycoprotein synthesized primarily in the liver. Fibrinogen is a major component of plasma, where it circulates at a concentration of 1.5 to 4.0 mg/mL. Because it also is an acute-phase protein, its circulating levels increase significantly in several infections and inflammatory diseases. Fibrinogen circulates in blood as a head-to-head dimer, with 2 external D-domains connected to one central E-domain by a coiled segment (see **Fig. 3**). Each ~170-kDa monomer is composed of 3 nonidentical α, β, and γ chains.[78–80] The γ chain is the largest, and its more extended C-terminus is not cross-linked to the other domains in the 3-chained protein. Conversion of fibrinogen to fibrin during vascular damage is a multistep process (see **Fig. 3**).[78] Initially, thrombin cleaves the N-termini of fibrinogen's α and β chains.[81,82] The newly formed N-terminal ends of these chains interact with complementary sequences in the neighboring fibrinogen molecules, resulting in double-stranded fibrils.[83,84] Fibrils also establish lateral junctions to create multiple-stranded fibrils.[85,86] The development of insoluble fibrin depends on the cross-linking activity of Factor XIIIa, which is a transglutaminase.[87,88] Less clear is the role of the large C-terminal domain of the α chain in the conversion process. Nevertheless, platelets express integrin $\alpha_{2b}\beta_3$, which recognizes fibrin, thereby creating the fibrin-platelet clot. Efficient blood coagulation does not occur when the plasma concentration of fibrinogen is less than 1 mg/mL, if its E- or D-domains are proteolytically damaged, or if the levels of enzymatically active thrombin are low.

HEPARIN-DEPENDENT ANTICOAGULATION

Sodium cromoglycate prevents MC degranulation, and Samoszuk and Corwin[89] noted that tumor-bearing BALB/c mice that were given the drug intraperitoneally contained lakes of blood in and around their tumors. These data and others suggested the presence of a potent anticoagulation factor in the MC's secretory granules. Heparin resides in that intracellular location, and some fragments of this MC-derived GAG and endothelial cell–derived heparan sulfate have anticoagulant activity in vivo (reviewed in Ref.[90]). These anticoagulant oligosaccharides catalyze the anti-thrombin-III/SERPINC1-dependent inactivation of thrombin by inducing a conformational change in the latter protease inhibitor, which causes the expulsion of residues Gly[14] and Ser[15] in the hinge region of the serpin at the base of its reactive-site loop. This change in the tertiary structure of serpin allows the serpin to accelerate the inactivation of thrombin approximately 3,000-fold, ultimately resulting in the generation of less fibrin and a delayed blood-coagulation time.[91,92]

Commercial low molecular weight oligosaccharides generated from bovine or porcine heparin following a depolymerization step (eg, by exposure to crude heparin preparations to heparin lyase I) are routinely used pharmacologically to hinder blood coagulation in humans. Despite the value of these manufactured preparations, there is very little free heparin glycosaminoglycan or its low molecular weight oligosaccharides in the human body because of the preference of heparin-containing SGPGs for hTryptase-β and the other proteases stored in the secretory granules of human MCs. In addition, approximately 70% of the naturally occurring heparin purified from in vivo differentiated MCs has no anticoagulant activity. It is now believed that the endogenous anticoagulant physiologically relevant GAG at the blood-endothelium interface in the human body is endothelial cell–derived heparan sulfate from syndecan and glycipan proteoglycans rather than MC-derived heparin.[93] In support of this conclusion, MC-deficient[94] and heparin-deficient[63,64] mice do not constitutively have coagulation disorders. It therefore remained to be determined how MCs physiologically prevent fibrin deposition in edema tissue sites when these immune cells degranulate and release their vasopermeability factors.

ANTICOAGULANT ACTIVITY OF MC TRYPTASES

When the V3 mastocytosis BALB/c mouse underwent systemic anaphylaxis, substantial amounts of enzymatically active mMCP-7 was detected in the plasma within 15 minutes.[69] Sodium dodecyl sulfate–polyacrylamide gel electrophoresis (SDS-PAGE) and N-terminal sequence analyses of the plasma from these mice revealed the presence of appreciable amounts of peptides that were derived from the C-terminus of the α chain of mFibrinogen. It was then shown that recombinant mMCP-7 was able to cleave the α chain of mouse and human fibrinogen in vitro, even if the digestion reactions were carried out in the presence of the diverse array of protease inhibitors in mouse serum or plasma.[71] These in vitro and in vivo data were unexpected because of the large size of the circulating fibrinogen dimer. The biological significance of the V3 mastocytosis data obtained in the 1990s also was not clear because mMCP-7-deficient WT B6 mice[49,50] constitutively had no defect in fibrinogen metabolism during an MC-dependent anaphylactic reaction.

Samoszuk and colleagues[95] concluded that the anticoagulant activity of the recombinant hTryptase-β–heparin complexes used in their in vitro study probably was due to the heparin component because its activity was inhibited by protamine and heparinase. Nevertheless, in support of the mMCP-7 data, Thomas and colleagues[96] reported that the α chain of hFibrinogen was highly susceptible in vitro to an undefined hTryptase-β in preparations from their human lung biopsies. No in vivo experiment was carried out to determine the physiologic relevance of the data published in this and other in vitro studies. Moreover, recombinant hTryptase-β was not used to eliminate the possibility that the fibrinogen-degrading activity originated from a minor allelic isoform of the TPSAB1 or TPSB2 gene (see Fig. 2).[97,98] Nevertheless, Thomas and colleagues[96] tentatively concluded that their enzymatic preparation preferentially cleaved the α chain of hFibrinogen at Arg[591].

SELECTIVE PROTEOLYSIS OF THE C-TERMINUS OF THE α CHAIN OF HUMAN FIBRINOGEN BY hTRYPTASE-β–HEPARIN COMPLEXES

Prieto-García and colleagues[14] showed that the α chain of hFibrinogen also was preferentially cleaved by a recombinant hTryptase-β–heparin complex in vitro at neutral pH (**Fig. 4**). The generated fragment had a slightly lower molecular weight than the native α chain. Using an SDS-PAGE immunoblot approach, it was discovered that proteolysis selectively occurred in the C-terminus of the α chain. Tandem mass spectrometry (MS/MS) and C-terminal sequence analysis of the generated fragment revealed that hTryptase-β cleaved the α chain of hFibrinogen at Lys[575], 69 amino acids from its C-terminus.

These data were supported by the identification of a 7-kDa peptide in the SDS-PAGE immunoblot analysis of the digestion reactions. MS/MS analysis of the liberated peptide confirmed that it originated from the C-terminus of the α chain. The finding that the liberated peptide was only weakly recognized by an anti-hFibrinogen antibody in some assays indicated that hTryptase-β–heparin complexes subsequently cleaved the initially formed 69-mer peptide to smaller peptides.

PREFERENTIAL PROTEOLYSIS OF MOUSE FIBRINOGEN'S α CHAIN BY hTRYPTASE-β–HEPARIN, mMCP-6–HEPARIN, AND MMCP-6–SGPG COMPLEXES

In contrast to the results reported in the Prieto-Garcia and colleagues study,[14] Thomas and colleagues[96] concluded that hTryptase-β preferentially cleaved the α chain of hFibrinogen at Arg[591]. A comparison of the amino acid sequences of the protein expressed in different species revealed that Arg[591] resides in a 14-mer amino acid sequence that is not present in the corresponding α chain of mFibrinogen. Thus, if proteolysis preferentially occurred in humans at this nonconserved amino acid sequence, the α chain of mFibrinogen could not be cleaved by hTryptase-β or by its murine orthologue mMCP-6. That mFibrinogen was efficiently cleaved by both recombinant hTryptase-β–heparin and mMCP-6–heparin complexes in follow-up studies[14] raised questions as to where mouse and human tetramer-forming tryptases initially cleaved the α chain of fibrinogen.

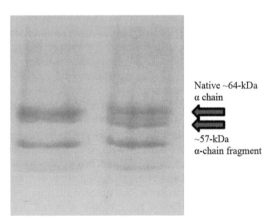

Native ~64-kDa
α chain

~57-kDa
α-chain fragment

Fig. 4. The α chain of hFibrinogen is a preferred target of hTryptase-β-heparin complexes. hFibrinogen was incubated with a recombinant hTryptase-β-heparin complex, and the resulting digest was analyzed by sodium dodecyl sulfate–polyacrylamide gel electrophoresis in the presence of β-mercaptoethanol to disrupt the protein's intrachain and interchain disulfide bonds. The position of the protein's native α chain and its prominent, slightly smaller fragment in the digest are highlighted. (*Adapted from* Prieto-Garcia A, Zheng D, Adachi R, et al. Mast cell restricted mouse and human tryptase-heparin complexes hinder thrombin-induced coagulation of plasma and the generation of fibrin by proteolytically destroying fibrinogen. J Biol Chem 2012;287(11):7837. © the American Society for Biochemistry and Molecular Biology; with permission.)

hTryptase-β and mMCP-6 are stored in MC secretory granules ionically bound to SGPGs instead of the GAGs used in aforementioned experiments. For this reason, the susceptibility of the α chain of mFibrinogen to the native mMCP-6–SGPG complexes present in interleukin (IL)-3/IL-33–developed mMCP-6$^+$/mMCP-7$^-$ mouse bone marrow–derived MCs was evaluated. As occurred with the recombinant mMCP-6–heparin complex, the α chain of mFibrinogen was preferentially cleaved by a heat-sensitive neutral protease present in these cells bound to SGPG.

IN VITRO ANTICOAGULANT ACTIVITY OF mMCP-6–HEPARIN AND hTRYPTASE-β–HEPARIN COMPLEXES

The finding that α chains of mouse and human fibrinogen were rapidly cleaved by mMCP-6–heparin and hTryptase-β–heparin complexes in vitro (even if the digestions were carried out in the presence of serum protease inhibitors) raised the possibility that these MC mediators could hinder thrombin-dependent coagulation of plasma.[14] The clotting-time measurement in a fibrometer of plasma samples before and after incubation with tryptase-heparin complexes showed that the time required by thrombin to clot plasma was markedly delayed when plasma samples were exposed to the human or mouse tryptase-heparin complexes. This delay in the clotting time was longer than that induced by heparin at a dose of 100 μg, much higher than the amount present in the enzymatic complexes (0.5–4.5 μg). It therefore was concluded that the primary anticoagulant factor present in these complexes was the tryptase rather than heparin.

IN VIVO ANTICOAGULANT ACTIVITY OF mMCP-6–HEPARIN SGPG COMPLEXES

To confirm the aforementioned in vitro data, the anticoagulant activity of mMCP-6 was next investigated in vivo.[14] Like WT mice, mMCP-6-null B6 mice underwent a passive cutaneous anaphylaxis (PCA) reaction. However, more fibrin deposits accumulated in the skin of mMCP-6–deficient B6 mice 1 to 6 hours after these animals had been subjected to the PCA reaction than in the skin of the similarly treated WT B6 mice (**Fig. 5**). Thus, mMCP-6 has a critical role in preventing the accumulation of fibrin deposits in tissues when the cutaneous MCs in mice degranulate in response to the PCA reaction. The observation that the α chain of human and mouse fibrinogen were similarly cleaved by recombinant hTryptase-β–heparin complex at neutral pH suggested that the in vivo data from WT mice reflects what occurs in humans at inflammation sites.[14]

Less clear is why tryptase-treated plasma cannot clot efficiently. Loss of the C-terminal 69-mer domain in the fibrinogen's α chain could result in a structural change in those regions of the protein's γ and β chains that are recognized by the N-termini of the α and β chains formed when the precursor protein encounters thrombin. MS/MS and amino acid sequence analyses of hTryptase-β–heparin treated human fibrinogen failed to reveal proteolysis of the N-terminus of the protein's α chain. Nevertheless, the possibility that the enzyme damages the β chain of human fibrinogen was not ruled out. Whatever the mechanism, the MCs in mMCP-6$^-$/mMCP-7$^-$ B6 mice have no defect in heparin expression.[4] Thus, the accumulated data suggest the primary way whereby activated MCs physiologically prevent fibrin formation in vivo is through their exocytosed tryptases proteolytically damaging fibrinogen.

CLINICAL IMPLICATIONS

The findings that mMCP-6, mMCP-7, and hTryptase-β are more effective anticoagulants than many heparin preparations have important clinical implications that change

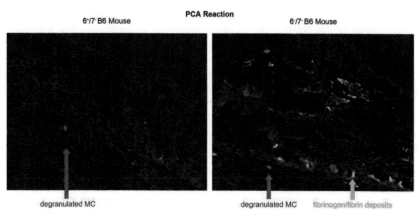

Fig. 5. Fibrin immunohistochemistry after inducing a passive cutaneous anaphylaxis (PCA) reaction. Anti-dinitrophenol (DNP)–immunoglobulin E was injected into the ears of a WT B6 mouse (*left panel*) and an mMCP-6-null B6 mouse (*right panel*). DNP-albumin was then injected into the tail veins of both sensitized animals. Six hours later, the animals were euthanized and processed for immunohistochemistry using fluorescein-labeled antimouse fibrinogen/fibrin antibody (*green color; arrow*). The tissue sections also were stained with Hoechst 33342, a dye that binds the DNA in the nucleus of cells (*blue*), as well as with Texas red–labeled avidin (*red color; arrows*), which recognizes heparin to identify MCs and their exocytosed protease-heparin complexes. The presence of these complexes outside of the activated MCs and the presence of edema that results from exocytosed histamine confirmed that the cutaneous MCs in both animal populations had degranulated. Six hours after the induction of the PCA reaction, the ear of the mMCP-6-null B6 mouse contained noticeably more fibrin (*green color*) than the corresponding ear of the treated WT B6 mouse. (*From* Prieto-Garcia A, Zheng D, Adachi R, et al. Mast cell restricted mouse and human tryptase-heparin complexes hinder thrombin-induced coagulation of plasma and the generation of fibrin by proteolytically destroying fibrinogen. J Biol Chem 2012;287(11):7842. © the American Society for Biochemistry and Molecular Biology; with permission.)

the paradigm as to how mouse and human MCs prevent blood coagulation and fibrin accumulation. Formation of fibrin deposits and fibrin-platelet clots internally could have devastating consequences in vivo. Thus, these data provide an explanation as to why no hTryptase-β–null human has been identified and why mammals possess 2 genes that encode MC-restricted serine proteases able to recognize fibrinogen. The findings also account for the apparent strong evolutionary pressure to prevent the expression of circulating protease inhibitors that could efficiently inactivate mouse and human tetramer-forming MC tryptases. The accumulated data raise the possibility that an hTryptase-β–null human cannot be born, because of an excess of fibrin deposits and/or fibrin-platelet clots in the developing fetus. Finally, the data explain why some pediatric patients with a diffuse cutaneous form of mastocytosis have excessive bleeding of their skin and gastrointestinal tract,[99,100] why some women have menstrual-like bleeding[101,102] shortly after they experience a severe anaphylactic event, and why some patients with systemic mastocytosis or anaphylactic shock show prolongation of activated partial thromboplastin time or prothrombin time with or without bleeding.[103–108]

FUTURE CONSIDERATIONS

The finding that mMCP-6, mMCP-7, and hTryptase-β are potent anticoagulants raise the possibility that the next generation of tryptase inhibitors that are more specific than those currently available might be useful in hindering the bleeding abnormalities that sometimes occur in patients with systemic mastocytosis and/or anaphylaxis. The use of the recombinant hTryptase-β–heparin complexes[1,24,109] also might be a more effective way to prevent blood coagulation in the clinic in the prevention and treatment of thromboembolic disease, than by using heparin alone. Finally, the in vivo detection of the fragments released from hTryptase-β digestion of hFibrinogen (eg, the 2–7 kDa peptides derived from the C-terminus of fibrinogen α chain) possibly could be used as a biomarker to identify and evaluate the effectiveness of treatment of patients with mastocytosis (see **Fig. 1**) or the MC activation syndrome.[110–112] However, more investigations are needed to clarify the participation of different allelic isoforms of hTryptase-β in the coagulation system and the compensatory mechanisms that avoid bleeding as a frequent manifestation in mastocytosis and anaphylaxis. The role of MCs as reparative cells in thromboembolic events is another area of future investigation.

REFERENCES

1. Huang C, De Sanctis GT, O'Brien PJ, et al. Evaluation of the substrate specificity of human mast cell tryptase β1 and demonstration of its importance in bacterial infections of the lung. J Biol Chem 2001;276(28):26276–84.
2. Marshall JS. Mast-cell responses to pathogens. Nat Rev Immunol 2004;4(10): 787–99.
3. Galli SJ, Nakae S, Tsai M. Mast cells in the development of adaptive immune responses. Nat Immunol 2005;6(2):135–42.
4. Thakurdas SM, Melicoff E, Sansores-García L, et al. The mast cell-restricted tryptase mMCP-6 has a critical immunoprotective role in bacterial infections. J Biol Chem 2007;282:20809–15.
5. McNeil HP, Adachi R, Stevens RL. Mast cell-restricted tryptases: structure and function in inflammation and pathogen defense. J Biol Chem 2007;282(29): 20785–9.
6. Shin K, Watts GF, Oettgen HC, et al. Mouse mast cell tryptase mMCP-6 is a critical link between adaptive and innate immunity in the chronic phase of *Trichinella spiralis* infection. J Immunol 2008;180(7):4885–91.
7. Irani AM, Craig SS, DeBlois G, et al. Deficiency of the tryptase+, chymase- mast cell type in gastrointestinal mucosa of patients with defective T lymphocyte function. J Immunol 1987;138(12):4381–6.
8. Li Y, Li LL, Wadley R, et al. Mast cells/basophils in the peripheral blood of allergic individuals who are HIV-1 susceptible due to their surface expression of CD4 and the chemokine receptors CCR3, CCR5, and CXCR4. Blood 2001;97(11): 3484–90.
9. Bannert N, Farzan M, Friend DS, et al. Human mast cell progenitors can be infected by macrophage tropic human–immunodeficiency virus type 1 and retain virus with maturation in vitro. J Virol 2001;75(22):10808–14.
10. Lagunoff D, Benditt EP. Proteolytic enzymes of mast cells. Ann N Y Acad Sci 1963;103:185–98.
11. Schwartz LB, Metcalfe DD, Miller JS, et al. Tryptase levels as an indicator of mast-cell activation in systemic anaphylaxis and mastocytosis. N Engl J Med 1987;316(26):1622–6.
12. Schwartz LB, Yunginger JW, Miller J, et al. Time course of appearance and disappearance of human mast cell tryptase in the circulation after anaphylaxis. J Clin Invest 1989;83(5):1551–5.

13. Leach L, Eaton BM, Westcott ED, et al. Effect of histamine on endothelial permeability and structure and adhesion molecules of the paracellular junctions of perfused human placental microvessels. Microvasc Res 1995;50(3): 323–37.

14. Prieto-García A, Zheng D, Adachi R, et al. Mast cell restricted mouse and human tryptase-heparin complexes hinder thrombin-induced coagulation of plasma and the generation of fibrin by proteolytically destroying fibrinogen. J Biol Chem 2012;287(11):7834–44.

15. Schwartz LB, Lewis RA, Austen KF. Tryptase from human pulmonary mast cells: purification and characterization. J Biol Chem 1981;256(22):11939–43.

16. Schwartz LB, Lewis RA, Seldin D, et al. Acid hydrolases and tryptase from secretory granules of dispersed human lung mast cells. J Immunol 1981; 126(4):1290–4.

17. Pallaoro M, Fejzo MS, Shayesteh L, et al. Characterization of genes encoding known and novel human mast cell tryptases on chromosome 16p13.3. J Biol Chem 1999;274(6):3355–62.

18. Miller JS, Westin EH, Schwartz LB. Cloning and characterization of complementary DNA for human tryptase. J Clin Invest 1989;84(4):1188–95.

19. Huang C, Li L, Krilis SA, et al. Human tryptases α and β2 are functionally distinct due, in part, to a single amino acid difference in one of the surface loops that forms the substrate-binding cleft. J Biol Chem 1999;274(28):19670–6.

20. Marquardt U, Zettl F, Huber R, et al. The crystal structure of human α1-tryptase reveals a blocked substrate-binding region. J Mol Biol 2002;321(3):491–502.

21. Selwood T, Wang ZM, McCaslin DR, et al. Diverse stability and catalytic properties of human tryptase α and β isoforms are mediated by residue differences at the S1 pocket. Biochemistry 2002;41(10):3329–40.

22. Schwartz LB, Min HK, Ren S, et al. Tryptase precursors are preferentially and spontaneously released, whereas mature tryptase is retained by HMC-1 cells, Mono-Mac-6 cells, and human skin-derived mast cells. J Immunol 2003; 170(11):5667–73.

23. Miller JS, Moxley G, Schwartz LB. Cloning and characterization of a second complementary DNA for human tryptase. J Clin Invest 1990;86(3):864–70.

24. Vanderslice P, Ballinger SM, Tam EK, et al. Human mast cell tryptase: multiple cDNAs and genes reveal a multi-gene serine protease family. Proc Natl Acad Sci U S A 1990;87(10):3811–5.

25. Harris JL, Niles A, Burdick K, et al. Definition of the extended substrate specificity determinants for β tryptases I and II. J Biol Chem 2001;276(37):34941–7.

26. Badge RM, Yardley J, Jeffreys AJ, et al. Crossover breakpoint mapping identifies a subtelomeric hotspot for male meiotic recombination. Hum Mol Genet 2000;9(8):1239–44.

27. Peng Q, McEuen AR, Benyon RC, et al. The heterogeneity of mast cell tryptase from human lung and skin. Eur J Biochem 2003;270(2):270–83.

28. Sakai K, Ren S, Schwartz LB. A novel heparin-dependent processing pathway for human tryptase: autocatalysis followed by activation with dipeptidyl peptidase I. J Clin Invest 1996;97(4):988–95.

29. Almeida RP, Melchior M, Campanelli D, et al. Complementary DNA sequence of human neutrophil azurocidin, an antibiotic with extensive homology to serine proteases. Biochem Biophys Res Commun 1991;177(2):688–95.

30. Campanelli D, Detmers PA, Nathan CF, et al. Azurocidin and a homologous serine protease from neutrophils: differential antimicrobial and proteolytic properties. J Clin Invest 1990;85(3):904–15.

31. Pereira HA. CAP37, a neutrophil-derived multifunctional inflammatory mediator. J Leukoc Biol 1995;57(6):805–12.
32. Soto D, Malmsten C, Blount JL, et al. Genetic deficiency of human mast cell a tryptase. Clin Exp Allergy 2002;32(7):1000–6.
33. Trivedi NN, Tong Q, Raman K, et al. Mast cell α and β tryptases changed rapidly during primate speciation and evolved from γ-like transmembrane peptidases in ancestral vertebrates. J Immunol 2007;179(9):6072–9.
34. Trivedi NN, Tamraz B, Chu C, et al. Human subjects are protected from mast cell tryptase deficiency despite frequent inheritance of loss-of-function mutations. J Allergy Clin Immunol 2009;124(5):1099–105.
35. Wong GW, Foster PS, Yasuda S, et al. Biochemical and functional characterization of human transmembrane tryptase (TMT)/tryptase γ: TMT is an exocytosed mast cell protease that induces airway hyperresponsiveness in vivo via an IL-13/IL-4Rα/STAT6-dependent pathway. J Biol Chem 2002;277:41906–15.
36. Yuan J, Beltman J, Gjerstad E, et al. Expression and characterization of recombinant γ-tryptase. Protein Expr Purif 2006;49(1):47–54.
37. McNeil HP, Shin K, Campbell IK, et al. The mouse mast cell-restricted tetramer-forming tryptases mouse mast cell protease 6 and mouse mast cell protease 7 are critical mediators in inflammatory arthritis. Arthritis Rheum 2008;58(8):2338–46.
38. Shin K, Gurish MF, Friend DS, et al. Lymphocyte-independent connective tissue mast cells populate murine synovium. Arthritis Rheum 2006;54(9):2863–71.
39. Shin K, Nigrovic PA, Crish J, et al. Mast cells contribute to autoimmune inflammatory arthritis via their tryptase/heparin complexes. J Immunol 2009;182(1):647–56.
40. Beckett EL, Stevens RL, Jarnicki AG, et al. A new short-term mouse model of chronic obstructive pulmonary disease identifies a role for mast cell tryptase in pathogenesis. J Allergy Clin Immunol 2013;131(3):752–62.
41. Caughey GH. Tryptase genetics and anaphylaxis. J Allergy Clin Immunol 2006;117(6):1411–4.
42. Wong GW, Yasuda S, Morokawa N, et al. Mouse chromosome 17A3.3 contains thirteen genes that encode functional tryptic-like serine proteases with distinct tissue and cell expression patterns. J Biol Chem 2004;279:2438–52.
43. Reynolds DS, Gurley DS, Austen KF, et al. Cloning of the cDNA and gene of mouse mast cell protease 6: transcription by progenitor mast cells and mast cells of the connective tissue subclass. J Biol Chem 1991;266(6):3847–53.
44. McNeil HP, Reynolds DS, Schiller V, et al. Isolation, characterization, and transcription of the gene encoding mouse mast cell protease 7. Proc Natl Acad Sci U S A 1992;89(23):11174–8.
45. Wong GW, Tang Y, Feyfant E, et al. Identification of a new member of the tryptase family of mouse and human mast cell proteases that possesses a novel C-terminal hydrophobic extension. J Biol Chem 1999;274(43):30784–93.
46. Huang C, Morales G, Vagi A, et al. Formation of enzymatically active, homotypic, and heterotypic tetramers of mouse mast cell tryptases: dependence on a conserved Trp-rich domain on the surface. J Biol Chem 2000;275(1):351–8.
47. Stevens RL, Friend DS, McNeil HP, et al. Strain-specific and tissue-specific expression of mouse mast cell secretory granule proteases. Proc Natl Acad Sci U S A 1994;91(1):128–32.
48. Caughey GH, Raymond WW, Blount JL, et al. Characterization of human γ tryptases, novel members of the chromosome 16p mast cell tryptase and prostasin gene families. J Immunol 2000;164(12):6566–75.

49. Ghildyal N, Friend DS, Freelund R, et al. Lack of expression of the tryptase mouse mast cell protease 7 in mast cells of the C57BL/6J mouse. J Immunol 1994;153(6):2624–30.

50. Hunt JE, Stevens RL, Austen KF, et al. Natural disruption of the mouse mast cell protease 7 gene in the C57BL/6 mouse. J Biol Chem 1996;271(5):2851–5.

51. Ugajin T, Kojima T, Mukai K, et al. Basophils preferentially express mouse mast cell protease 11 among the mast cell tryptase family in contrast to mast cells. J Leukoc Biol 2009;86(6):1417–25.

52. Stevens RL, Otsu K, Austen KF. Purification and analysis of the core protein of the protease-resistant intracellular chondroitin sulfate E proteoglycan from the interleukin 3-dependent mouse mast cell. J Biol Chem 1985;260(26):14194–200.

53. Bourdon MA, Oldberg A, Pierschbacher M, et al. Molecular cloning and sequence analysis of a chondroitin sulfate proteoglycan cDNA. Proc Natl Acad Sci U S A 1985;82(5):1321–5.

54. Stevens RL, Avraham S, Gartner MC, et al. Isolation and characterization of a cDNA that encodes the peptide core of the secretory granule proteoglycan of human promyelocytic leukemia HL-60 cells. J Biol Chem 1988;263(15):7287–91.

55. Humphries DE, Nicodemus CF, Schiller V, et al. The human serglycin gene: nucleotide sequence and methylation pattern in human promyelocytic leukemia HL-60 cells and T-lymphoblast Molt-4 cells. J Biol Chem 1992;267(19):13558–63.

56. Yurt RW, Leid RW Jr, Austen KF. Native heparin from rat peritoneal mast cells. J Biol Chem 1977;252(2):518–21.

57. Lane DA, Bjork I, Lindahl U. Heparin and related polysaccharides. Adv Exp Med Biol 1992;313:1–374.

58. Razin E, Stevens RL, Akiyama F, et al. Culture from mouse bone marrow of a subclass of mast cells possessing a distinct chondroitin sulfate proteoglycan with glycosaminoglycans rich in N-acetylgalactosamine-4,6-disulfate. J Biol Chem 1982;257(12):7229–36.

59. Seldin DC, Austen KF, Stevens RL. Purification and characterization of protease-resistant secretory granule proteoglycans containing chondroitin sulfate diB and heparin-like glycosaminoglycans from rat basophilic leukemia cells. J Biol Chem 1985;260(20):11131–9.

60. Stevens RL, Lee TD, Seldin DC, et al. Intestinal mucosal mast cells from rats infected with Nippostrongylus brasiliensis contain protease-resistant chondroitin sulfate diB proteoglycans. J Immunol 1986;137(1):291–5.

61. Enerbäck L, Kolset SO, Kusche M, et al. Glycosaminoglycans in rat mucosal mast cells. Biochem J 1985;227(2):661–8.

62. Stevens RL, Fox CC, Lichtenstein LM, et al. Identification of chondroitin sulfate E proteoglycans and heparin proteoglycans in the secretory granules of human lung mast cells. Proc Natl Acad Sci U S A 1988;85(7):2284–7.

63. Humphries DE, Wong GW, Friend DS, et al. Heparin is essential for the storage of specific granule proteases in mast cells. Nature 1999;400(6746):769–72.

64. Forsberg E, Pejler G, Ringvall M, et al. Abnormal mast cells in mice deficient in a heparin-synthesizing enzyme. Nature 1999;400(6746):773–6.

65. Abrink M, Grujic M, Pejler G. Serglycin is essential for maturation of mast cell secretory granule. J Biol Chem 2004;279(39):40897–905.

66. Johnson DA, Barton GJ. Mast cell tryptases: examination of unusual characteristics by multiple sequence alignment and molecular modeling. Protein Sci 1992;1(3):370–7.

67. Šali A, Matsumoto R, McNeil HP, et al. Three-dimensional models of four mouse mast cell chymases: identification of proteoglycan binding regions and protease-specific antigenic epitopes. J Biol Chem 1993;268(12):9023–34.

68. Matsumoto R, Šali A, Ghildyal N, et al. Packaging of proteases and proteoglycans in the granules of mast cells and other hematopoietic cells: a cluster of histidines on mouse mast cell protease 7 regulates its binding to heparin serglycin proteoglycans. J Biol Chem 1995;270(33):19524–31.

69. Ghildyal N, Friend DS, Stevens RL, et al. Fate of two mast cell tryptases in V3 mastocytosis and normal BALB/c mice undergoing passive systemic anaphylaxis: prolonged retention of exocytosed mMCP-6 in connective tissues, and rapid accumulation of enzymatically active mMCP-7 in the blood. J Exp Med 1996;184(3):1061–73.

70. Pereira PJ, Bergner A, Macedo-Ribeiro S, et al. Human β-tryptase is a ring-like tetramer with active sites facing a central pore. Nature 1998;392(6673):306–11.

71. Huang C, Wong GW, Ghildyal N, et al. The tryptase, mouse mast cell protease 7, exhibits anticoagulant activity in vivo and in vitro due to its ability to degrade fibrinogen in the presence of the diverse array of protease inhibitors in plasma. J Biol Chem 1997;272(50):31885–93.

72. Huang C, Friend DS, Qiu WT, et al. Induction of a selective and persistent extravasation of neutrophils into the peritoneal cavity by tryptase mouse mast cell protease 6. J Immunol 1998;160(4):1910–9.

73. Schwartz LB, Bradford TR. Regulation of tryptase from human lung mast cells by heparin: stabilization of the active tetramer. J Biol Chem 1986;261(16):7372–9.

74. Alter SC, Kramps JA, Janoff A, et al. Interactions of human mast cell tryptase with biological protease inhibitors. Arch Biochem Biophys 1990;276(1):26–31.

75. Gurish MF, Pear WS, Stevens RL, et al. Tissue-regulated differentiation and maturation of a v-abl-immortalized mast cell-committed progenitor. Immunity 1995;3(2):175–86.

76. Fukuoka Y, Schwartz LB. Human β-tryptase: detection and characterization of the active monomer and prevention of tetramer reconstitution by protease inhibitors. Biochemistry 2004;43(33):10757–64.

77. Fabian I, Bleiberg I, Aronson M. Increased uptake and desulphation of heparin by mouse macrophages in the presence of polycations. Biochim Biophys Acta 1978;544(1):69–76.

78. Mosesson MW. Fibrinogen and fibrin structure and functions. J Thromb Haemost 2005;3(8):1894–904.

79. Huang S, Cao Z, Davie EW. The role of amino-terminal disulfide bonds in the structure and assembly of human fibrinogen. Biochem Biophys Res Commun 1993;190(2):488–95.

80. Zhang JZ, Redman CM. Identification of β chain domains involved in human fibrinogen assembly. J Biol Chem 1992;267(30):21727–32.

81. Blomback B, Hessel B, Hogg D, et al. A two-step fibrinogen-fibrin transition in blood coagulation. Nature 1978;275(5680):501–5.

82. Siebenlist KR, DiOrio JP, Budzynski AZ, et al. The polymerization and thrombin-binding properties of des-(β1-42)-fibrin. J Biol Chem 1990;265(30):18650–5.

83. Pratt KP, Cote HC, Chung DW, et al. The primary fibrin polymerization pocket: three-dimensional structure of a 30-kDa C-terminal γ chain fragment complexed with the peptide Gly-Pro-Arg-Pro. Proc Natl Acad Sci U S A 1997;94(14):7176–81.

84. Everse SJ, Spraggon G, Veerapandian L, et al. Crystal structure of fragment double-D from human fibrin with two different bound ligands. Biochemistry 1998;37(24):8637–42.

85. Muller MF, Ris H, Ferry JD. Electron microscopy of fine fibrin clots and fine and coarse fibrin films: observations of fibers in cross-section and in deformed states. J Mol Biol 1984;174(2):369–84.

86. Mosesson MW, Siebenlist KR, Amrani DL, et al. Identification of covalently linked trimeric and tetrameric D domains in crosslinked fibrin. Proc Natl Acad Sci U S A 1989;86(4):1113–7.

87. Siebenlist KR, Meh DA, Mosesson MW. Protransglutaminase (factor XIII) mediated crosslinking of fibrinogen and fibrin. Thromb Haemost 2001;86(5):1221–8.

88. Mosesson MW, Siebenlist KR, Hernandez I, et al. Fibrinogen assembly and crosslinking on a fibrin fragment E template. Thromb Haemost 2002;87(4):651–8.

89. Samoszuk M, Corwin MA. Mast cell inhibitor cromolyn increases blood clotting and hypoxia in murine breast cancer. Int J Cancer 2003;107(1):159–63.

90. Rosenberg RD. Heparin, antithrombin, and abnormal clotting. Annu Rev Med 1978;29:367–78.

91. Jin L, Abrahams JP, Skinner R, et al. The anticoagulant activation of antithrombin by heparin. Proc Natl Acad Sci U S A 1997;94(26):14683–8.

92. Skinner R, Abrahams JP, Whisstock JC, et al. The 2.6 Å structure of antithrombin indicates a conformational change at the heparin binding site. J Mol Biol 1997; 266(3):601–9.

93. Marcum JA, Atha DH, Fritze LM, et al. Cloned bovine aortic endothelial cells synthesize anticoagulantly active heparan sulfate proteoglycan. J Biol Chem 1986;261(16):7507–17.

94. Marcum JA, McKenney JB, Galli SJ, et al. Anticoagulantly active heparin-like molecules from mast cell-deficient mice. Am J Phys 1986;250(5 Pt 2):H879–88.

95. Samoszuk M, Corwin M, Yu H, et al. Inhibition of thrombosis in melanoma allografts in mice by endogenous mast cell heparin. Thromb Haemost 2003;90(2): 351–60.

96. Thomas VA, Wheeless CJ, Stack MS, et al. Human mast cell tryptase fibrinogenolysis: kinetics, anticoagulation mechanism, and cell adhesion disruption. Biochemistry 1998;37(8):2291–8.

97. Schwartz LB, Bradford TR, Littman BH, et al. The fibrinogenolytic activity of purified tryptase from human lung mast cells. J Immunol 1985;135(4):2762–7.

98. Ren S, Lawson AE, Carr M, et al. Human tryptase fibrinogenolysis is optimal at acidic pH and generates anticoagulant fragments in the presence of the anti-tryptase monoclonal antibody B12. J Immunol 1997;159(7):3540–8.

99. Kettelhut BV, Metcalfe DD. Pediatric mastocytosis. J Invest Dermatol 1991; 96(3):15S–8S.

100. Smith TF, Welch TR, Allen JB, et al. Cutaneous mastocytosis with bleeding: probable heparin effect. Cutis 1987;39(3):241–4.

101. Gonzalo-Garijo MA, Perez-Rangel I, Alvarado-Izquierdo MI, et al. Metrorrhagia as an uncommon symptom of anaphylaxis. J Investig Allergol Clin Immunol 2010;20(6):540–1.

102. Toubi E, Kessel A, Golan TD. Vaginal bleeding, a rare complication of immunotherapy. Allergy 1997;52(7):782–3.

103. Mazzi G, Raineri A, Lacava E, et al. Primary hyperfibrinogenolysis in a patient with anaphylactic shock. Haematologica 1994;79(3):283–5.

104. Wang JL, Shen EY, Ho MY. Isolated prolongation of activated partial thromboplastin time following wasp sting. Acta Paediatr Taiwan 2005;46(3):164–5.

105. Sucker C, Mansmann G, Steiner S, et al. Fatal bleeding due to a heparin-like anticoagulant in a 37-year-old woman suffering from systemic mastocytosis. Clin Appl Thromb Hemost 2008;14(3):360–4.
106. Koenig M, Morel J, Reynaud J, et al. An unusual cause of spontaneous bleeding in the intensive care unit—mastocytosis: a case report. Cases J 2008;1(1):100.
107. Lombardini C, Helia RE, Boehlen F, et al. "Heparinization" and hyperfibrinogenolysis by wasp sting. Am J Emerg Med 2009;27(9):1176.e1–3.
108. Black JS, Feldmann M, Leon S. Systemic mastocytosis as a rare cause of diffuse gastrointestinal hemorrhage. Am Surg 2009;75(5):429–30.
109. Niles AL, Maffitt M, Haak-Frendscho M, et al. Recombinant human mast cell tryptase β: stable expression in *Pichia pastoris* and purification of fully active enzyme. Biotechnol Appl Biochem 1998;28(Pt 2):125–31.
110. Valent P, Horny H, Escribano L, et al. Diagnostic criteria and classification of mastocytosis: a consensus proposal. Leuk Res 2001;25(7):603–25.
111. Valent P, Akin C, Sperr WR, et al. Aggressive systemic mastocytosis and related mast cell disorders: current treatment options and proposed response criteria. Leuk Res 2003;27(7):635–41.
112. Valent P. Mast cell activation syndromes: definition and classification. Allergy 2013;68(4):417–24.

Epidemiology, Prognosis, and Risk Factors in Mastocytosis

Knut Brockow, MD

KEYWORDS

- Mastocytosis • Mast cell activity syndrome
- Monoclonal mast cell activation syndrome • Epidemiology • Prognosis • Risk factors

KEY POINTS

- The prevalence of overt mastocytosis has been estimated to be about 10 cases per 100,000 inhabitants. That of monoclonal mast cell activation syndrome and of idiopathic mast cell activation syndrome remains unknown.
- Adult patients with mastocytosis predominantly exhibit indolent systemic mastocytosis (ISM) and in children cutaneous mastocytosis (CM) is assumed.
- Regression of mastocytosis in children is common and chronic persistence of skin mastocytosis in adults is typical.
- Evolution of ISM into more advanced forms of disease is an exceptional event.
- The life expectancy in patients with CM or ISM is not reduced.

EPIDEMIOLOGY OF MASTOCYTOSIS AND MAST CELL ACTIVATION SYNDROMES
Prevalence of Mastocytosis

Mastocytosis is considered to be an orphan disease (affecting <200,000 people in the United States). There are no epidemiologic studies to define the precise incidence, point prevalence, or cumulative prevalence of mastocytosis in the general population (**Box 1**). Because of its rarity many doctors were unfamiliar with this disease and did not recognize it. Thus, until recently, the number of recognized patients per single center was not sufficient and not reliable to estimate incidence and prevalence. In 1997, it was estimated that 1 in 1000 to 8000 new patients seen in dermatology outpatient clinics may have some form of mastocytosis.[1] Fortunately, this situation has improved greatly during the last two decades and this diagnosis has become more recognized.[2,3] Another reason for missing data is that firm criteria for the diagnosis of mastocytosis have only been defined in 2001 and that the methods and experience to detect mastocytosis have improved, but continue to differ between departments.[4]

The author has nothing to disclose.
Department of Dermatology and Allergy Biederstein, Technische Universität München, Biedersteiner Strasse 29, Munich 80802, Germany
E-mail address: knut.brockow@lrz.tum.de

Immunol Allergy Clin N Am 34 (2014) 283–295
http://dx.doi.org/10.1016/j.iac.2014.01.003   immunology.theclinics.com

---

Box 1
Prevalence of mastocytosis

- There is a lack of data to define the exact prevalence
- Prevalence for suspected or confirmed mastocytosis of 13 cases in 100,00 inhabitants is given in one study
- It remains unclear if and how the inclusion of patients with anaphylaxis, but without skin involvement, will increase the prevalence
- The prevalence of monoclonal mast cell activation syndrome is unknown
- Only a few patients with idiopathic mast cell activation syndrome have been described

---

The European Competence Network on Mastocytosis attempts to ensure a good quality of diagnosis by defining reference and excellence centers for mastocytosis.[3,5]

In the only available study giving prevalence data in the general population, cases with confirmed indolent systemic mastocytosis (ISM) or presumed ISM based on either the presence of maculopapular cutaneous mastocytosis (MPCM) plus tryptase levels greater than 20 ng/mL or on MPCM together with elevated tryptase levels (>10 ng/mL) or on clinical suspicion together with elevated mediator levels, were collected.[6] The home address was verified and the number of patients was divided by the number of the total adult population living in this Dutch region. In this study, ISM prevalence in the adult population in the Netherlands has been estimated to be 13 cases per 100,000 inhabitants. Of those, 31 patients had MPCM and 10 patients were seen because of anaphylaxis without skin involvement. When the number of patients in this competence center was analyzed, a steep increase in the number of ISM patients was noted from 1998 to 2010, which is very likely the result of increased experience and recognition of the disease in this area during these years. At the consensus meeting of mastocytosis experts in Boston 2010, a general cumulative prevalence of approximately 1 in 10,000 persons was also estimated by other centers (Luis Escribano, Patrizia Bonadonna, personal communication, 2012).

Mastocytosis in Different Age and Gender Groups

Mastocytosis can occur in children and adults.[7] Although mastocytosis can occur at any age, the onset of mastocytosis is in the first 2 years of life in 50% or more of cases.[8] Congenital mastocytosis at birth is exceptional.[9] In adults, most patients are diagnosed in middle age between 20 and 50 years of age.[8] Because of a chronic nature and low regression rate of adult-age mastocytosis the cumulative prevalence of adult patients of mastocytosis rises with age. Gender distribution is approximately equal.

Systemic Mastocytosis Without Skin Lesions

It was previously believed that more than 95% of patients with mastocytosis would be detectable by the presence of typical skin lesions.[10] A few years ago, it was discovered that approximately 10% of patients with Hymenoptera sting anaphylaxis had elevated serum tryptase levels greater than 11.4 ng/mL. Of these patients, a substantial proportion had ISM without skin lesions (ISM−).[11] In one center that recruited patients with classical skin lesions and patients with Hymenoptera sting and idiopathic anaphylaxis for further assessment, the number of patients without skin lesions (ISM−; N = 46) was nearly as high as that with mastocytosis in the skin (MIS; ISM+; N = 51) indicating that isolated bone marrow mastocytosis may be an underestimated subvariant of SM.[12]

Patients with insect-sting anaphylaxis and no MIS had male predominance (78%), less common cutaneous and abdominal symptoms of anaphylaxis, but more often syncope, lower baseline tryptase values, less frequently bone marrow mast cell aggregates, and a mast cell–restricted KIT mutation pattern in comparison with ISM+.[13] Thus, it has to be assumed that there is an additional specific subpopulation of patients with SM, but without MIS, which may still be underdiagnosed.

Incidence of Monoclonal Mast Cell Activation Syndrome

By consensus classification, mastocytosis is only diagnosed if a set of major and minor criteria is present.[3,4] Patients with anaphylaxis and clonal mast cells expressing the D816V mutation in KIT and expressing the α-chain of the interleukin-2 receptor CD25, but without the full set of criteria needed to diagnose mastocytosis, have been described.[14,15] The diagnosis for these patients has been named monoclonal mast cell activation syndrome (MMAS).[14,16] The prevalence of patients with other symptoms of MMAS is yet unknown. In patients with anaphylaxis and systemic mast cell activation symptoms but without skin lesions where clonal mast cells could be detected, the most patients fulfilled the criteria for SM.[17] Because the frequency of MMAS varies among different study groups between 6% and 27%, it may be assumed that the distinction between ISM without skin lesions (ISM−) and MMAS also depends on the methods used and the experience of the analyzers.[11,17]

Incidence of Idiopathic Mast Cell Activation Syndrome

An idiopathic mast cell activation syndrome recently has been defined.[16,18] To give this diagnosis, patients have to exhibit symptoms indicating mast cell mediator release; the involvement of mast cells has to be documented by biochemical measurements, preferably by the increase in tryptase during a symptomatic period; symptoms should respond to therapies with mast cell stabilizing agents or drugs directed against mast cell mediator production, mediator release, or mediator effects; and other known mast cell diseases should have been excluded.[16] Different physicians in varied disciplines have seen an increased number of subjects who presented with signs and symptoms potentially indicating mast cell activation, such as flushing, abdominal pain, diarrhea, and more nonspecific symptoms, but where an extensive medical evaluation has failed to result in a definitive diagnosis.[18] Up to now only one study has convincingly presented patients with idiopathic mast cell activation syndrome and studied the clinical manifestation of the disease in this cohort of 18 patients.[19] About three-quarters of the patients presented with a combination of abdominal pain, dermatographism, and flushing with or without additional symptoms. Of note, only in five of these patients were increased levels of total or mature tryptase measured; in most patients this increased mediator release was detected by histamine or prostaglandin D_2 measurements, which are more sensitive but less standardized and less specific compared with tryptase measurements. Thus, the prevalence of patients with idiopathic mast cell activation syndrome presenting with otherwise unexplained clinical symptoms resembling mast cell diseases remains unknown, but seems to be low.

EPIDEMIOLOGY OF DIFFERENT FORMS OF MASTOCYTOSIS
Prevalence of Systemic Disease in Patients with Mastocytosis

The prevalence of systemic disease in patients with mastocytosis depends greatly on the definition of SM, which has been changed in 2001, on the associated development of more sensitive methods for detecting mast cells and clonality (eg, use of the tryptase stain to highlight mast cells), and on the experience of physicians. The extracutaneous tissue that shows the highest numbers of mast cell in systemic involvement and that is still easily available is the bone marrow.[20] Whereas in older studies mast cell infiltrates were detected in less than half of all patients with MPCM,[21] this frequency did increase over the years,[22] and with the availability of newer methods and criteria, the prevalence of SM in adult patients with MPCM has recently been reported to be more than 95% when the most sensitive methods are used by experienced physicians (**Box 2**).[23,24] In children, bone marrow biopsies are rarely performed. In an older study, often more subtle nondiagnostic abnormalities have been reported in the bone marrow biopsy specimens of children.[25] SM in children does exist, but overall the diagnosis is seldom made.[26,27] Newer studies on the exact prevalence of SM in children are lacking because of ethical reasons, but available evidence indicates that SM in children is rare.

Prevalence of Different Forms of SM

Mastocytosis is subclassified into cutaneous mastocytosis (CM), ISM, aggressive SM (ASM), SM with an associated hematologic non–mast cell disorder (SM-AHNMD), mast cell leukemia (MCL), mast cell sarcoma, and extracutaneous mastocytosis[28] with differing typical clinical characteristics (**Fig. 1**). CM without systemic involvement is assumed but not proven in most children with MIS and seems to be seldom in adults with mastocytosis.[3] In adults and in the small majority of those children with internal involvement, ISM is the most common form. The exact frequency of this form depends strongly on the specialty of the department seeing the patients. It is prudent to assume that 90% to 95% of all patients with mastocytosis exhibit ISM. After CM and ISM, SM-AHNMD is the most frequent form of mastocytosis and predominantly seen in hematology departments. In one large study of the Mayo Clinic analyzing 342 consecutive patients, 89% of patients with SM-AHNMD had an associated myeloid neoplasm, such as myeloproliferative neoplasm, chronic myelocytic leukemia, and myelodysplastic syndrome.[29] Diagnoses in the remainder were lymphoma, myeloma, chronic lymphocytic leukemia, or primary amyloidosis. Aggressive SM is rare and often associated with SM-AHNMD.[30] Whereas in specialized hematology departments the frequency of ASM, SM-AHNMD, and MCL has been reported to be up to 40%, 12%, and 1% of patients,[29] respectively, in our and most other dermatology and allergy departments less than 5% of patients fulfill the criteria for these subtypes (Brockow, unpublished observation, 2014). Patients with ISM are significantly more likely to have MIS and less likely to exhibit constitutional symptoms or hepatomegaly compared with patients with advanced SM.[29] MCL is rare even in hematology departments.[29] Of interest, MCL is associated normally with no MIS and it has been speculated that in aggressive SM and in SM-AHNMD the frequency of cutaneous signs of

---

Box 2
Epidemiology of different forms of mastocytosis

- More than 95% of adults but only a minority of children with mastocytosis has systemic involvement

- In adults, indolent systemic mastocytosis is predominant, whereas more advanced forms are infrequent

- Maculopapular cutaneous mastocytosis is the most commonly reported form of mastocytosis in the skin in children and adults

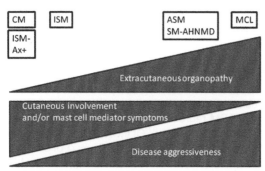

Fig. 1. Typical clinical characteristics of patients with different forms of mastocytosis. ASM, aggressive systemic mastocytosis; CM, cutaneous mastocytosis; ISM, indolent systemic masto-cytosis; ISM−/Ax+, patients with anaphylaxis and isolated bone marrow mastocytosis; MCL, mast cell leukemia; SM-AHNMD, systemic mastocytosis with associated hematologic non–mast cell disease. (*Modified from* Pardanani A. Systemic mastocytosis in adults: 2013 update on diagnosis, risk stratification, and management. Am J Hematol 2013 Jul;88:612–24; with permission.)

mastocytosis is only approximately 50%.[16] Mast cell sarcoma and extracutaneous mastocytomas are exceedingly rare.[4,31]

Prevalence of Different Forms of MIS

The characteristics of MIS differ between childhood- and adult-onset mastocytosis.[32] In pediatric mastocytosis, different forms of skin involvement exist. In our department and some other studies, mostly children with MPCM are seen,[8,33] whereas a different study states that mastocytomas would be more prevalent.[34] Because children with mastocytomas may be less likely to be presented at specialty departments, it remains unclear which manifestation may occur more often. Nodular and plaque forms of MIS in children are less common.[33] The distinction between MPCM and the plaque form may be difficult, because skin lesions are sometimes only minimally elevated and have variable sizes. Diffuse CM is the least common form of childhood MIS and most reference centers only see a few of these patients. In adults, all patients have MPCM with more or less pigmentation and erythema. The extreme depigmented telangiectatic spectrum of this form may also be called telangiectasia macularis erup-tiva perstans, but has to be differentiated from essential telangiectasias.[35,36] Because there is no clear distinction, the percentage of patients with MPCM called telangiec-tasia macularis eruptiva perstans varies among different physicians in different studies.

PROGNOSIS FOR REGRESSION OR PROGRESSION OF DISEASE
Prognosis for Resolution of CM in Children

Data on the natural history of childhood-onset mastocytosis come mostly from studies where the analysis depended on retrospective chart reviews and reporting on skin ex-aminations.[26] Although it often has been stated that resolution of the disease would happen in more than 50% of patients, there are only a small number of studies on which this conclusion was based. A recent study attempted to analyze patients with a longer duration of follow-up and re-examined 15 individuals who had been diag-nosed with mastocytosis as children 20 years earlier.[26] Complete regression was seen in 67%, major regression in 20%, and partial regression in 13%. Initial bone marrow examinations in three patients with SM were associated with later persistent disease. Thus, mast cell aggregates in the bone marrow biopsies were prognostic for persistent disease.

Prognosis for Resolution of CM in Adults

For patients with adult-onset mastocytosis, persistence of disease is typical and regression of skin lesions only occurs in a subset of patients. In a study investigating clinical correlates of MPCM regression in adult patients with SM, 106 patients were followed up for a minimum of 10 years.[37] Of those, regression was noted in 12 patients with complete clearance (N = 5) or a decrease (N = 7) of skin lesions. An age older than 50 years was the only prognostic feature for regression of MPCM. Regression of MIS was not indicative for the clinical course of disease because two patients with SM-AHNMD experienced deterioration of their clinical condition, whereas in all 10 patients with ISM severity and frequency of symptoms decreased. The regression of MPCM also did not indicate total clearance from mastocytosis because in all patients in whom bone marrow biopsy results were available at different time points, the later did not differ significantly from the initial findings in patients undergoing the procedure.

Prognosis for Progression of Disease and Survival

After initial occurrence and deterioration of MIS and clinical symptoms, a stable phase is seen in most children and adults with mastocytosis.[10] The prognosis of patients with adult ISM has been studied in a long-term follow-up of 145 consecutive adult patients observed for a median of 147 months.[24] The results show that the disease was stable in most patients. There were signs for biologic progression indicating an increased proliferation of mast cells, such as an increase in serum tryptase greater than 200 ng/mL, osteoporosis, or organomegalies in 27% of patients. Only five patients (3%) showed progression from ISM to a more advanced form of SM. One patient developed ASM, three patients SM-AHNMD, and one patient MCL. The cumulative probability of disease progression in ISM was calculated to be 1.7% in 10 years. Multivariate analysis showed that serum β_2-microglobulin in combination with the presence of KIT-mutation in all hematopoietic lineages was the best combination of independent parameters for predicting disease progression from ISM into a more aggressive form (**Box 3**). Regarding overall survival, most patients with initial ISM had a normal life expectancy and death was directly related to mastocytosis in only two cases.

Thus, evolution of ISM into an aggressive form of the disease has to be considered to be an exceptional event. The results are in contrast to a retrospective study with 58 cases of SM where only 45.5% remained alive after a median follow-up of 7.6 years,[38] but in agreement with a later study from the same institution that discriminated between patients with ISM (N = 24) and ASM (N = 16). Eight patients (20%) in this study with ASM died during the observation period, but none with ISM.[39] Apart from the specific subtype of mastocytosis, anemia, increased serum alkaline phosphatase, and the degree of bone marrow involvement assessed by histopathology had been discussed as predictors for overall survival of mastocytosis in these older studies.[39] In the study by Escribano and coworkers,[24] the association between these parameters and overall survival in patients with ISM was confirmed. The variables with the highest predicted value for a shorter overall survival in the multivariable analysis were age at diagnosis greater than 60 years, increased serum alkaline phosphatase, and development of SM-AHNMD. The cumulative probability of death in patients with ISM was 2.2% at 5 years and 11% at 25 years.

Box 3
Prognostic factors for mastocytosis

Factors	May Indicate
Mast cell aggregates in the initial bone marrow biopsy	Persistence of pediatric mastocytosis into adulthood
Advanced age	Regression of cutaneous mastocytosis in adults
Presence of *KIT* mutation in all hematopoietic lineages; elevated β_2 microglobulin levels	Progression from indolent systemic mastocytosis to more advanced forms of SM
Immature bone marrow mast cell phenotype (CD25$^+$/FCεR1^{low}/FSC^{low}/SSC^{low}/CD45^{low}) in absence of coexisting normal mast cells	Presence of *KIT* mutation in all hematopoietic lineages
Advanced subtypes of SM, anemia, hypoalbuminemia, serum alkaline phosphatase, blasts in and degree of bone marrow involvement, advanced age, age at diagnosis, weight loss, high allele burden, additional genetic mutations in hematopoietic cells	Decreased survival

---

In a retrospective study on 342 consecutive adult patients seen at the Mayo Clinic, where more than half of the patients had advanced forms of SM, life expectancy in ISM was superior and not significantly different from that of the age and gender-matched population.[40] However, the survival of the smoldering form of ISM, which is characterized by high mast cell numbers in the tissue, was associated with a shorter survival compared with the rest of ISM. The overall median survival in SM-AHNMD was 24 months, in patients with ASM 41 months, and in the four patients with MCL only 2 months. Multivariable analysis identified advanced age, weight loss, anemia, thrombocytopenia, hypoalbuminemia, and excess bone marrow blasts as independent prognostic factors for survival.

Increased plasma CD25 levels have been reported to be associated with inferior overall survival in a mixed cohort of patients with advanced and indolent SM, which were independent of other risk factors.[41] Immunophenotyping may also be of value as a prognostic marker for disease progression. An immature bone marrow mast cell phenotype (CD25$^+$/FCεR1^{low}/FSC^{low}/SSC^{low}/CD45^{low}) in absence of coexisting normal mast cells correlates with multilineage hematopoietic *KIT* D816V mutations more frequently seen in cases with SM-AHNMD, ASM, and MCL.[42] In contrast, in ISM bone marrow mast cells display a more mature activated MC phenotype (CD63$^+$/CD69$^+$/CD203$^+$).

In a study measuring *KIT* D816V–expressed allele burden by quantitative polymerase chain reaction, the allele burden was strongly correlated with disease activity, disease subtype (ISM vs advanced SM), and survival in 63 patients with ISM, 8 patients with a smoldering type of ISM, 16 patients with AS-AHNMD, and 60 patients with ASM or MCL ± AHNMD.[30] The prognosis of SM was also related to the pattern of mutated genes that were acquired during disease evolution.[43] In 39 patients with different forms of indolent and advanced SM, additional molecular aberrations were found in 24 of 27 patients with advanced SM but only in 3 of 12 patients (25%) with ISM. Most frequently affected genes were TET2, SRSF2, ASXL1, CBL, and RUNX1. Most patients with advanced SM carried greater than or equal to 3 mutations. The overall survival was shorter in patients with additional aberration compared with those with only *KIT* D816V mutations.

RISK FACTORS FOR MAJOR COMPLICATIONS OF MASTOCYTOSIS
Risk Factors for More Severe Clinical Disease

In a prospective study of 48 adults and 19 children with MPCM the extent and density of cutaneous lesions were compared with symptomatology, tryptase levels, and bone marrow pathology.[32] In children, possibly because of a low number of included patients, symptoms, and available bone marrow pathologies, the extent of cutaneous disease was not associated with systemic involvement or symptomatology. There was a borderline correlation between the extent of cutaneous disease and serum tryptase levels (P<.06). Because it is known that patients with diffuse CM involving the whole body tend to have more severe symptoms and sometimes also positive bone marrow pathologies,[44] it has been discussed that inclusion of a higher number of children with more severe disease would have been more likely to show a significant association. This is in agreement with a study of 111 patients with MIS to identify predictors for severe mast cell activation episodes.[45] The results showed that all 12 children (11% of total) who suffered symptoms requiring hospitalization also exhibited extensive cutaneous disease involving greater than 90% of the body surface area. These patients also had higher serum tryptase levels compared with those of the rest of the children with skin involvement of less than 90% (45 vs 5 ng/mL). Thus, a high extent of cutaneous disease involvement and elevated tryptase levels identified patients at risk for severe and sometimes life-threatening mast cell activation events. Receiver operating characteristic curve analysis showed that serum tryptase levels of 7, 16, and 31 ng/mL were the best cut-off values for the risk of daily antimediator therapy, hospitalization, and the management in an intensive care unit, respectively. When the data were reanalyzed, it was emphasized that all of the patients who had to be treated in the intensive care unit had extensive blistering, which should be regarded as a predictor for severe complications in children with mastocytosis.[46] This is in agreement with rare fatal complications in children with mastocytosis that were reported together with severe blistering episodes.[47,48]

In adults with skin lesions, the extent of lesions correlated to disease duration, pruritus, flushing, fatigue, splenomegaly, hepatomegaly, serum tryptase levels, and bone marrow pathology.[32] Thus, an examination of the extent of cutaneous lesions in adults helps to identify those with more extensive extracutaneous disease.

MIS itself may be diagnostic for SM. When new sensitive methods were applied to analyze the presence of World Health Organization–defined diagnostic criteria for SM in 95 patients with MIS, it was shown that in all 58 bone marrow biopsies investigated an SM could be detected.[49] Thus, adult-onset MIS itself was highly predictive of systemic involvement in mastocytosis. Baseline serum tryptase and elevated urinary histamine metabolites have been reported to be surrogate markers for SM.[50,51]

In a study of 39 adult patients with ISM, the *KIT* D816V mutation burden as detected by a sensitive quantitative polymerase chain reaction in peripheral blood cells shows that mutation levels were associated with baseline serum tryptase levels.[52] Baseline serum tryptase levels greater than 20 ng/mL are a minor criterion for SM.[4] However, within the group of patients with ISM, the *KIT* D816V mutation burden in peripheral blood and bone marrow aspirate cells was not correlated with the grade of symptoms of mast cell activation episodes with and without anaphylaxis or with and without osteoporosis and normal bone mineral density.[53]

Other predictors for an increased disease severity described in the literature and related to baseline serum tryptase levels were soluble CD25, soluble CD117 (*KIT*), and interleukin-6.[54,55]

Risk Factors for Anaphylaxis in Patients with Mastocytosis

In children with mastocytosis, a significantly increased risk to develop anaphylaxis seems to be restricted to those with extensive skin involvement and high serum tryptase levels.[45] In adults with mastocytosis, depending on the study population, a cumulative prevalence of anaphylaxis has been reported to be between 22% and 49% of patients.[56–58] Those with systemic disease had an increased risk of anaphylaxis compared with those with cutaneous disease, especially when atopy was present.[56,58] Anaphylaxis in patients with mastocytosis with but not without skin involvement was associated with higher basal serum tryptase levels.[56,58]

The most frequently reported elicitors of anaphylaxis in patients with mastocytosis are Hymenoptera venoms.[56–58] The severity of reactions in patients with mastocytosis seems to be increased compared with those without mastocytosis.[59] The level of basal serum tryptase is the strongest predictor for a higher severity in insect sting anaphylaxis.[60] In contrast to this general principle, a more complex association between serum tryptase levels and the prevalence of insect sting anaphylaxis has been reported with the prevalence initially rising but subsequently falling in relation to increasing serum tryptase levels.[61]

Whereas there is a strong association between mastocytosis and insect sting anaphylaxis, and whereas not uncommonly patients with idiopathic anaphylaxis have been described in this patient group, the association between mastocytosis and drug or food anaphylaxis does not seem to be strong.[62,63] In one study of 137 patients with drug- or food-induced anaphylaxis, only two patients were diagnosed with mastocytosis.[62]

Risk Factors for Osteoporosis in Patients with Mastocytosis

Vertebral osteoporosis and fractures are frequent in adult patients with SM. In a study of 75 patients with SM who underwent skeletal radiographs and bone mineral density assessment, 37 patients (48%) had bone involvement including osteoporosis (N = 23; 31%) with vertebral fractures in 13 patients (17%).[64] In one retrospective study in 157 patients with ISM, 235 lifetime fractures including 140 osteoporotic fractures were recorded, of which 62% were vertebral.[65] Osteoporotic fractures and osteoporosis were reported to be present in 37% and 28% of patients, respectively. The prevalence of these manifestations was higher in men than in women. Predictors for osteoporotic manifestations were older age, male gender, and higher urinary methylhistamine.[65] There seems to be no significant correlation between serum tryptase levels and T or Z scores for bone mineral density,[66] and in one publication elevated tryptase levels were associated with an even greater bone density in one cohort of patients.[67]

REFERENCES

1. Golkar L, Bernhard JD. Mastocytosis. Lancet 1997;349:1379–85.
2. Metcalfe DD. Classification and diagnosis of mastocytosis: current status. J Invest Dermatol 1991;96(Suppl 3):2S–4S.
3. Valent P, Akin C, Escribano L, et al. Standards and standardization in mastocytosis: consensus statements on diagnostics, treatment recommendations and response criteria. Eur J Clin Invest 2007;37:435–53.
4. Valent P, Horny HP, Escribano L, et al. Diagnostic criteria and classification of mastocytosis: a consensus proposal. Leuk Res 2001;25:603–25.
5. Valent P, Arock M, Bonadonna P, et al. European Competence Network on Mastocytosis (ECNM): 10-year jubilee, update, and future perspectives. Wien Klin Wochenschr 2012;124:807–14.

6. van Doormaal JJ, Arends S, Brunekreeft KL, et al. Prevalence of indolent systemic mastocytosis in a Dutch region. J Allergy Clin Immunol 2013;131: 1429–31.
7. Brockow K, Metcalfe DD. Mastocytosis. Chem Immunol Allergy 2010;95:110–24.
8. Kettelhut BV, Metcalfe DD. Pediatric mastocytosis. J Invest Dermatol 1991;96: 15S–8S.
9. Kuint J, Bielorai B, Gilat D, et al. C-kit activating mutation in a neonate with in-utero presentation of systemic mastocytosis associated with myeloproliferative disorder [letter]. Br J Haematol 1999;106:838–9.
10. Brockow K, Metcalfe D. Mastocytosis. In: Rich R, Fleischer T, Shearer W, et al, editors. Clinical immunology. Vol. 1. 2nd edition. London: Mosby International Ltd; 2001. p. 55.1–.9.
11. Bonadonna P, Perbellini O, Passalacqua G, et al. Clonal mast cell disorders in patients with systemic reactions to Hymenoptera stings and increased serum tryptase levels. J Allergy Clin Immunol 2009;123:680–6.
12. Zanotti R, Bonadonna P, Bonifacio M, et al. Isolated bone marrow mastocytosis: an underestimated subvariant of indolent systemic mastocytosis. Haematologica 2011;96(3):482–4.
13. Alvarez-Twose I, Zanotti R, Gonzalez-de-Olano D, et al. Nonaggressive systemic mastocytosis (SM) without skin lesions associated with insect-induced anaphylaxis shows unique features versus other indolent SM. J Allergy Clin Immunol. pii: S0091-6749(13)00988-3. http://dx.doi.org/10.1016/j.jaci.2013.06.020. Accessed August 3, 2013. [Epub ahead of print].
14. Sonneck K, Florian S, Mullauer L, et al. Diagnostic and subdiagnostic accumulation of mast cells in the bone marrow of patients with anaphylaxis: monoclonal mast cell activation syndrome. Int Arch Allergy Immunol 2007;142:158–64.
15. Akin C, Scott LM, Kocabas CN, et al. Demonstration of an aberrant mast-cell population with clonal markers in a subset of patients with "idiopathic" anaphylaxis. Blood 2007;110:2331–3.
16. Valent P, Akin C, Arock M, et al. Definitions, criteria and global classification of mast cell disorders with special reference to mast cell activation syndromes: a consensus proposal. Int Arch Allergy Immunol 2012;157:215–25.
17. Alvarez-Twose I, Gonzalez de Olano D, Sanchez-Munoz L, et al. Clinical, biological, and molecular characteristics of clonal mast cell disorders presenting with systemic mast cell activation symptoms. J Allergy Clin Immunol 2010;125: 1269–78.
18. Akin C, Valent P, Metcalfe DD. Mast cell activation syndrome: proposed diagnostic criteria. J Allergy Clin Immunol 2010;126:1099–104.
19. Hamilton MJ, Hornick JL, Akin C, et al. Mast cell activation syndrome: a newly recognized disorder with systemic clinical manifestations. J Allergy Clin Immunol 2011;128:147–52.
20. Parker RI. Hematologic aspects of mastocytosis: I: bone marrow pathology in adult and pediatric systemic mast cell disease. J Invest Dermatol 1991;96: 47S–51S.
21. Czarnetzki BM, Kolde G, Schoemann A, et al. Bone marrow findings in adult patients with urticaria pigmentosa. J Am Acad Dermatol 1988;18:45–51.
22. Topar G, Staudacher C, Geisen F, et al. Urticaria pigmentosa: a clinical, hematopathologic, and serologic study of 30 adults. Am J Clin Pathol 1998;109: 279–85.
23. Brockow K, Ring J. Update on diagnosis and treatment of mastocytosis. Curr Allergy Asthma Rep 2011;11:292–9.

24. Escribano L, Alvarez-Twose I, Sanchez-Munoz L, et al. Prognosis in adult indolent systemic mastocytosis: a long-term study of the Spanish Network on Mastocytosis in a series of 145 patients. J Allergy Clin Immunol 2009;124:514–21.
25. Kettelhut BV, Parker RI, Travis WD, et al. Hematopathology of the bone marrow in pediatric cutaneous mastocytosis. A study of 17 patients. Am J Clin Pathol 1989;91:558–62.
26. Uzzaman A, Maric I, Noel P, et al. Pediatric-onset mastocytosis: a long term clinical follow-up and correlation with bone marrow histopathology. Pediatr Blood Cancer 2009;53:629–34.
27. Carter MC, Uzzaman A, Scott LM, et al. Pediatric mastocytosis: routine anesthetic management for a complex disease. Anesth Analg 2008;107:422–7.
28. Valent P, Arock M, Akin C, et al. The classification of systemic mastocytosis should include mast cell leukemia (MCL) and systemic mastocytosis with a clonal hematologic non-mast cell lineage disease (SM-AHNMD). Blood 2010; 116:850–1.
29. Lim KH, Tefferi A, Lasho TL, et al. Systemic mastocytosis in 342 consecutive adults: survival studies and prognostic factors. Blood 2009;113:5727–36.
30. Erben P, Schwaab J, Metzgeroth G, et al. The KIT D816V expressed allele burden for diagnosis and disease monitoring of systemic mastocytosis. Ann Hematol 2014;93(1):81–8.
31. Bautista-Quach MA, Booth CL, Kheradpour A, et al. Mast cell sarcoma in an infant: a case report and review of the literature. J Pediatr Hematol Oncol 2013;35:315–20.
32. Brockow K, Akin C, Huber M, et al. Assessment of the extent of cutaneous involvement in children and adults with mastocytosis: relationship to symptomatology, tryptase levels, and bone marrow pathology. J Am Acad Dermatol 2003;48:508–16.
33. Brockow K. Urticaria pigmentosa. Immunol Allergy Clin North Am 2004;24: 287–316, vii.
34. Hannaford R, Rogers M. Presentation of cutaneous mastocytosis in 173 children. Australas J Dermatol 2001;42:15–21.
35. Weber FP. Telangiectasia macularis eruptiva perstans: probably a telangiectatic variety of urticaria pigmentosa in an adult. Proc R Soc Med 1930;24:96–7.
36. Moursund MP, Hirschmann VR. Telangiectasia macularis eruptiva perstans: review of the literature, report of a case and discussion of the etiology and pathology of generalized telangiectasia. AMA Arch Derm Syphilol 1951;63:232–49.
37. Brockow K, Scott LM, Worobec AS, et al. Regression of urticaria pigmentosa in adult patients with systemic mastocytosis: correlation with clinical patterns of disease. Arch Dermatol 2002;138:785–90.
38. Travis WD, Li CY, Bergstralh EJ, et al. Systemic mast cell disease. Analysis of 58 cases and literature review. Medicine (Baltimore) 1988;67:345–68 [Erratum appears in Medicine (Baltimore) 1990;69(1):34].
39. Pardanani A, Baek JY, Li CY, et al. Systemic mast cell disease without associated hematologic disorder: a combined retrospective and prospective study. Mayo Clin Proc 2002;77:1169–75.
40. Lim KH, Pardanani A, Butterfield JH, et al. Cytoreductive therapy in 108 adults with systemic mastocytosis: outcome analysis and response prediction during treatment with interferon-alpha, hydroxyurea, imatinib mesylate or 2-chlorodeoxyadenosine. Am J Hematol 2009;84:790–4.
41. Pardanani A, Finke C, Abdelrahman RA, et al. Increased circulating IL-2Ralpha (CD25) predicts poor outcome in both indolent and aggressive forms of mastocytosis: a comprehensive cytokine-phenotype study. Leukemia 2013;27:1430–3.

42. Teodosio C, Garcia-Montero AC, Jara-Acevedo M, et al. An immature immuno-phenotype of bone marrow mast cells predicts for multilineage D816V KIT mutation in systemic mastocytosis. Leukemia 2012;26:951–8.
43. Schwaab J, Schnittger S, Sotlar K, et al. Comprehensive mutational profiling in advanced systemic mastocytosis. Blood 2013;122:2460–6.
44. Waxtein LM, Vega-Memije ME, Cortes-Franco R, et al. Diffuse cutaneous mastocytosis with bone marrow infiltration in a child: a case report. Pediatr Dermatol 2000;17:198–201.
45. Alvarez-Twose I, Vano-Galvan S, Sanchez-Munoz L, et al. Increased serum baseline tryptase levels and extensive skin involvement are predictors for the severity of mast cell activation episodes in children with mastocytosis. Allergy 2012;67:813–21.
46. Brockow K, Ring J, Alvarez-Twose I, et al. Extensive blistering is a predictor for severe complications in children with mastocytosis. Allergy 2012;67:1323–4.
47. Murphy M, Walsh D, Drumm B, et al. Bullous mastocytosis: a fatal outcome. Pediatr Dermatol 1999;16:452–5.
48. Golitz LE, Weston WL, Lane AT. Bullous mastocytosis: diffuse cutaneous mastocytosis with extensive blisters mimicking scalded skin syndrome or erythema multiforme. Pediatr Dermatol 1984;1:288–94.
49. Berezowska S, Flaig MJ, Rueff F, et al. Adult-onset mastocytosis in the skin is highly suggestive of systemic mastocytosis. Mod Pathol 2014;27(1):19–29.
50. Schwartz LB. Diagnostic value of tryptase in anaphylaxis and mastocytosis. Immunol Allergy Clin North Am 2006;26:451–63.
51. van Doormaal JJ, van der Veer E, van Voorst Vader PC, et al. Tryptase and histamine metabolites as diagnostic indicators of indolent systemic mastocytosis without skin lesions. Allergy 2012;67:683–90.
52. Kristensen T, Broesby-Olsen S, Vestergaard H, et al. Serum tryptase correlates with the KIT D816V mutation burden in adults with indolent systemic mastocytosis. Eur J Haematol 2013;91:106–11.
53. Broesby-Olsen S, Kristensen T, Vestergaard H, et al. KIT D816V mutation burden does not correlate to clinical manifestations of indolent systemic mastocytosis. J Allergy Clin Immunol 2013;132:723–8.
54. Akin C, Schwartz LB, Kitoh T, et al. Soluble stem cell factor receptor (CD117) and IL-2 receptor alpha chain (CD25) levels in the plasma of patients with mastocytosis: relationships to disease severity and bone marrow pathology. Blood 2000;96:1267–73.
55. Brockow K, Akin C, Huber M, et al. IL-6 levels predict disease variant and extent of organ involvement in patients with mastocytosis. Clin Immunol 2005;115:216–23.
56. Brockow K, Jofer C, Behrendt H, et al. Anaphylaxis in patients with mastocytosis: a study on history, clinical features and risk factors in 120 patients. Allergy 2008;63:226–32.
57. Gonzalez de Olano D, de la Hoz Caballer B, Nunez Lopez R, et al. Prevalence of allergy and anaphylactic symptoms in 210 adult and pediatric patients with mastocytosis in Spain: a study of the Spanish network on mastocytosis (REMA). Clin Exp Allergy 2007;37:1547–55.
58. Gulen T, Hagglund H, Dahlen B, et al. High prevalence of anaphylaxis in patients with systemic mastocytosis: a single-center experience. Clin Exp Allergy 2014;44(1):121–9.
59. Ludolph-Hauser D, Rueff F, Fries C, et al. Constitutively raised serum concentrations of mast-cell tryptase and severe anaphylactic reactions to Hymenoptera stings. Lancet 2001;357:361–2.

60. Rueff F, Przybilla B, Bilo MB, et al. Predictors of severe systemic anaphylactic reactions in patients with Hymenoptera venom allergy: importance of baseline serum tryptase. A study of the European Academy of Allergology and Clinical Immunology Interest Group on Insect Venom Hypersensitivity. J Allergy Clin Immunol 2009;124:1047–54.
61. van Anrooij B, van der Veer E, de Monchy JG, et al. Higher mast cell load decreases the risk of Hymenoptera venom-induced anaphylaxis in patients with mastocytosis. J Allergy Clin Immunol 2013;132:125–30.
62. Bonadonna P, Zanotti R, Pagani M, et al. How much specific is the association between Hymenoptera venom allergy and mastocytosis? Allergy 2009;64: 1379–82.
63. Brockow K, Bonadonna P. Drug allergy in mast cell disease. Curr Opin Allergy Clin Immunol 2012;12:354–60.
64. Barete S, Assous N, de Gennes C, et al. Systemic mastocytosis and bone involvement in a cohort of 75 patients. Ann Rheum Dis 2010;69(10):1838–41.
65. van der Veer E, van der Goot W, de Monchy JG, et al. High prevalence of fractures and osteoporosis in patients with indolent systemic mastocytosis. Allergy 2012;67:431–8.
66. Rossini M, Zanotti R, Bonadonna P, et al. Bone mineral density, bone turnover markers and fractures in patients with indolent systemic mastocytosis. Bone 2011;49:880–5.
67. Kushnir-Sukhov NM, Brittain E, Reynolds JC, et al. Elevated tryptase levels are associated with greater bone density in a cohort of patients with mastocytosis. Int Arch Allergy Immunol 2006;139:265–70.

Flow Cytometry in Mastocytosis
Utility as a Diagnostic and Prognostic Tool

Laura Sánchez-Muñoz, MD, PhD[a,b,*], Cristina Teodosio, PhD[b,c],
Jose Mario T. Morgado, MSc[a,b], Omar Perbellini, MD[d],
Andrea Mayado, PhD[b,c], Ivan Alvarez-Twose, MD[a,b],
Almudena Matito, MD, PhD[a,b], María Jara-Acevedo, MSc[b,c],
Andrés C. García-Montero, PhD[b,c], Alberto Orfao, MD, PhD[b,c],
Luis Escribano, MD, PhD[b,c]

KEYWORDS

- Mast cells • Mastocytosis • Flow cytometry • Bone marrow • Cell purification
- Diagnosis • Classification • Prognosis

KEY POINTS

- Multiparametric flow cytometry is an essential technique applied in the diagnosis of systemic mastocytosis (SM).
- The application of specific protocols for the analysis of rare samples is mandatory when studying bone marrow (BM) aspirates to establish a correct diagnosis.
- To establish the prognosis of each patient, BM cell populations should be purified to study the degree of BM hematopoiesis involvement by the *KIT* mutation.

INTRODUCTION

Mastocytosis is a heterogeneous disease characterized by the accumulation of pathological mast cells (MCs) in different tissues.[1,2] Because the prevalence of Mastocytosis disease is low and, consequently, knowledge regarding the management of the disease is restricted to few professionals, patients are usually referred to specialized

No potential conflicts of interest.

This work was supported by grants from the Fondo de Investigaciones Sanitarias (FIS) of the Instituto de Salud Carlos III, Ministerio de Economía y Competitividad of Spain (PS09/00032); Fundación Sociosanitaria de Castilla-La Mancha (2010/008); Fundación Española de Mastocitosis (FEM 2013).

[a] Mastocytosis Unit of Castilla La-Mancha, Hospital Virgen del Valle, Toledo, Spain; [b] Spanish Network on Mastocytosis (REMA), Toledo, Spain; [c] Departments of Cytometry and Medicine, Centro de Investigación del Cáncer, (IBMCC-CSIC/USAL and IBSAL) University of Salamanca, Salamanca, Spain; [d] Section of Hematology, Department of Medicine, University of Verona, Verona, Italy

* Corresponding author. Mastocytosis Unit of Castilla La-Mancha, Hospital Virgen del Valle, Toledo, Spain.

E-mail address: lsmunoz@sescam.jccm.es

reference centers, where their diagnosis and follow-up are performed using the most sensitive and specific techniques.

In practice, diagnosis of SM is typically suspected in patients having mastocytosis in the skin[1,3] or in patients without skin lesions presenting with systemic symptoms of MC activation (systemic MC activation syndrome)[3,4] and it is currently based on clinical, biochemical, morphologic, histopathologic, immunophenotypical, and molecular data. With the exception of the more aggressive categories of SM (eg, aggressive SM [ASM] and MC leukemia [MCL]), MCs represent only a small proportion of all nucleated BM cells. Such a low MC burden raises the need for applying highly sensitive and specific methodological approaches for the study of MCs in routine laboratory diagnosis.[5,6]

In the following sections, readers are provided with information about the methodological approaches that should be applied to perform an objective and reproducible diagnosis and classification of SM, with particular emphasis on BM studies. Additionally, the importance of flow cytometry for the establishment of long-term prognosis for patients individually is explored.

METHODOLOGICAL APPROACH FOR THE IDENTIFICATION, ENUMERATION, AND CHARACTERIZATION OF BONE MARROW MAST CELLS

Although other techniques, such as immunohistochemistry and immunocytochemistry, can be used for analysis of the expression of specific antigens on MCs, flow cytometry is currently the recommended method for this analysis, because it allows sensitive detection and quantitative evaluation of the expression of multiple antigens simultaneously in large numbers of MCs, even when they are present in a sample at low frequencies.[5] To accomplish optimal results, however, several issues need to be taken into account. Among these issues, several critical parameters have been identified regarding the immunophenotypical analysis of BM MCs (reviewed by Escribano and colleagues[5] and Sanchez-Munoz colleagues[6] and in **Box 1**).

First, the BM aspirate should contain sufficient numbers of BM particles; because MCs are firmly attached to the stromal cells, BM samples should be executed firmly and quickly in the posterior iliac crest by a 14G to 8G biopsy needle. Samples obtained without BM particles could be adequate for other immunophenotypical studies but not for MC enumeration. In addition, only fresh samples with high cell viability (>95%) should be used for the enumeration of BM MCs; this parameter is especially critical for the enumeration of MCs from ascitic fluid and other body fluids, where MC viability rapidly decreases with time (Sanchez-Muñoz, personal communication).

After the collection, BM samples should be disaggregated through 25G needles to separate MCs from BM stroma for obtaining a homogeneous cell suspension.

A critical parameter when a low BM MC burden is expected, and preferably always used as a routine technique, is performing a 0.5% toluidine blue (pH 0.5 or 3) stain of a BM smear prior to immunophenotyping, to get an overall impression on the percentage of MCs in the sample. This stain provide a chance to stain duplicates or even triplicates of each tube to get enough number of MCs to analyze (**Fig. 1**).

Another technical factor that may have an impact on the results relates to the specific monoclonal antibody (mAb) clones, fluorochrome reagents, and combinations used, which should be carefully selected for optimal performance.[5–8] Human MCs strongly express CD117, CD203c, and the high-affinity receptor for immunoglobulin E (FcεRI) (reviewed in Refs.[5,9–11]). Nevertheless, none of these proteins is specific for MCs and, therefore, at least 2 antigens are needed for the accurate identification

---

Box 1
Critical parameters in the protocol of identification of bone marrow mast cells by flow cytometry

- Collection of samples
  - Always perform both BM aspiration and biopsy.
  - Perform BM aspiration firmly and quickly to obtain a sufficient number of BM fragments.
  - 1–2 mL of heparinized or EDTA anticoagulated BM should be obtained for immunophenotypical purposes.
  - Process BM within 24 hours of collection.
  - Only use fresh samples with high cell viability for the enumeration of BM MCs.
- Staining of samples
  - Stain a BM smear containing BM particles with 0.5% toluidine blue prior to immunophenotyping.
  - Assess the nucleated cell count before staining.
  - Stain at least $1–2 \times 10^6$ cells per tube.
  - Use a stain-and-then-lyse technique for membrane antigens.
  - Staining for CD45 and CD117 is mandatory; counterstaining with CD33, FcεRI, or CD203c is desirable.
- Acquisition and analysis
  - Assess the basal MC autofluorescence levels either by using an unstained tube or by using fluorochrome-matched isotype controls.
  - Use of a double-step acquisition procedure.
  - Run a short panel of screening of mastocytosis and a larger one for further characterization of MC immunophenotype when aberrant MCs are detected.

---

of these cells; in the authors' experience, BM MCs are clearly identifiable on the basis of their light scatter properties and their CD117/CD45 pattern of expression.[5,9,10,12,13]

A single mAb combination, including CD45, CD117, CD34, CD25, and CD2, can be sufficient to identify the clonal MCs in most SM cases. Furthermore, the simultaneous

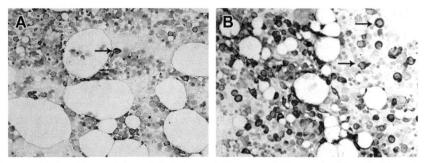

Fig. 1. Toluidine blue staining of 2 different BM smears. MCs may be identified based on their characteristic reddish violet color (*arrows*). The visual evaluation of a BM smear using this stain is of great help in determining the amount of sample to be stained for immunophenotyping by flow cytometry (original magnification ×400). (*A*) BM smear with a low MC burden. (*B*) BM smear with a high MC burden.

analysis of different markers using a polychromatic strategy allows for better evaluation of the effective coexpression of such markers on BM MCs, improves the standardization of diagnostic procedures, and reduces the costs of the analysis.

A lyse-wash procedure is recommended instead of density gradient centrifugation procedure for eliminating the red cells, because it minimizes the selective loss or enrichment of different cell populations. Evaluation of nonspecific and autofluorescence levels of human MCs must be performed prior to the definition of the levels of expression of individual markers on BM MCs. Isotype-matched immunoglobulins or MC autofluorescence can be used as a negative control.

A double-step acquisition approach is suitable to overcome the problems related to the acquisition and storage of multiparameter information on a large number of events. This strategy has been widely applied for the detection of small populations of leukemic cells in complete remission human BM samples, even when their frequency is as low as 1 leukemic cell in 10^6 normal cells,[5,6,14] allowing for a systematic analysis of the immunophenotypic features of infrequent cell populations. Briefly, in the first step, 50 to 100 × 10^3 nucleated cells are acquired. In the second step, only the CD117[+] events are selectively stored. This approach has proved well suited for analysis of rare cells with frequencies below 0.01% (**Fig. 2**).

Once identified, the enumeration of BM MCs is an important factor in the diagnosis of the disease. Although patients with SM display increased BM MC counts, low and overlapping frequencies are still found on these patients, compared to normal BM [0.21± 0.27% (range: 0.001–1.7%) vs 0.02± 0.02% (range: 0.001–0.09%), respectively].[10,12] Furthermore, increased BM MC burden can also be detected in reactive BM (0.087 ± 0.12% [range 0.0021%–0.54%])[8,10,15] or in patients with other hematological disorders, such as Waldenström macroglobulinemia (0.095 ± 0.11% [range: 0.01%–0.47%]) or myelodysplastic syndromes (0.099 ± 0.12% [range 0.002%–0.47%]).[10,16] For that reason, it is mandatory to analyze a high number of cells (>2 × 10^6 cells) to obtain information from sufficient MCs to correctly interpret their phenotypic characteristics, which is the only way to get an accurate diagnosis.[16]

IMMUNOPHENOTYPIC FEATURES OF NORMAL BONE MARROW MAST CELLS
The MC-Committed Progenitor Cell

Human MCs can be generated from a CD34[+] hematopoietic progenitor cell (HPC) in response to stimulation with stem cell factor/kit-ligand. Early reports, using in vitro MC differentiation models, revealed that these progenitors circulate as CD34[+], c-kit[+], CD14[−], CD17[−],[17,18] FcεRI[−],[19] CD38 often positive, HLA-DR often negative,[20] and CD13[+21] cells. Later ex vivo studies, using BM from both healthy controls and patients with myelodysplastic syndrome, suggested that MC-committed precursors may be identified within the BM CD34[+] human progenitor cell compartment as CD117[hi]/HLA-DR[−/int].[22] Nevertheless, because these precursors are infrequent in normal BM, representing less than 0.001% to 0.02% of the CD34[+] HPC compartment,[22] most knowledge about the normal patterns of MC maturation is based on in vitro differentiation studies.[23–27] Using this strategy, it is now known that both immature MC-committed progenitors and mature MCs express CD117, CD58, CD63, CD147, CD151, CD203c, and CD172a but that the expression of interleukin (IL)-3Rα (CD123) and of the granulocyte-macrophage colony-stimulating factor receptor is restricted to early MC precursors.[25] Conversely, proteins typically associated with MC function, such as FcεRI, MC proteases chymase and tryptase, and histamine, are only expressed in late stages of the maturation process and are absent in the CD34[+] MC precursors.[19,24,27,28] The exception seems to be tryptase, which, based

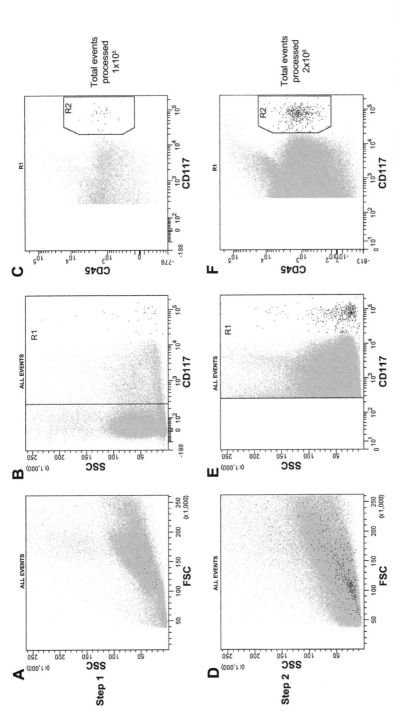

Fig. 2. Two-step acquisition procedure in a BM sample to study MCs. Representative bivariate dot plots illustrating the light scatter (graphs A and D) and immunophenotypical characteristics (SSC vs. CD117 expression: graphs B, C) (CD45 and CD117 expression: graphs E, F) of BM MCs. In step 1, the information on all the events processed is stored to provide general information on the sample studied. In step 2, only the information on CD117+ events is stored. R1: identifies CD117 high positive expression events; R2: identifies CD117 high positive and CD45 intermediate positive events, where MC should be identified.

on unpublished observations of the authors' group from ex vivo studies, may be dimly expressed in a small susbset of MC-committed CD34[+] precursors (Teodosios, personal communication).

Immunophenotypic Characteristics of Normal/Reactive Mature BM MCs

BM MCs from both healthy subjects and patients with distinct hematologic and non-hematologic non–MC-related disorders display typical high forward light scatter and sideward light scatter characteristics associated with a variable degree of autofluorescence.[10] Moreover, these cells also express overlapping levels of a wide range of molecules, such as MC-related markers (eg, CD117 and FcεRI) and MC proteases (eg, cytoplasmic carboxypeptidase [CyCPA]) and cytoplasmic total tryptase (CyB12).[8] Furthermore, although the expression of adhesion-related proteins, such as CD11c, CD29, and CD33; tetraspanins (eg CD9 and CD63); and the CD55 and CD59 complement receptors, or of activation markers, such as CD69 and CD203c, are also consistently expressed by BM MCs, other molecules are only detected in a restricted number of the cases (eg, the IgG Fc receptors CD16 or CD64 or the HLA-DR and HLA-DQ molecules) (**Table 1**).[8,10,29,30] Normal/reactive BM MCs constantly lack the expression of several proteins, including molecules that are relevant for SM diagnosis, such as CD2 or CD25.[10,12,29,30]

UTILITY OF FLOW CYTOMETRY FOR THE DIAGNOSIS OF SYSTEMIC MASTOCYTOSIS

In 1996, Orfao and colleagues[12] demonstrated that BM MCs may be clearly identifiable by flow cytometry on the basis of their light scatter properties and strong CD117 expression; this technical advance was revealed of major value in the study of MC-related disorders, such as mastocytosis and other clonal MC diseases. During the past few years, multiparametric flow cytometry has been shown a powerful tool for the study of mastocytosis.[9,29–32,40,41]

In contrast to normal MCs, and with the exception of patients with a well-differentiated form of SM (WDSM), MCs from mastocytosis aberrantly express high levels of the low-affinity IL-2R alpha (CD25)[5,8,29,30,33,34]; in turn, CD2 is also aberrantly expressed by BM MCs from most SM patients. Despite previous reports on individual cases or small series of patients indicating that it is a good marker for SM MCs,[30,33,34] in a variable percentage of the cases, expression of CD2 is not detected.[8] Thus, at present it seems more appropriate to use the CD25[+] and either CD2[+] or CD2[−] BM, blood, or other extracutaneous organs' MC immunophenotypical criteria for SM instead of the traditional CD25[+] and/or CD2[+] criterion.[42] A prospective analysis of BM MCs from a large series of normal subjects and individuals with reactive and other non-MC neoplastic conditions showed that this criterion is highly specific for SM, with CD25[+] BM MCs additionally found only in patients with hypereosinophilic syndrome and platelet-derived growth factor receptor α gene rearrangements.[42]

Apart from the aberrant expression of CD2 and CD25, SM BM MCs show other distinctive phenotypes, because they display abnormally high expression of CD33[13,35] and of the CD2 ligand, CD58.[9] Increased expression for activation markers, such as CD69[31] and CD63 lysosomal membrane antigen,[36] and complement-associated molecules, such as CD11c and CD35,[36] the CD59 complement regulatory molecule, and CD88, is also found in SM BM MCs.[41] In contrast, expression of CD117,[9] the CD71 transferrin receptor, and CD29 integrin is abnormally down-regulated in these patients (see **Table 1**).[9]

Although only the CD25 expression on BM MCs is now considered a diagnostic criterion, it is advisable to completely analyze the immunophenotype of BM MCs to

Table 1
Qualitative and semiquantitative antigen expression on bone marrow mast cells from controls and patients with mastocytosis, as analyzed by multiparameter flow cytometry

Functional Group	Protein	Controls	Systemic Mastocytosis
Fc receptors	CD16	−/+ (13%)	−/+ (69%)
	CD23	−	a
	CD32	+	+/++
	CD64	−/+ (5%)	−/+ (84%)
	FcεRI	+	+[b]
MHC-associated molecules	CD1a	−	a
	HLA-I	+	+
	HLA-DR	−/+ (25%)	−/+ (85%)
	HLA-DQ	−/+ (13%)	−/+ (58%)
Integrin	CD11a	−/+ (20%)	−
	CD11b	−/+ (50%)	−/+ (50%)
	CD11c	−/+ (71%)	+/++
	CD18	−/+ (65%)	−/+ (44%)
	CD29	+	+
	CD41a	−	−/+ (45%)
	CD49d	+	+ (80%)
	CD49e	+	−/+ (30%)
	CD51	+	−/+ (45%)
	CD54	−/+ (75%)	++ (100%)
Tetraspanin	CD9	+	+
	CD37	−	a
	CD53	+	a
	CD81	+	a
	CD82	+	a
	CD151	+	a
Cell adhesion	CD2	−	−/+ (72%)
	CD6	−	−
	CD15	−	−
	CD22	−/+ (50%)	−/+ (96%)
	CD33	+	+/++
	CD34	−	−
	CD44	+	+
	CD61	−/+ (66%)	−/+ (22%)
	CD66b	−	a
	CD146	+	a
Protease	CD13	−/+ (33%)	−/+ (75%)
	Carboxypeptidase A3 (CPA)	+	+/+++[b]
	Total tryptase (B12)	+	+/+++[b]
	Mature tryptase (G5)	−/+ (75%)	+/++
Cytokine receptor	CD25	−	−/+ (93%)
	CD117	+	+[b]
	CD123	−	−/+ (73%)
	CD124	+/−	a
Complement-associated molecules	CD21	−	a
	CD35	−	+
	CD59	+	+/++
	CD88	−/+ (18%)	−/+ (54%)
Tumor necrosis factor receptor family	CD30	−	a
	CD40	−/+ (65%)	−/+ (65%)

(continued on next page)

Table 1
(continued)

Functional Group	Protein	Controls	Systemic Mastocytosis
Immune response	CD3	−	a
	CD4	−/+ (60%)	−/+ (60%)
	CD5	−	a
	CD8	−	−
	CD14	−	−
	CD19	−	−
	CD20	−	−
	CD43	+	+
Ectoenzyme	CD38	−	−
	CD157	+	a
Activation marker	CD63	+	+/++
	CD69	−/+ (88%)	+/++
	CD203c	+	+/++
Other	CD10	−	−
	CD42b	−	−/+ (45%)
	CD45	+	+
	CD65	−	a
	CD71	+	−/+ (38%)
	CD116	−	a
	CD138	−	−
	CD147	+	a
	bcl2	−/+ (94%)	−/+ (87%)

−/+, expressed in a subset of patients (percentage of positive cases); +, expressed on 100% of the cases analyzed; −, absent in all cases analyzed; ++, increased expression compared with normal/reactive BM MCs.

[a] Expression has not been systematically described for SM BM MCs.
[b] In some SM patients, expression is decreased compared with normal/reactive BM MCs.
Data from Refs.[8–10,12,13,29–39]

get the whole profile of these cells and help in subclassification of the disease. Recent work from the authors' group[8] described 3 clearly different maturation-associated immunophenotypic profiles for BM MCs that are related in both genetic markers of the disease and clinical behavior.

UTILITY OF FLOW CYTOMETRY FOR THE SUBCLASSIFICATION OF SYSTEMIC MASTOCYTOSIS
Immunophenotypic Profiles of BM MCs in SM

Although SM patients share some clinical, histopathological, and biochemical features and typically show BM involvement, the clinical presentation of the disease is diverse, and distinct variants with different biologic, clinical, and prognostic features as well as distinct therapeutic requirements are currently defined.[1]

In line with this heterogeneity, reports from of the authors' group have recently established the existence of different immunophenotypic profiles on BM MCs from the distinct subtypes of SM[8,43]; in these analyses, 3 different patterns were identified, which correlate with distinct prognostic and molecular subtypes of SM and, at the same time, reflect the maturation status of clonal MCs (**Fig. 3**).[8]

The most frequently detected profile corresponded to the category of indolent SM (ISM), with skin lesions (s+) or without skin lesions (s−); in these patients, a mature (CD34−, CD117$^{+/hi}$, and FcεRI$^{+/hi}$) MC with aberrant expression of CD25 and CD2

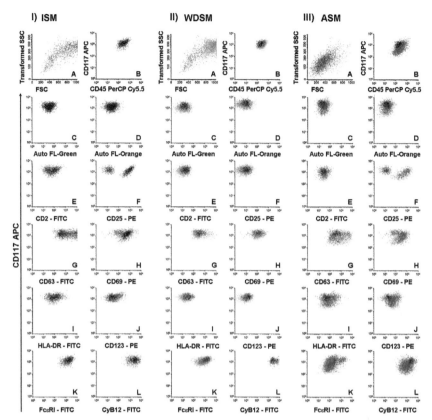

Fig. 3. Representative bivariate dot plots illustrating the light scatter (graphs A) and immunophenotypical characteristics (graphs C–L) of BM MCs from healthy donors (*black dots*) and BM MCs from patients with ISM (*blue dots in column I*), WDSM (*green dots in column II*), and ASM (*red dots in column III*), identified on the basis of their strong reactivity for CD117 and positivity for CD45 (graphs B). APC, Allophycocyanin; FITC, fluorescein isothiocyanate; FL, fluorescence; FSC, forward scatter; PE, Phycoerythrin; PerCP, Peridinin chlorphyll protein; SSC, side scatter.

is detected. This aberrant phenotype is associated with features compatible with MC activation, including the overexpression of the CD63, CD69, and CD203c activation markers and of the CD35 and CD59 complement regulatory proteins. Decreased cytoplasmic content of tryptase (CyB12) is also detected in this group of patients.

Conversely, a mature, resting MC phenotype defined by the lack of expression of both CD25 and CD2, normal levels of expression of activation-associated markers, and abnormally increased light scatter is found on BM MCs from WDSM patients. This high light scatter is typically associated with increased cytoplasmic protease content, such as CyB12 and cyCPA.

A more immature immunophenotypical profile, defined by the aberrant expression of CD25, usually in the absence of CD2; altered expression of MC maturation-related molecules, including decreased expression of CD117, FcεRI, and cytoplasmic proteases; and increased positivity for CD123, HLA-DQ, and HLA-DR is typically observed in poor-prognosis SM patients (ASM and MCL patients).

These 3 distinct immunophenotypic patterns are typically observed at variable frequencies among the different diagnostic subtypes of SM. Accordingly, an activated

MC phenotype is characteristic of ISM (s+ or s−), whereas a mature resting pattern and an immature profile are typical of WDSM and of the poor-prognosis variants of SM (ASM and MCL), respectively; in the latter cases (poor prognosis variants), MCs with an immature phenotype are usually found in association with clonal involvement of all myeloid lineages by the *KIT* D816V mutation. These aberrant immunophenotypic features are of great relevance for the assessment of tissue involvement in mastocytosis with consequences in the diagnosis, classification, and follow-up of the disease as well as in its differential diagnosis with other entities (**Fig. 4**).[8]

Expression of Novel Antigens: CD30

Recently, diverse antigens have been evaluated for their utility in the diagnosis of SM[44]; one of the most promising is CD30. This molecule is typically expressed on the surface of Hodgkin disease Reed-Sternberg cells, on tumor cells from some World Health Organization subtypes of non-Hodgkin lymphomas, and in embryonic carcinomas.[45–47] In non-neoplastic conditions, expression of CD30 is restricted to a small subset of activated B and T lymphocytes and to a small proportion of eosinophils.[45–47] In a recent work, it has been shown, by means of immunohistochemisty, that CD30 expression on BM MCs is associated with advanced forms of SM.[48,49]

In a recent study, the authors' group investigated the potential diagnostic and prognostic value of CD30 expression in the largest series of SM patients studied to date, using flow cytometry.[43] This study revealed an up-regulation of CD30 expression on BM MCs from SM patients. The authors' approach did not find higher levels of CD30 in aggressive forms of SM; nonetheless, unlike in ISM patients, all ASM cases expressed this marker. These results support previous reports, which suggest an association between CD30 expression and more aggressive forms of SM.[48]

Furthermore, and most importantly, unlike CD25, aberrant CD30 expression, detected using flow cytometry, was observed in most WDSM cases.[43]

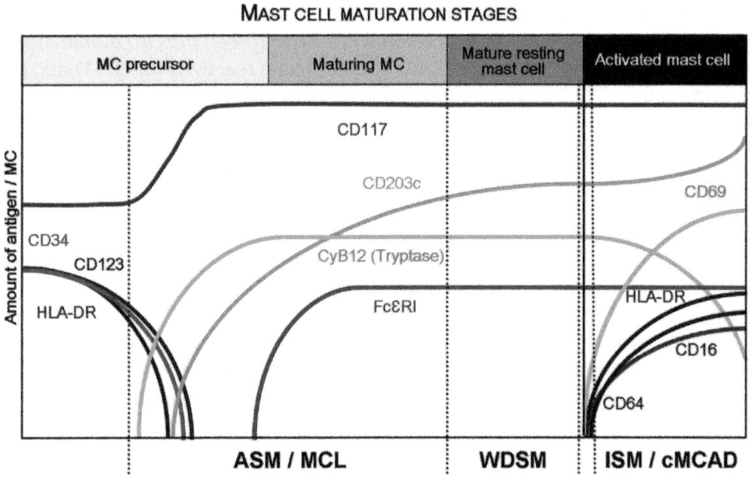

Fig. 4. Schematic representation of the phenotypic changes that occur during normal MC differentiation[19,22,25,35,61] and activation of mature MCs[35,62–64] and their correlation with the different immunophenotypic profiles of BM MCs observed among patients with different subtypes of systemic mastocytosis. (*Data from* Teodosio C, Garcia-Montero AC, Jara-Acevedo M, et al. Mast cells from different molecular and prognostic subtypes of systemic mastocytosis display distinct immunophenotypes. J Allergy Clin Immunol 2010;125:719–26.)

Coexistence of Normal and Pathologic BM MCs

Although the BM MC burden in ISM patients can be extremely low (0.07% [range 0.04%–1.4%] in ISM s– and 0.06 [range 0.00001%–1.7%] in ISM s+ cases), the coexistence of normal and pathologic MCs in the same patient is frequent in specific disease categories (33% of ISM s– and 18% of ISM s+ patients).[4] Furthermore, the coexistence of normal and aberrant BM MC populations is restricted to SM patients with *KIT* mutation limited to the BM MC compartment.[50]

In line with these findings, and although this cannot be considered a general rule, the detection of a double population, normal and pathologic, of BM MCs should be considered a good prognosis factor due to its association with indolent forms of disease and BM MCs' compartment-restricted *KIT* mutation.

In the authors' experience, aberrant MCs can be as few as 20% of the total BM MCs, which raises the need to study many cells so as to have enough sensitivity to avoid false-negative results.

Identification of MCs in Peripheral Blood, Organic Fluids, or Tissues

Identification of MCs in tissues other than BM can be necessary in some cases to stage the exact subtype of the disease or to evaluate the presence of MC infiltration in other tissues. Although flow cytometry is mainly indicated for the study of cells and other particles in suspension, when appropriate methods are used to create cell suspensions from solid tissues, these may be efficiently studied by this technique.

Identification of circulating MCs in peripheral blood

The same approach used for the analysis of BM MCs can be applied for the study of the presence of circulating MCs in peripheral blood. Nevertheless, counterstaining with CD203c or FcεRI and CD25 is advisable in these cases to correctly determine the presence of circulating mature pathologic MCs, and a large number of events (preferably $>3 \times 10^6$) should be analyzed. In the authors' experience, the demonstration of circulating MCs has been associated with aggressive subtypes of the disease, further indicating the need to perform this test in the follow-up of mastocytosis patients[52] (data not published).

Identification of MCs in organic fluids or tissues

In cases of fluid samples as ascitic fluid or pleural effusions, a first step of centrifugation is necessary to concentrate the sample. Before staining, assessment of the nucleated cell count of the sample is necessary, and from this point on the same protocol as for BM can be applied.

A modified protocol can be used for the identification of MCs in solid tissues as lymph nodes or tonsils. To obtain a cell suspension appropriate for flow cytometric analysis, the fragment of fresh tissue must be cut into small pieces (1–2 mm) using surgical blades and tweezers. Although mechanical disaggregation procedures can be applied, manual or enzymatic disaggregation is preferred, especially in lymphoid tissues, and yields a high number of single cells in a few minutes. It is recommended to filter the suspension of cells obtained to eliminate the aggregates. After assessing the nucleated cell count in a hematological cell analyzer, stain samples follow protocol for isolated cell staining.

Time parameter is especially critical for the enumeration of MCs from ascitic fluid as well as from lymph nodes, for which both the MC count and the immunophenotypical characterization studies should be performed immediately after drainage of ascitic fluid or lymph node biopsy. Samples obtained from tonsils or other solid tissues could be considered adequate for the identification and immunophenotypical characterization of MCs but probably not for their enumeration. At present, information on this subject is lacking in the literature.

UTILITY OF FLOW CYTOMETRY FOR THE PROGNOSTIC STRATIFICATION OF SYSTEMIC MASTOCYTOSIS PATIENTS

Given the special characteristics and the heterogeneity of this disease, it is mandatory to establish the prognosis of each patient at the moment of the diagnosis, to identify those patients at high risk of progression to a more aggressive form. Currently, one of the most important prognostic factors is the degree of clonal hematopoiesis in individual patients, assessed by analysis of BM involvement by the *KIT* mutation typically detected in SM patients (D816V), because patients with a more extensive BM involvement by this mutation show a higher probability of disease progression.[51,52]

Purification of BM cell lineages by FACS. Because most SM patients (>93%), except those with WDSM, carry the same D816V *KIT* mutation on BM MCs,[51] the detection of this mutation on other BM cell populations is mandatory for the prognostic stratification of SM patients. Although several methods can be used for purification of different populations, currently fluorescence-activated cell sorting (FACS) is the approach recommended by the Spanish Network on Mastocytosis (REMA).[51–53] In SM cases carrying the *KIT* mutation in BM MCs, the REMA recommends performing the *KIT* mutation assays in at least one other highly purified (>97%) myeloid cell population (eg, BM monocytes and/or maturing neutrophils) and a population of lymphoid cells (eg, total lymphocytes or CD3+ cells), apart from MCs (**Fig. 5**).[52,54]

Because the percentage of BM MCs is low in the most common ISM cases, the BM MCs yield should also be taken into account. It is also important to rule out cross-contamination of the purified cell populations by mutated MCs, because some of the molecular methods used to detect *KIT* mutation show a high sensitivity (<1%) and, therefore, even a small cross-contamination by clonal MCs could lead to false-positive results.

Analysis of KIT Mutation on BM Purified Cells

Different approaches have been applied to detect *KIT* mutations in enriched or purified cell compartments; because virtually all mature myeloid and lymphoid hematopoietic cells lack the expression of the c-kit receptor, only those methods targeting genomic DNA[51,53,55–59] are informative for the detection of the presence of the *KIT* mutations in

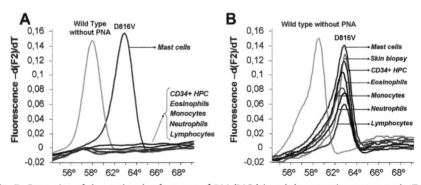

Fig. 5. Examples of the molecular features of BM (MCs) in adult systemic mastocytosis. Two illustrative cases, one showing the *KIT* D816V mutation only in BM MCs (*A*) and one showing it in MCs as well as other myeloid and lymphoid BM hematopoietic cell compartments (*B*). CD34 HPC, human progenitor cells; PNA, peptide nucleic acid.

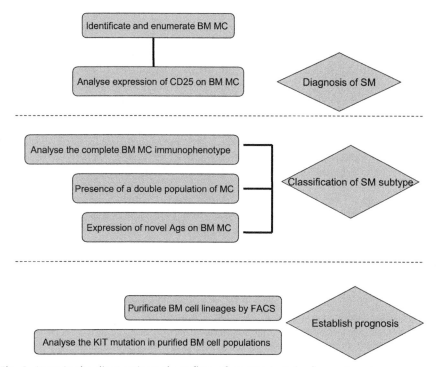

Fig. 6. Steps in the diagnostic work-up flow of mastocytosis by flow cytometry.

mature non-MC hematopoietic cells. Nevertheless, in SM with multilineage involvement by the D816V *KIT* somatic mutation, the disease emerges from early pluripotent mutated stem cells that coexist with normal stem cells, and, consequently, each hematopoietic population (eg, the monocytes) typically consists of a mixture at different proportions of mutated and nonmutated cells.[60] Thus, the selected method should have enough sensitivity to detect low numbers of mutated cells. New genomic DNA–based methods have been recently described that are associated with good sensitivity (<0.03%) and quantitative polymerase chain reaction estimation of the percentage of mutated allele dosage[59] in whole peripheral blood samples from aleukemic SM patients.

SUMMARY

The diagnostic work-up of patients with mastocytosis should be routinely performed in experienced reference centers where highly sensitive and specific diagnostic procedures are routinely applied by experts in this field. All the data, protocols, and information provided in this review support the role of multiparameter flow cytometry as the most sensitive and useful technique in the diagnosis and classification of patients with SM (**Fig. 6**).

In addition, a prognosis-based classification of adult mastocytosis, coupling flow cytometry with molecular biology techniques, allows for investigation of the presence of *KIT* mutations in all hematopoietic cell lineages within the BM, and, therefore, currently represents the best approach to predict outcome of ISM patients.

REFERENCES

1. Horny HP, Metcalfe DD, Bennet JM, et al. Mastocytosis. In: Swerdlow SH, Campo E, Harris NL, et al, editors. WHO classification of tumours of haemato-poietic and lymphoid tissues. Lyon (France): IARC; 2008. p. 54–63.
2. Metcalfe DD. Mast cells and mastocytosis. Blood 2008;112:946–56.
3. Valent P, Akin C, Escribano L, et al. Standards and standardization in mastocytosis: consensus statements on diagnostics, treatment recommendations and response criteria. Eur J Clin Invest 2007;37:435–53.
4. Alvarez-Twose I, Gonzalez de Olano D, Sanchez-Munoz L, et al. Clinical, biological and molecular characteristics of systemic mast cell disorders presenting with severe mediator-related symptoms. J Allergy Clin Immunol 2010;125: 1269–78.
5. Escribano L, Diaz-Agustin B, López A, et al. Immunophenotypic analysis of mast cells in mastocytosis: when and how to do it. Proposals of the Spanish network on mastocytosis (REMA). Cytometry B Clin Cytom 2004;58:1–8.
6. Sanchez-Munoz L, Teodosio C, Morgado JM, et al. Immunophenotypic characterization of bone marrow mast cells in mastocytosis and other mast cell disorders. Methods Cell Biol 2011;103:333–59.
7. Escribano L, Navalón R, Núñez R, et al. Flow cytometry immunophenotypic analysis of human mast cells. In: Robinson JP, Darzynkiewicz Z, Dean P, et al, editors. Current protocols in cytometry. New York: John Wiley & Sons Inc; 2000. p. 6.6.1–6.6.18.
8. Teodosio C, Garcia-Montero AC, Jara-Acevedo M, et al. Mast cells from different molecular and prognostic subtypes of systemic mastocytosis display distinct immunophenotypes. J Allergy Clin Immunol 2010;125:719–26.
9. Escribano L, Diaz-Agustin B, Nunez R, et al. Abnormal expression of CD antigens in mastocytosis. Int Arch Allergy Immunol 2002;127:127–32.
10. Escribano L, Garcia Montero AC, Nunez R, et al. Flow cytometric analysis of normal and neoplastic mast cells: role in diagnosis and follow-up of mast cell disease. Immunol Allergy Clin North Am 2006;26:535–47.
11. Hauswirth AW, Escribano L, Prados A, et al. CD203c is overexpressed on neoplastic mast cells in systemic mastocytosis and is upregulated upon IgE receptor cross-linking. Int J Immunopathol Pharmacol 2008;21:797–806.
12. Orfao A, Escribano L, Villarrubia J, et al. Flow cytometric analysis of mast cells from normal and pathological human bone marrow samples. Identification and enumeration. Am J Pathol 1996;149:1493–9.
13. Escribano L, Díaz Agustín B, Bravo P, et al. Immunophenotype of bone marrow mast cells in indolent systemic mast cell disease in adults. Leuk Lymphoma 1999;35:227–35.
14. Nieto WG, Almeida J, Romero A, et al. Increased frequency (12%) of circulating chronic lymphocytic leukemia-like B-cell clones in healthy subjects using a highly sensitive multicolor flow cytometry approach. Blood 2009;114: 33–7.
15. Escribano L, Garcia-Montero A, Sanchez-Munoz L, et al. Diagnosis of adult mastocytosis: role for bone marrow analysis. In: Kottke-Marchant K, Davis B, editors. Laboratory hematology practice. London: Wiley-Blackwell; 2012. p. 388–98.
16. Sanchez-Munoz L, Morgado JM, Alvarez-Twose I, et al. Flow cytometry criteria for systemic mastocytosis: bone marrow mast cell counts do not always count. Am J Clin Pathol 2013;139:404–6.

17. Agis H, Willheim M, Sperr WR, et al. Monocytes do not make mast cells when cultured in the presence of SCF: characterization of the circulating mast cell progenitor as a c-*kit*+, CD34+, Ly⁻, CD14⁻, CD17⁻, colony- forming cell. J Immunol 1993;151:4221–7.

18. Agis H, Fureder W, Bankl HC, et al. Comparative immunophenotypic analysis of human mast cells, blood basophils and monocytes. Immunology 1996;87: 535–43.

19. Rottem M, Okada T, Goff JP, et al. Mast cells cultured from the peripheral blood of normal donors and patients with mastocytosis originate from a CD34+/Fc epsilon RI⁻ cell population. Blood 1994;84:2489–96.

20. Kempuraj D, Saito H, Kaneko A, et al. Characterization of mast cell-committed progenitors present in human umbilical cord blood. Blood 1999;93:3338–46.

21. Kirshenbaum AS, Goff JP, Semere T, et al. Demonstration that human mast cells arise from a progenitor cell population that is CD34+, c-*kit*+, and expresses aminopeptidase N (CD13). Blood 1999;94:2333–42.

22. Matarraz S, Lopez A, Barrena S, et al. The immunophenotype of different immature, myeloid and B-cell lineage-committed CD34+ hematopoietic cells allows discrimination between normal/reactive and myelodysplastic syndrome precursors. Leukemia 2008;22:1175–83.

23. Dahl C, Hoffmann HJ, Saito H, et al. Human mast cells express receptors for IL-3, IL-5 and GM-CSF; a partial map of receptors on human mast cells cultured in vitro. Allergy 2004;59:1087–96.

24. Shimizu Y, Suga T, Maeno T, et al. Detection of tryptase-, chymase plus cells in human CD34+ bone marrow progenitors. Clin Exp Allergy 2004;34: 1719–24.

25. Schernthaner GH, Hauswirth AW, Baghestanian M, et al. Detection of differentiation- and activation-linked cell surface antigens on cultured mast cell progenitors. Allergy 2005;60:1248–55.

26. Yokoi H, Myers A, Matsumoto K, et al. Alteration and acquisition of Siglecs during in vitro maturation of CD34+ progenitors into human mast cells. Allergy 2006;61:769–76.

27. Tedla N, Lee CW, Borges L, et al. Differential expression of leukocyte immunoglobulin-like receptors on cord-blood-derived human mast cell progenitors and mature mast cells. J Leukoc Biol 2008;83:334–43.

28. Shimizu Y, Sakai K, Miura T, et al. Characterization of 'adult-type' mast cells derived from human bone marrow CD34+ cells cultured in the presence of stem cell factor and interleukin-6. Interleukin-4 is not required for constitutive expression of CD54, Fc epsilon RI alpha and chymase, and CD13 expression is reduced during differentiation. Clin Exp Allergy 2002;32:872–80.

29. Escribano L, Orfao A, Villarrubia J, et al. Immunophenotypic characterization of human bone marrow mast cells. A flow cytometric study of normal and pathological bone marrow samples. Anal Cell Pathol 1998;16:151–9.

30. Escribano L, Orfao A, Diaz-Agustin B, et al. Indolent systemic mast cell disease in adults: immunophenotypic characterization of bone marrow mast cells and its diagnostic implications. Blood 1998;91:2731–6.

31. Diaz-Agustin B, Escribano L, Bravo P, et al. The CD69 early activation molecule is overexpressed in human bone marrow mast cells from adults with indolent systemic mast cell disease. Br J Haematol 1999;106:400–5.

32. Valent P, Schernthaner GH, Agis H, et al. Variable expression of activation-linked surface antigens on human mast cells in health and disease. Immunol Rev 2001; 179:74–81.

33. Escribano L, Orfao A, Villarrubia J, et al. Expression of lymphoid-associated antigens in mast cells: report of a case of systemic mast cell disease. Br J Haematol 1995;91:941–3.

34. Escribano L, Orfao A, Villarrubia J, et al. Sequential immunophenotypic analysis of mast cells in a case of systemic mast cell disease evolving to a mast cell leukemia. Cytometry 1997;30:98–102.

35. Escribano L, Díaz Agustín B, Bellas C, et al. Utility of flow cytometric analysis of mast cells in the diagnosis and classification of adult mastocytosis. Leuk Res 2001;25:563–70.

36. Escribano L, Orfao A, Díaz Agustín B, et al. Human bone marrow mast cells from indolent systemic mast cell disease constitutively express increased amounts of the CD63 protein on their surface. Cytometry 1998;34:223–8.

37. Nuñez R, Escribano L, Schernthaner G, et al. Overexpression of complement receptors and related antigens on the surface of bone marrow mast cells in patients with systemic mastocytosis. Br J Haematol 2002;120:257–65.

38. Bodni RA, Sapia S, Galeano A, et al. Indolent systemic mast cell disease: immunophenotypic characterization of bone marrow mast cells by flow cytometry. J Eur Acad Dermatol Venereol 2003;17:160–6.

39. Pardanani A, Kimlinger T, Reeder T, et al. Bone marrow mast cell immunophenotyping in adults with mast cell disease: a prospective study of 33 patients. Leuk Res 2004;28:777–83.

40. Cerveró C, Escribano L, Orfao A, et al. Expression of bcl-2 by human bone marrow mast cells and its overexpression in mast cell leukemia. Am J Hematol 1999;60:191–5.

41. Núñez R, Akin C, Díaz Agustín B, et al. Immunophenotypical profile of CD25-expressing Mast Cells in Mastocytosis. Clin Cytometry 2003;56B(1):72–3 Ref Type: Abstract.

42. Morgado JM, Sanchez-Munoz L, Teodosio CG, et al. Immunophenotyping in systemic mastocytosis diagnosis: 'CD25 positive' alone is more informative than the 'CD25 and/or CD2' WHO criterion. Mod Pathol 2012;25(4):516–21.

43. Morgado JM, Perbellini O, Johnson RC, et al. CD30 expression by bone marrow mast cells from different diagnostic variants of systemic mastocytosis. Histopathology 2013;63:780–7.

44. Valent P, Cerny-Reiterer S, Herrmann H, et al. Phenotypic heterogeneity, novel diagnostic markers, and target expression profiles in normal and neoplastic human mast cells. Best Pract Res Clin Haematol 2010;23:369–78.

45. Durkop H, Latza U, Hummel M, et al. Molecular cloning and expression of a new member of the nerve growth factor receptor family that is characteristic for Hodgkin's disease. Cell 1992;68:421–7.

46. Falini B, Pileri S, Pizzolo G, et al. CD30 (Ki-1) molecule: a new cytokine receptor of the tumor necrosis factor receptor superfamily as a tool for diagnosis and immunotherapy. Blood 1995;85:1–14.

47. Matsumoto K, Terakawa M, Miura K, et al. Extremely rapid and intense induction of apoptosis in human eosinophils by anti-CD30 antibody treatment in vitro. J Immunol 2004;172:2186–93.

48. Sotlar K, Cerny-Reiterer S, Petat-Dutter K, et al. Aberrant expression of CD30 in neoplastic mast cells in high-grade mastocytosis. Mod Pathol 2010;24(4):585–95.

49. Valent P, Sotlar K, Horny HP. Aberrant expression of CD30 in aggressive systemic mastocytosis and mast cell leukemia: a differential diagnosis to consider in aggressive hematopoietic CD30-positive neoplasms. Leuk Lymphoma 2011;52:740–4.

50. Teodosio C, Garcia-Montero AC, Jara-Acevedo M, et al. An immature immuno-phenotype of bone marrow mast cells predicts for multilineage D816V KIT mutation in systemic mastocytosis. Leukemia 2011;26(5):951–8.

51. Garcia-Montero AC, Jara-Acevedo M, Teodosio C, et al. KIT mutation in mast cells and other bone marrow haematopoietic cell lineages in systemic mast cell disorders. A prospective study of the Spanish Network on Mastocytosis (REMA) in a series of 113 patients. Blood 2006;108:2366–72.

52. Escribano L, Alvarez-Twose I, Sanchez-Munoz L, et al. Prognosis in adult indo-lent systemic mastocytosis: a long-term study of the Spanish Network on Mastocytosis in a series of 145 patients. J Allergy Clin Immunol 2009;124:514–21.

53. Kocabas CN, Yavuz AS, Lipsky PE, et al. Analysis of the lineage relationship between mast cells and basophils using the *c-kit* D816V mutation as a biologic signature. J Allergy Clin Immunol 2005;115:1155–61.

54. Sanchez-Munoz L, Alvarez-Twose I, Garcia-Montero AC, et al. Evaluation of the WHO criteria for the classification of patients with mastocytosis. Mod Pathol 2011;24:1157–68.

55. Nagata H, Worobec AS, Oh CK, et al. Identification of a point mutation in the cat-alytic domain of the protooncogene *c-kit* in peripheral blood mononuclear cells of patients who have mastocytosis with an associated hematologic disorder. Proc Natl Acad Sci U S A 1995;92:10560–4.

56. Sotlar K, Escribano L, Landt O, et al. One-step detection of c-kit point mutations using PNA-mediated PCR-clamping and hybridization probes. Am J Pathol 2003;162:737–46.

57. Tan A, Westerman D, McArthur GA, et al. Sensitive detection of KIT D816V in patients with mastocytosis. Clin Chem 2006;52:2250–7.

58. Schumacher JA, Elenitoba-Johnson KS, Lim MS. Detection of the c-kit D816V mutation in systemic mastocytosis by allele-specific PCR. J Clin Pathol 2007; 61(1):109–14.

59. Kristensen T, Vestergaard H, Moller MB. Improved detection of the KIT D816V mutation in patients with systemic mastocytosis using a quantitative and highly sensitive real-time qPCR assay. J Mol Diagn 2011;13:180–8.

60. Yavuz AS, Lipsky PE, Yavuz S, et al. Evidence for the involvement of a hemato-poietic progenitor cell in systemic mastocytosis from single-cell analysis of mu-tations in the c-*kit* gene. Blood 2002;100:661–5.

61. Schwartz LB, Min HK, Ren SL, et al. Tryptase precursors are preferentially and spontaneously released, whereas mature tryptase is retained by HMC-1 cells, mono-mac-6 cells, and human skin-derived mast cells. J Immunol 2003;170: 5667–73.

62. Henz BM, Maurer M, Lippert U, et al. Mast cells as initiators of immunity and host defense. Exp Dermatol 2001;10:1–10.

63. Marshall JS, Jawdat DM. Mast cells in innate immunity. J Allergy Clin Immunol 2004;114:21–7.

64. Galli SJ, Nakae S, Tsai M. Mast cells in the development of adaptive immune responses. Nat Immunol 2005;6:135–42.

Mastocytosis
Immunophenotypical Features of the Transformed Mast Cells Are Unique Among Hematopoietic Cells

Hans-Peter Horny, MD[a],*, Karl Sotlar, MD[a], Peter Valent, MD[b]

KEYWORDS

- Mastocytosis • Systemic mastocytosis • Immunophenotype • Mast cell
- Mast cell leukemia • CD30 • CD117 • Tryptase

KEY POINTS

- Mastocytosis is a hematologic disorder of bone marrow origin. The disease exhibits an unusual broad heterogeneity regarding clinical, morphologic, and immunologic features.
- Mast cells in reactive and neoplastic states almost always coexpress the antigens CD117 (*KIT*) and tryptase, irrespective of the stage of maturation or activation.
- Aberrant immunophenotypical features of mast cells are very common in mastocytosis, but only expression of the antigens CD2, CD25, and CD30 is used in the routine diagnostic work-up of the disease.
- The aberrant expression of various myelomonocytic, lymphoid, natural killer, and stem cell associated antigens by mast cells is unique among hematopoietic cells and not seen in other myelogenous neoplasms.
- Mastocytosis is not a myeloproliferative disorder as stated in the World Health Organization classification of tumors of hematopoietic origin but deserves a separate disease category.

INTRODUCTION

Mastocytosis is regarded as a disease of bone marrow origin and is histologically characterized by compact tissue infiltrates of atypical mast cells that are never seen in reactive states.[1] Most patients with mastocytosis, in particular those with systemic disease, have transformed mast cells carrying an activating point mutation at codon 816 of *KIT*, usually *KIT*D816V, and also show an elevated serum tryptase level.[2] The

The authors have nothing to disclose.
[a] Institute of Pathology, Ludwig-Maximilians-Universität, Thalkirchnerstrasse 36, D-80337 Munich, Germany; [b] Division of Hematology and Hemostaseology, Department of Internal Medicine, Medical University of Vienna, Währinger Gürtel 18 – 20, A-1090 Vienna, Austria
* Corresponding author. Europäisches Referenzzentrum für Mastozytose (ECNM), Institut für Pathologie, LMU, Thalkirchnerstrasse 36, München 80337, Germany.
E-mail address: Hans-Peter.Horny@med.uni-muenchen.de

Immunol Allergy Clin N Am 34 (2014) 315–321
http://dx.doi.org/10.1016/j.iac.2014.01.005
0889-8561/14/$ – see front matter © 2014 Elsevier Inc. All rights reserved.

disease shows a broad spectrum of clinical features, including the typical skin lesion of urticaria pigmentosa, which are not found in all patients. Mastocytosis is listed among myeloproliferative neoplasms according to the World Health Organization classification.[3] In this article the immunophenotypical features of mast cells are described. Based on these features, it is obvious that mast cells are not closely related to other myeloid cells. Using the knowledge on aberrantly expressed antigens by mast cells, the hematopathologist should be able to recognize the disease even in the presence of unusual morphologic findings or an associated hematologic non–mast cell lineage disease.

CLASSIFICATION AND DIAGNOSIS OF SYSTEMIC MASTOCYTOSIS

Mastocytosis basically presents in two major variants: pure cutaneous disease usually occurring in children; and systemic mastocytosis (SM) showing infiltration of at least one extracutaneous organ, commonly the bone marrow, occurring in adults. Diagnosis of SM is based on the presence of one major and one or more out of four minor criteria. The central role of the hematopathologist is reflected by the fact that the only major diagnostic SM criterion is the demonstration of compact mast cell infiltrates in various extracutaneous tissues. Moreover, minor criteria include two that can also be assessed by the hematopathologist: demonstration of prominent spindling of mast cells, and an aberrant immunophenotype of mast cells with expression of the lymphocyte-associated antigens CD2 and/or CD25. Because compact mast cell infiltrates can be absent in a significant proportion of patients with suspected SM, it is necessary to demonstrate at least three minor criteria to be able to establish a final diagnosis of SM.

IMMUNOHISTOCHEMISTRY

Immunohistochemical analysis is strongly recommended in all patients with suspected SM for several reasons.[4] First, detection and quantification of loosely scattered mast cells that often are difficult to count in conventional stains, such as Giemsa or toluidine blue, because of significant decrease or even absence of metachromatic granules, in particular in spindle-shaped or fibroblast-like mast cells. Second, detection of even very small compact mast cell infiltrates to demonstrate the major diagnostic SM criterion. Finally, detection of an atypical immunophenotype of mast cells, in particular expression of CD25, which can be found in more than 90% of cases of SM, in particular in indolent SM.

The following antibodies should be applied in every case of suspected mastocytosis, in particular when bone marrow trephine specimens are investigated: tryptase, CD117 (*KIT*), and CD25.[5] Expression of CD2 is listed also as a minor diagnostic criterion but has proved to be of minor relevance for two reasons. First, CD2 has a significantly lower sensitivity compared with CD25; is not expressed in most cases with advanced disease, such as aggressive SM or mast cell leukemia; and is expressed only in about 50% to 60% of cases of indolent SM. Second, it is of minor relevance because of the constant presence of CD2-positive T cells within compact mast cell infiltrates, with the possibility of false-positive results.

All normal/reactive and neoplastic mast cells coexpress the antigens tryptase and CD117 (*KIT*), with a few exceptions regarding tryptase.[6] Tryptase expression may be very low or even missing in about 1% to 5% of patients with mastocytosis resulting in an incomplete "CD117-only" immunophenotype of mast cells and the possibility of an erroneous diagnosis of a non–mast cell tumor with expression of CD117 (**Fig. 1**). A cell not expressing CD117 is not a mast cell.

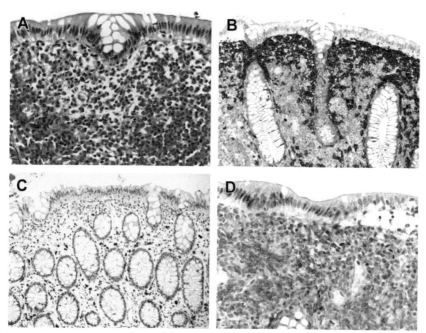

Fig. 1. Systemic mastocytosis (intestinal type). (*A*) Giemsa staining shows the typical picture of eosinophilic colitis with an abundance of mature eosinophils diffusely infiltrating the lamina propria mucosae (Giemsa, original magnification ×40). (*B*) Immunostaining, however, reveals a compact band-like infiltrate consisting of medium-sized CD117-expressing round mast cells beneath the surface epithelium, which is intact (anti-CD117; ABC method, original magnification ×40). (*C*) Most CD117-expressing cells, in particular those forming the band-like infiltrate, do not react with an antibody against tryptase. Note the presence of loosely scattered partly spindle-shaped tryptase-expressing cells, which are mast cells probably not belonging to the neoplastic clone (antitryptase/AA1; ABC method, original magnification ×20). (*D*) The mast cell nature of the CD117-expressing cells is further underlined by the coexpression of CD25 (and the demonstration of the activating point mutation *KIT*D816V) (anti-CD25; ABC method, original magnification ×40). Diagnosis in this unusual case could read as follows: systemic (intestinal) mastocytosis associated with (obscured by) eosinophilic colitis, or systemic (intestinal) mastocytosis with marked eosinophilia mimicking eosinophilic colitis.

The aberrant expression of various other hematopoietic antigens by the transformed mast cells in SM is of minor importance for the correct diagnosis but may easily lead to misdiagnoses of hematologic tumors other than mastocytosis.[7] The following antigens may be expressed, although in varying frequency and intensity:

1. Myelomonocytic antigens: CD14, CD33, CD61, CD63, CD68, CD203c, 2D7, myeloperoxidase, naphthol AS-D chloroacetate esterase
2. Lymphoid antigens: CD2, CD9, CD25, CD26, CD30 (**Fig. 2**), CD52, CD79a
3. Stem cell–associated antigens: CD44
4. Natural killer cell–associated antigen: CD57 (**Fig. 2**)
5. Dendritic cell–associated antigens: CD35, CD123
6. Other antigens: CD99, SDF-1 (**Fig. 3**)

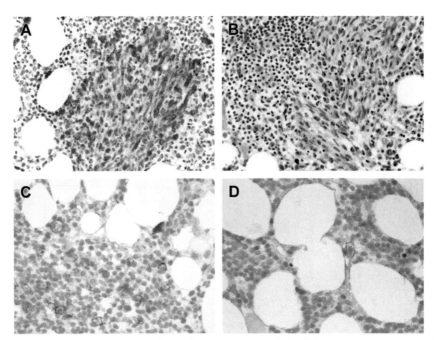

Fig. 2. Systemic mastocytosis involving the bone marrow. (*A*) Indolent systemic mastocytosis exhibiting a typical compact infiltrate consisting of densely packed spindle-shaped mast cells with strong expression of tryptase (antitryptase/AA1; ABC method, original magnification ×20). (*B*) The same case shows mast cells with an aberrant immunophenotype and coexpression of the natural killer/T cell–associated antigen CD57 (anti-CD57; ABC method, original magnification ×20). (*C*) Isolated bone marrow mastocytosis exhibiting a compact infiltrate of mixed cellularity consisting of eosinophils, lymphocytes, and medium-to-large size atypical mast cells with strong aberrant expression of CD30. These histologic findings initially were interpreted as involvement of the bone marrow by Hodgkin disease in a patient with known Hodgkin disease of an axillary lymph node (anti-CD30; ABC method, original magnification ×40). (*D*) The same case shows some loosely scattered CD30-expressing mast cells within the bone marrow stroma (anti-CD30; ABC method, original magnification ×40). Hodgkin cells never occur as single cells but invariably show the typical cellular microenvironment with attraction of eosinophils, lymphocytes, and other "inflammatory" cells. Based on this picture alone a diagnosis of systemic mastocytosis could be established by an experienced hematopathologist.

Regarding these above-mentioned aberrantly expressed antigens, the following differential diagnoses have to be considered:

1. CD14, CD68: Monocytic leukemias, histiocytoses
2. CD63, CD203c, 2D7: Basophilic leukemias
3. CD33, MPO, CAE: Myeloid neoplasms
4. CD2: T-cell neoplasms
5. CD9, CD25, CD37, CD52, CD79a: B-cell lymphomas (hairy cell leukemia)
6. CD30: Hodgkin lymphoma, ALK+ anaplastic large cell lymphoma, embryonal carcinoma
7. CD57: Natural killer cell neoplasms
8. CD35, CD123: Dendritic cell tumors
9. CD99: Ewing sarcoma, acute lymphoblastic leukemia

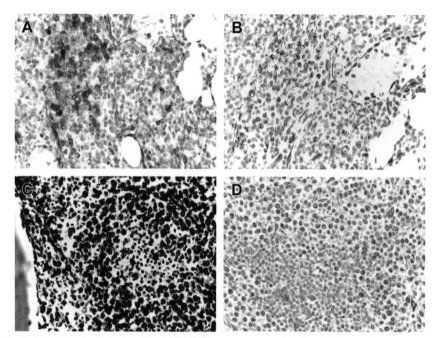

Fig. 3. Systemic mastocytosis involving the bone marrow. (*A, B*) Indolent systemic mastocytosis with multifocal bone marrow involvement. The mast cells in the compact and the diffuse infiltrate exhibit an aberrant immunophenotype with expression of two antigens: CD26 and SDF-1. Note the CD26/SDF-1 expression can also be seen on endothelial cells but not on hematopoietic cells other than mast cells. (*C, D*) Mast cell leukemia with diffuse-compact infiltration of the bone marrow by small-to-medium sized mast cells containing large numbers of metachromatic granules (*C*) but also expressing SDF-1. Normal blood cell precursors and fat cells are virtually absent (*A*, anti-CD26, ABC method, original magnification ×20; *B* and *D*, anti–SDF-1, ABC method, original magnification ×20; *C*, Giemsa, original magnification ×20).

It has to be emphasized that immunophenotypical features exhibited by transformed mast cells may easily lead to wrong diagnoses. The cytomorphologic aspects of mast cells including features like broad pale nongranulated cytoplasm and bilobated or monocytoid nuclei primarily may raise suspicion of a monocytic or histiocytic tumor, a hairy cell leukemia, or even a clear cell carcinoma. The expression of such markers as CD14, CD68, or CD25 (in cases of suspected hairy cell leukemia) confirms the suspicion and the underlying SM is not detected. Moreover, the presence of metachromatic granules is not unique to mast cells but also is seen in basophilic granulocytes. Because the secondary metachromatic granules of basophils are water-soluble these cells cannot be seen in routinely processed tissue. The aberrant expression of basophil-associated antigens, such as 2D7, CD63, and CD203c, therefore is not of major significance in diagnostic hematopathology, in particular regarding that basophilic leukemias are extremely rare.

CD30⁺ SM

Expression of the activation antigen CD30 by transformed mast cells is intriguing and one of the major pitfalls in this field.[8] CD30 is commonly known as a highly specific marker for Hodgkin lymphoma but is also seen in other hematopoietic and nonhematopoietic neoplasms, such as anaplastic large cell lymphoma, lymphomatoid papulosis, and embryonal carcinoma. The recent description of CD30 expression in a considerable number of mastocytoses enables one to assess or exclude this disease by application of diagnostic relevant markers, such as tryptase or CD117. In advanced SM including aggressive SM and mast cell leukemia the expression of CD30 is seen more often, in more mast cells, and in stronger intensity than in the more common SM subvariants with no or only low-grade malignant potential. In the following a prototypical case is briefly reported.

A 32-year-old man suffered from a Hodgkin lymphoma (mixed type) diagnosed in an axillary lymph node. Staging investigation of the bone marrow revealed disseminated nodular infiltrates consisting of lymphocytes, eosinophils, and large atypical cells expressing CD30 (see **Fig. 2**C, D). Thus, a diagnosis of generalized lymphoma (stage IV) was established. A slightly elevated serum tryptase led to reinvestigation of the bone marrow histology. The CD30-expressing cells reacted with antibodies against CD25, CD117, and tryptase, and a point mutation at codon 816 of *KIT* was also detected. This point mutation, however, was not found in the lymph node and morphologic investigation did not reveal nodal infiltrates of SM. Accordingly, the final diagnoses had to read as follows: localized Hodgkin lymphoma in an axillary lymph node, and isolated bone marrow mastocytosis with *KIT*D816T (which is a novel hitherto not described point mutation of *KIT*).

Some diagnostic relevant antigens in hematopathology have been found to be never expressed by mast cells and therefore can be used as cell markers in microdissection experiments, for example in cases of associated SM and non–mast cell hematologic neoplasm (SM-AHNMD) to determine whether or not the *KIT*D816V mutation is restricted to the mast cell compartment or has spread to other lineages. These antigens are the following: TdT, glycophorin A/C, CD3, CD7, CD10, CD15, CD20, CD34, CD38, and CD56.

SUMMARY

Mastocytosis comprises an extremely heterogeneous group of diseases ranging from the absolutely benign solitary mastocytoma of the skin to the life-threatening mast cell leukemia. All variants of mastocytosis have been assigned to the group of myeloproliferative neoplasms in the World Health Organization classification system of tumors of the hematopoietic tissues. In neoplastic states, mast cells show an unusually broad spectrum of immunophenotypical aberrancies. The most important mast cell–related antigens used for diagnosis in histologic sections are tryptase and CD117 (*KIT*). In normal and reactive states all mast cells coexpress tryptase and CD117, but tryptase expression may be strongly decreased or even lost in rare cases of mastocytosis, thus leading to an incomplete "CD117-only" immunophenotype. Cells not expressing CD117 are not mast cells. CD25 is not expressed by normal/reactive but by transformed mast cells and has been found to be the most reliable immunohistochemical marker for diagnosis of mastocytosis. Moreover, mast cells may express a great variety of myeloid (eg, MPO, 2D7, CD203c, naphthol AS-D chloroacetate esterase), monohistiocytic (eg, CD14, CD68), stem cell–related (eg, CD44), and lymphoid (eg, CD2, CD30, CD52, CD79a) antigens in varying frequencies and intensities. Such immunophenotypical features of transformed mast cells may lead to severe diagnostic problems for the hematopathologist. This high degree of immunophenotypical atypia is not seen in myeloid cells even in neoplastic states and therefore strongly argues against the assumption that mastocytosis is a true myeloproliferative neoplasm.

REFERENCES

1. Valent P, Horny H-P, Escribano L, et al. Diagnostic criteria and classification of mastocytosis: a consensus proposal. Leuk Res 2001;25:603–25.
2. Valent P, Akin C, Escribano L, et al. Standards and standardization in mastocytosis: consensus statements on diagnostics, treatment recommendations and response criteria. Eur J Clin Invest 2007;37:435–53.
3. Horny H-P, Metcalfe DD, Bennett JM, et al. Mastocytosis (Mast cell disease). In: Swerdlow SH, Campo E, Harris NL, et al, editors. WHO Classification of Tumours of Haematopoietic and Lymphoid Tissues. Geneva, Switzerland: IARCPress; 2008. p. 54–63.
4. Horny H-P, Sotlar K, Valent P. Mastocytosis: state of the art. Pathobiology 2007; 74:121–32.
5. Sotlar K, Horny H-P, Simonitsch I, et al. CD25 indicates the neoplastic phenotype of mast cells: a novel immunohistochemical marker for the diagnosis of systemic mastocytosis (SM) in routinely processed bone marrow biopsy specimens. Am J Surg Pathol 2004;28:1319–25.
6. Valent P, Cerny-Reiterer S, Herrmann H, et al. Phenotypic heterogeneity, novel diagnostic markers, and target expression profiles in normal and neoplastic human mast cells. Best Pract Res Clin Haematol 2010;23:369–78.
7. Horny H-P, Sotlar K, Valent P. Differential diagnoses of systemic mastocytosis in routinely processed bone marrow biopsy specimens: a review. Pathobiology 2010;77:169–80.
8. Sotlar K, Cerny-Reiterer S, Petat-Dutter K, et al. Aberrant expression of CD30 in neoplastic mast cells in high-grade mastocytosis. Mod Pathol 2011;24:585–95.

Pathology of Extramedullary Mastocytosis

Leona A. Doyle, MD[a], Jason L. Hornick, MD, PhD[a,b,*]

KEYWORDS

- Mast cells • Mastocytosis • Urticaria pigmentosa • Mast cell sarcoma • KIT

KEY POINTS

- Histopathologic findings of mastocytosis have distinguishing features at different anatomic locations, but at all sites mast cell infiltrates may be subtle and easily overlooked.
- Useful immunohistochemical markers of mast cell lineage include KIT and tryptase; aberrant expression of CD25 is a marker of neoplasia in mast cell infiltrates.
- Gastrointestinal involvement by mastocytosis is increasingly recognized; endoscopic gastrointestinal biopsies can be used to establish a diagnosis of systemic mastocytosis in some patients with cutaneous mastocytosis and gastrointestinal symptoms.
- Mast cell sarcoma is an extremely rare clinically and pathologically distinct aggressive variant of mast cell disease.

ANCILLARY MARKERS IN SURGICAL PATHOLOGY FOR THE EVALUATION OF MASTOCYTOSIS

Nonneoplastic mast cells are round in shape, and contain a central nucleus and variable amounts of cytoplasm, which contains hundreds of membrane-bound modified lysosomes.[1] These lysosomes contain a variety of pharmacologically active substances, such as histamine, leukotrienes B4, C4, and D, and prostaglandin D2, which are released in response to various stimuli. Mast cells also produce heparin and enzymes such as neutral proteases.[2] The wide range of substances produced by mast cells reflects the broad functions of these cells and their participation in diverse inflammatory disorders. Mast cells may also be increased in number in some neoplasms, such as neurofibroma and spindle cell lipoma. Mastocytosis includes a distinct group of clonal mast cell disorders that may be limited to the skin or may involve other sites.[2] Confirmation of mast cell lineage, and confirmation that a mast

The authors have no conflicts of interest to declare.
[a] Department of Pathology, Brigham and Women's Hospital, Harvard Medical School, 75 Francis Street, Boston, MA 02115 USA; [b] Mastocytosis Center, Brigham and Women's Hospital, 75 Francis Street, Boston, MA 02115, USA
* Corresponding author.
E-mail address: jhornick@partners.org

Immunol Allergy Clin N Am 34 (2014) 323–339
http://dx.doi.org/10.1016/j.iac.2014.01.010   immunology.theclinics.com
0889-8561/14/$ – see front matter © 2014 Elsevier Inc. All rights reserved.

cell infiltrate is neoplastic, is afforded by the use of certain histochemical and, more reliably, immunohistochemical stains.

Mast cell granules, which are difficult to appreciate on a routine hematoxylin and eosin stain but may appear lightly basophilic, stain metachromatically with toluidine blue and Giemsa stains, and orange-red with chloroacetate esterase.[3] Because these histochemical stains require the presence of mast cell granules, they may underestimate the number of mast cells in comparison with immunohistochemical staining for KIT or mast cell tryptase, as neoplastic mast cells often contain greatly reduced numbers of cytoplasmic granules.[4] Consequently, these histochemical markers have largely been replaced by immunohistochemical markers in surgical pathology practice (**Table 1**).

KIT

KIT (also known as CD117), a type III receptor tyrosine kinase that plays a crucial role in mast cell development, is a highly sensitive marker of mast cells. In contrast to mast cell tryptase, expression is localized to the cell membrane rather than the cytoplasm. In addition to its role in mast cell development, KIT also functions in the development of melanocytes, germ cells, hematopoietic stem cells, and the interstitial cells of Cajal within the gastrointestinal (GI) tract.[5] KIT is therefore expressed in some malignant melanomas, seminoma, some acute myeloid leukemias, and gastrointestinal stromal tumors (the latter reflecting differentiation toward the interstitial cell of Cajal lineage). However, although the overall specificity of KIT for mast cells is low, in the appropriate clinical context KIT is invaluable for the identification of mast cells, as relatively few normal cell types show expression of this marker.

Adult-onset mastocytosis is associated with somatic point mutations in exon 17 of KIT (codon 816) in most cases, which result in ligand-independent activation and autophosphorylation of KIT.[6] KIT mutations can be detected in peripheral blood, bone marrow aspirates, or tissue samples, which can help support a diagnosis of mastocytosis; the presence of codon 816 mutations in KIT is one of the minor criteria for the diagnosis of systemic mastocytosis.[7] The most common mutation, D816V (substitution of valine for aspartate), is detected in neoplastic mast cells of more than 95% of adult patients with systemic mastocytosis, and in approximately one-third of pediatric patients with cutaneous mastocytosis.[8–10] Because this particular mutation results in a conformational change in the kinase domain of KIT that renders it resistant to the effects of imatinib, a tyrosine kinase inhibitor effective in the treatment of chronic

Table 1	
Useful immunohistochemical markers in the evaluation of mastocytosis	
Antibody	**Comments**
KIT	Confirms mast cell lineage; highly sensitive for mast cells, but not entirely specific (melanocytes, interstitial cells of Cajal, hematopoietic stem cells also express KIT); stains both normal and neoplastic mast cells
Mast cell tryptase	Confirms mast cell lineage; highly specific for mast cells; may be less sensitive than KIT for neoplastic mast cells in the gastrointestinal tract; stains both normal and neoplastic mast cells
CD25	Stains only neoplastic mast cells; confirms neoplastic nature of mast cell infiltrate; also stains some T lymphocytes
CD30	Stains a subset of neoplastic mast cells; may be a marker of aggressive disease in bone marrow involved by mastocytosis; does not appear to be associated with aggressive disease in the gastrointestinal tract

myeloid leukemia and gastrointestinal stromal tumor, imatinib therapy is not effective treatment for most patients with mastocytosis.[11,12] Less commonly, alternate activating point mutations are detected, such as D816Y, D816H, and D816F. Of note, a large subset of pediatric patients with urticaria pigmentosa (UP) has *KIT* mutations in the extracellular domain (exons 8 or 9), at approximately the same rate as exon 17 mutations.[10]

Mast Cell Tryptase

Tryptase is a cytoplasmic serine protease that is expressed almost exclusively by mast cells.[13] In contrast to other mast cell proteases, cytoplasmic tryptase expression appears to be present at all stages of mast cell maturation.[14] Its superiority for the detection of mast cells over histochemical markers was established along with the observation that aggressive forms of mastocytosis, in which the neoplastic mast cells often have minimal cytoplasm, show less tryptase expression than mast cells of cutaneous mastocytosis.[4] Similarly, it has been observed that in comparison with KIT, mast cell tryptase shows more variable levels of expression in the neoplastic cells of GI mastocytosis.[15]

CD25

CD25 is a low-affinity receptor for interleukin-2, which is normally expressed on a subset of T lymphocytes. Aberrant expression of CD25 is a consistent finding of neoplastic mast cells; CD25 is not expressed in normal mast cells.[16–19] Expression of CD25 on mast cells therefore helps confirm that a mast cell infiltrate represents a neoplastic process rather than a reactive hyperplasia.[20] Prior studies have established the utility of CD25 in the evaluation of mast cell infiltrates at different anatomic sites, including bone marrow, skin, and GI tract.[18,19,21] Coexpression of KIT on mast cells, more abundant cytoplasm in mast cells, and stronger CD25 staining on T lymphocytes all help distinguish between mast cells and T cells on a CD25 immunostain.[21]

CD2

Aberrant expression of CD2 is common in neoplastic mast cells.[22,23] CD2, also known as LFA-2, is usually expressed in T cells and a subset of natural killer cells. However, not all cases of systemic mastocytosis show expression of CD2, and within individual cases expression may be highly variable. CD2 therefore has lower sensitivity than CD25 for the detection of neoplastic mast cells, and also has lower specificity, as CD2 stains nearly all T lymphocytes.[20] Although coexpression of CD2 is considered a minor diagnostic criterion for the diagnosis of systemic mastocytosis, its low sensitivity limits its clinical utility. Despite the role of CD2 expression in systemic mastocytosis being unknown, it has been hypothesized that because mast cells also express CD58 (LFA-3), a natural ligand of CD2, CD2-CD58 interactions may be involved in the accumulation of mast cells in patients with systemic mastocytosis.[23] Of note, mast cells may also express other less specific hematopoietic markers used in surgical pathology, such as CD45 and CD68, and other less specific diagnostic markers may be detected by flow cytometry (eg, CD9 and CD33).[16,23]

CD30

CD30 is a member of the tumor necrosis factor receptor superfamily whose expression is normally limited to a subset of activated lymphocytes. Expression of CD30 in neoplastic mast cells in bone marrow biopsies has been found to be significantly associated with advanced disease.[24] By contrast, in the GI tract, the finding of CD30 expression does not seem to predict aggressive disease.[15] Among other neoplasms,

CD30 is also expressed by tumor cells of Hodgkin lymphoma, anaplastic large cell lymphoma, and embryonal carcinoma.

CUTANEOUS MASTOCYTOSIS
Urticaria Pigmentosa

UP is the most common form of cutaneous mastocytosis (**Table 2**). UP typically presents as a generalized eruption of red-brown macules or sometimes papules, predominantly involving the trunk, and occasionally the extremities and head and neck region.[25,26] It is named for the tendency for lesions to urticate when stroked (Darier sign) and the reactive basal hyperpigmentation of the epidermis. Most patients are younger than 4 years old at presentation, and in children with UP the clinical course is usually self-limited with resolution of disease by puberty.[27] However, when UP arises in adults, disease tends to be persistent and often reflects the presence of underlying systemic mastocytosis.[28,29]

In normal skin, small numbers of dermal interstitial mast cells are observed, most prominent around blood vessels and skin adnexa.[30,31] Histologically, UP in children is characterized by sheets of mast cells within the papillary dermis, often with extension into the reticular dermis, sometimes with a perivascular and periadnexal distribution (**Fig. 1**).[32] The mast cells typically have a predominantly round morphology, with a subset of cells showing elongated cytoplasmic processes (spindle shaped). In adults with cutaneous mastocytosis, the density of mast cells is usually less than that seen in pediatric UP, and multiple biopsies may be needed to make a definitive diagnosis of mastocytosis; However, even in children the number of mast cells may be highly variable between patients, and in some cases consist of only sparse perivascular mast cells. Basal hyperpigmentation is a typical finding in UP, and scattered eosinophils may be present, particularly in adults; both of these features may be helpful clues to the diagnosis when the infiltrate is sparse (see **Fig. 1**). In children, subepidermal vesiculobullous changes may arise as a result of persistent superficial edema. The bullae may contain mast cells, eosinophils, and neutrophils, with an underlying typical dermal mast cell infiltrate.[33]

Normal skin is reported to contain up to 15 mast cells per high-power field, although the range is in fact variable. A wide range of inflammatory dermatoses are

Table 2 Subtypes of cutaneous mastocytosis		
Type	**Clinical Features**	**Histologic Features**
Urticaria pigmentosa	Most common in children; onset in adulthood is associated with systemic disease in nearly all patients; most common form of cutaneous disease	Aggregates and sheets of mast cells within dermis; often perivascular or periadnexal in distribution; cytology ranges from round to spindled cells; may be more subtle in adults
Telangiectasia macularis eruptiva perstans	Rare variant; occurs in adults; highly associated with systemic disease	Subtle increase in mast cells around slightly dilated superficial blood vessels
Solitary mastocytoma	Rare variant; virtually always in infants; predilection for trunk	Sheets of round to ovoid mast cells within the dermis, occasionally extending into subcutis
Diffuse cutaneous mastocytosis	Rare variant; virtually always in childhood; peau d'orange appearance	Sheets of mature-appearing mast cells or limited lichenoid infiltrate of mast cells in papillary dermis

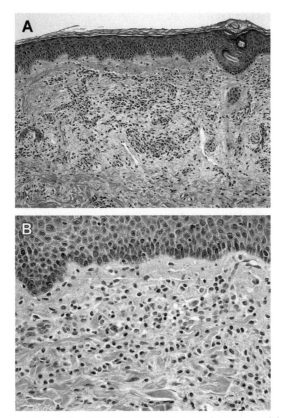

Fig. 1. Cutaneous mastocytosis. Urticaria pigmentosa is characterized by aggregates or sheets of mast cells within the dermis, sometimes showing a predominantly perivascular distribution (*A*) (H&E, original magnification ×100). The mast cells are typically round with moderate amounts of eosinophilic, vaguely granular cytoplasm; admixed eosinophils may be present, particularly in adults (*B*) (H&E, original magnification ×400). Note the characteristic hyperpigmentation of the basal layer of the epidermis.

accompanied by mast cell hyperplasia; therefore, mast cell density must be interpreted carefully in the context of the clinical presentation and other histologic findings. Given that some lesions, particularly those of telangiectasia macularis eruptiva perstans (TMEP), may be subtle, comparison with nonlesional skin in a given biopsy may be helpful.[1] As in other locations, mast cells express mast cell tryptase and KIT, both of which are invaluable in confirming a diagnosis of cutaneous mastocytosis. Expression of CD25 by mast cells in UP appears to be associated with systemic mastocytosis in adult patients.[34]

Telangiectasia Macularis Eruptiva Perstans

TMEP is a rare variant of UP that occurs in adults and is highly associated with systemic disease.[35–38] Clinically the skin lesions are lightly pigmented, telangiectatic and erythematous macules, usually few in number, which typically arise on the trunk and proximal extremities, and more rarely on the face. Histologically there is a subtle increase in mast cells, usually distributed around slightly dilated superficial dermal blood vessels.[1] The mast cells are predominantly spindle shaped, and an eosinophilic infiltrate is usually absent.

Solitary Mastocytoma of Skin

Cutaneous mastocytoma presents as a solitary skin lesion, virtually always in infants, over a wide anatomic distribution, with a predilection for the trunk and wrists.[39-41] Lesions may measure up to 3 cm, and usually involute spontaneously. Histologically, mastocytoma is composed of sheets of round to ovoid mast cells with abundant palely eosinophilic cytoplasm within the dermis, occasionally extending into underlying subcutis.[1] Without correlation with clinical findings, small examples of solitary mastocytoma cannot be distinguished on histologic grounds from UP. In contrast to mast cell sarcoma, the lesional cells lack atypia and their mast cell lineage is usually easily recognizable. Localized necrobiosis and stromal fibrosis may be present.[42,43]

Diffuse Cutaneous Mastocytosis

This clinical variant of cutaneous mastocytosis is uncommon and, similar to solitary mastocytoma, virtually always occurs in childhood.[44] Clinically the skin is diffusely thickened, erythematous or yellow-brown in color, and may have a peau d'orange appearance. Blistering, bullae, and nodule formation may occur.[45-49] Histologically the skin findings may resemble mastocytoma, containing sheets of mature-appearing mast cells, or may consist of a more limited lichenoid infiltrate of mast cells in the papillary dermis. Fibrosis is occasionally present.

MASTOCYTOSIS INVOLVING THE GASTROINTESTINAL TRACT

Involvement of the GI tract by mastocytosis is increasingly recognized, because of increasing awareness among pathologists and physicians involved in the care of patients with mastocytosis as well as the availability of sensitive and specific immunohistochemical markers to detect neoplastic mast cells. Key features of mastocytosis involving the GI tract are shown in **Box 1**.

GI symptoms are common in patients with mastocytosis, including patients without direct involvement of the GI tract, and include abdominal pain, nausea, and diarrhea. These symptoms are thought to be due to the release of mast cell mediators such as histamine and leukotrienes, and in patients with involvement of the GI tract may also be due to direct infiltration of the mucosa by mast cells, resulting in malabsorption or enhanced local effects of mediator release. The frequency of GI symptoms in patients with systemic mastocytosis is estimated at 70%,[50] diminishing in patients with UP (without known GI involvement) to 25%.[29] However, the true frequency of GI tract

---

Box 1
Key features: mastocytosis involving the gastrointestinal tract

- May be first presentation of systemic disease
- Colon and terminal ileum most commonly involved
- Endoscopically may be associated with mucosal erythema, granularity, or nodularity
- Lamina propria infiltrates of ovoid or spindle-shaped mast cells; superficial distribution underneath surface epithelium in colon is common
- Eosinophilic infiltrates may mask the mast cell infiltrate or lead to an erroneous diagnosis of eosinophilic gastroenteritis
- Disease is often focal; therefore multiple, systematic random biopsies are indicated
- Gastrointestinal involvement does not correlate with aggressive disease

involvement in patients with cutaneous mastocytosis or mastocytosis at other sites is not known, as many patients do not undergo endoscopic biopsy unless they have long-standing, persistent, or changing symptoms.

Detection of GI tract involvement by endoscopic biopsy is a useful method of confirming systemic disease in patients with GI symptoms; in a series of 24 patients with GI tract and liver mastocytosis, the first diagnosis of systemic disease was made based on GI/liver biopsy findings in 67% of patients.[15] However, interestingly 2 patients in this study were asymptomatic, and disease was only detected during colonoscopic screening for colorectal cancer. The median interval from the time of diagnosis of skin disease to the time of documented GI involvement in that study was 10 years. Endoscopic abnormalities are seen in approximately 60% of patients with GI mastocytosis, and include mucosal erythema/congestion, granularity, or nodularity.[51–53] GI mucosal involvement in the absence of malabsorption and weight loss does not appear to correlate with aggressive disease.[15]

Clinical and pathologic descriptions of mastocytosis in GI biopsies include case reports and small series,[21,51,52,54–58] as well as 2 recent large series of 23 and 24 patients with GI tract and liver mastocytosis.[15,59] When the GI tract is involved by mastocytosis, the most commonly involved sites are colon and ileum, followed by duodenum. The stomach is less often involved; only one-third of gastric biopsies from patients with other sites of GI tract involvement show involvement by mastocytosis.[15] Mastocytosis typically does not involve the esophagus.

The diagnosis of mastocytosis in mucosal biopsies can be difficult for several reasons; involvement can be very focal and subtle, making recognition of the infiltrate challenging. Histologically, mucosal biopsies involved by mastocytosis show lamina propria infiltrates of ovoid to spindle-shaped mast cells in aggregates or sheets. The mast cell aggregates usually show a predominantly superficial distribution in the lamina propria, with greatest density directly under the surface epithelium, especially in the colon (**Fig. 2**). Occasionally, aggregates are scattered randomly throughout the lamina propria. The mast cell infiltrate may extend into the muscularis mucosae. Mast cell morphology is variable, ranging from rounded cells with moderate amounts of palely eosinophilic cytoplasm to, more commonly, ovoid or spindled cells with more limited cytoplasm. As at other sites, mast cell density is highly variable, and in itself is not a useful diagnostic feature. Mast cell count is variable in normal biopsies and may be increased in other inflammatory disorders such as parasitic infection[15,21]; it is the presence of discrete aggregates or confluent sheets of mast cells, along with coexpression of CD25, that allow for a diagnosis of mastocytosis (see **Fig. 2**). Of importance is that involvement of the GI tract can be very focal in a given biopsy, consisting of a single discrete aggregate of mast cells. Heterogeneous, patchy involvement within biopsies taken from the same region can also be seen, with some biopsy fragments showing no or minimal involvement, and other fragments showing obvious sheets or aggregates of mast cells.[15] This feature emphasizes the need for multiple, systematic random biopsies at the time of endoscopy.

Prominent eosinophilic infiltrates frequently accompany GI involvement by mastocytosis, and may mask the mast cell infiltrate or lead to an erroneous diagnosis of eosinophilic gastroenteritis. Eosinophilic infiltrates appear to be more common in colonic biopsies than in upper GI tract biopsies involved by mastocytosis.[15] Other histologic findings that may be seen include architectural distortion in colonic biopsies, villous blunting in small intestinal biopsies, chronic duodenitis, and chronic inactive gastritis. In the colon, these findings may mimic inflammatory bowel disease.[55]

Neoplastic mast cells are highlighted by diffuse membranous staining for both KIT and CD25 (see **Fig. 2**). By contrast, expression of mast cell tryptase may be variable

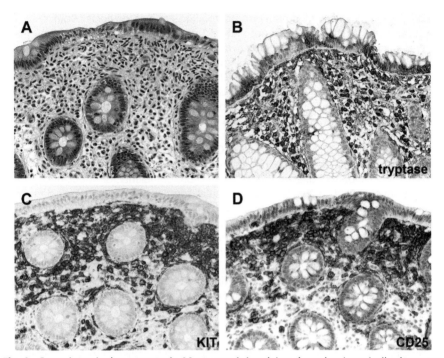

Fig. 2. Gastrointestinal mastocytosis. Mastocytosis involving the colon is typically character-ized by aggregates of spindle-shaped mast cells with limited cytoplasm, localized underneath the surface epithelium (*A*) (H&E, original magnification ×400). The mast cells are positive for tryptase (*B*) (original magnification ×400) and KIT (*C*) (original magnification ×400), and show aberrant membranous expression of CD25 (*D*) (original magnification ×400), confirming their neoplastic nature.

and may show positive staining in only a subset of mast cells.[15] In contrast to prior studies that have shown an association between CD30 expression and advanced disease in the bone marrow,[24] at least in the GI tract, the finding of reactivity for CD30 does not seem to predict aggressive disease: CD30 expression on GI mast cells has been reported in a subset of patients with an indolent clinical course, and was pre-sent in only 1 of 2 cases with aggressive features in a recent study, although the num-ber of cases examined was small.[15]

In general, the histologic differential diagnosis of mastocytosis in the GI tract is limited; perhaps the most difficult differential diagnosis is with normal colonic mucosa for those cases whereby the mast cell infiltrate is focal and subtle, followed by eosinophil-rich disorders such as primary eosinophilic gastroenteritis, parasitic dis-ease, and chronic inflammatory bowel disease.

MASTOCYTOSIS INVOLVING THE LIVER

In most cases, liver involvement by mastocytosis is associated with aggressive dis-ease. Patients with mastocytosis involving the liver may present with hepatomegaly, ascites, and other signs of portal hypertension such as bleeding varices.[15,60,61] Liver biopsies involved by mastocytosis typically show mast cell infiltrates in both a portal and sinusoidal distribution.[60,61] The sinusoidal component may be subtle, but can be highlighted by KIT or tryptase immunostaining (**Fig. 3**). The mast cells usually have

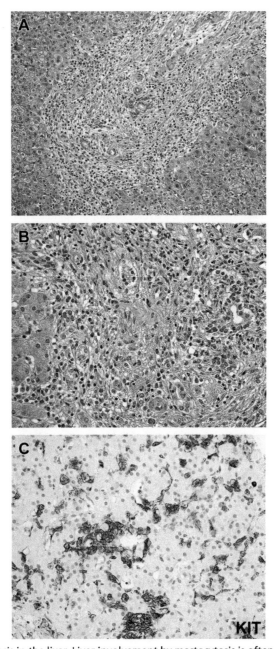

Fig. 3. Mastocytosis in the liver. Liver involvement by mastocytosis is often subtle, consisting of portal infiltrates (*A*) (H&E, original magnification ×100) of spindle-shaped mast cells with admixed eosinophils (*B*) (H&E, original magnification ×400). The mast cell infiltrate typically also involves sinusoidal spaces, which may be subtle and more readily appreciated with the aid of KIT immunohistochemical staining (*C*) (original magnification ×400).

spindle cell morphology. Admixed eosinophils are common and may mask the mast cell infiltrate. Periportal fibrosis may be present, but development of cirrhosis is rare.

MASTOCYTOSIS INVOLVING THE SPLEEN AND LYMPH NODES

The prevalence of splenic involvement by mastocytosis is uncertain, as splenectomy is rarely performed in patients with mastocytosis, except in the past in some patients whose aggressive disease included hypersplenism. Mastocytosis in the spleen may present as focal mast cell infiltrates in parafollicular areas, aggregates within follicles, or diffuse infiltration of the red pulp.[61,62] Similar to mastocytosis at other sites, an admixed eosinophilic infiltrate and fibrosis are common findings.

Involvement of lymph nodes by mastocytosis is rare, but can present as generalized lymphadenopathy. The paracortical region is most often involved (**Fig. 4**), either focally or diffusely, but any compartment can be infiltrated by mast cells. In addition to the presence of mast cells, which may be ovoid, round, or spindled in morphology, additional findings that may be seen include reactive follicular hyperplasia, eosinophilic infiltrates, fibrosis, and a plasma cell infiltrate (see **Fig. 4**).[61,63] In a subset of patients with nodal infiltrates of mast cells who present with lymphadenopathy and peripheral eosinophilia, *PDGFRA* rearrangements are detected; these patients are classified in the category of "myeloid neoplasm with eosinophilia and rearrangement of *PDGFRA*" (rather than systemic mastocytosis).[5,7]

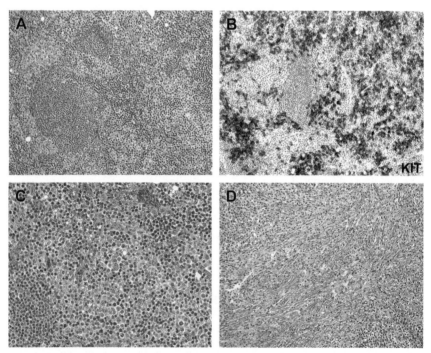

Fig. 4. Mastocytosis involving a retroperitoneal lymph node: the mast cell infiltrate shows a predominantly paracortical distribution (*A*) (H&E, original magnification ×100). KIT immunostaining highlights mast cells, and demonstrates sparing of follicles in this case (*B*) (original magnification ×100). The mast cells are variably ovoid to spindle-shaped; commonly associated features include a prominent eosinophilic infiltrate (*C*) (H&E, original magnification ×400) and fibrosis (*D*) (H&E, original magnification ×200).

MAST CELL SARCOMA

Mast cell sarcoma is characterized by cytologically malignant mast cells presenting as a destructive mass. Mast cell sarcoma may arise de novo (ie, in a patient with no history of mastocytosis) or, much more rarely, as a secondary (transformation) event in patients with cutaneous mastocytosis (see later discussion). Mast cell sarcoma is exceedingly rare in humans. Only 14 human cases of mast cell sarcoma have been reported to date in the English-language literature, either as single case reports or small series. Unlike cutaneous mastocytosis, which typically presents in infancy, mast cell sarcoma can arise at any age, with a reported range of 4 to 77 years. Mast cell sarcoma can also occur at a wide range of anatomic sites; tumors have been reported in oral/laryngeal mucosa,[64,65] gastrointestinal tract,[66,67] cranial bones and meninges,[68] extracranial skeleton,[69,70] somatic soft tissue,[70] uterus,[71] and skin.[55,72,73] Key features of mast cell sarcoma are listed in **Box 2**.

Histologically, mast cell sarcoma is composed of sheets of medium-sized to large pleomorphic epithelioid cells, usually with an infiltrative growth pattern. Tumor cells have abundant cytoplasm and well-defined cell borders. Nuclei often have prominent nuclear membrane irregularities and may be bilobed (**Fig. 5**). Bizarre multinucleated tumor giant cells are frequently present. Characteristically an eosinophilic infiltrate is present, and may be a helpful clue to the diagnosis. Similar to systemic mastocytosis, tumor cells are positive for KIT, CD25, and mast cell tryptase, but expression of histiocytic or myeloid lineage markers (CD68, CD4, CD43, lysozyme) has also been reported, which can lead to diagnostic confusion.[65] The cells of mast cell sarcoma do not closely resemble either normal tissue mast cells or the spindled mast cells typical of systemic mastocytosis, but show some similarity to the cytologically defined "atypical type II mast cells" or "promastocytes" reported in some cases of aggressive systemic mastocytosis, although the degree of nuclear atypia and pleomorphism are much more striking.[74] To date, the D816V mutation of the *KIT* kinase domain characteristic of systemic mastocytosis has not been detected in any case of mast cell sarcoma. However, 2 cases have shown other *KIT* mutations: a deletion mutation in exon 8 (D419del), similar to a common mutation in pediatric UP,[65] and an alternative exon 17 mutation (N822K).[66] Because the D816V mutation confers resistance to imatinib, the absence of this mutation in mast cell sarcoma has allowed treatment with imatinib to produce at least a temporary clinical response in a subset of patients.[65,71]

The histologic differential diagnoses of mast cell sarcoma include poorly differentiated carcinoma, melanoma, anaplastic large cell lymphoma (ALCL), Langerhans cell histiocytosis (or the exceptionally rare Langerhans cell sarcoma), and other myeloid or histiocytic neoplasms. Poorly differentiated carcinoma can usually be readily

---

Box 2
Key features: mast cell sarcoma

- Extremely rare malignant neoplasm composed of mast cells presenting as an isolated destructive mass
- Sheets of medium-sized to large pleomorphic epithelioid cells
- Tumor cells have abundant cytoplasm and well-defined cell borders
- Multinucleated tumor giant cells and eosinophilic infiltrates often present
- May mimic poorly differentiated carcinoma, melanoma, or anaplastic large cell lymphoma
- Lack D816V KIT mutations and may respond to imatinib in some cases

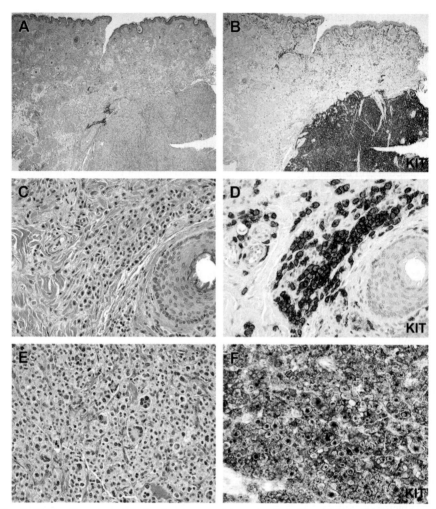

Fig. 5. Mast cell sarcoma. Mast cell sarcoma arising as a discrete nodule in the deep dermis (*lower right*) of the lip in a patient with a long-standing history of urticaria pigmentosa (*A*) (H&E, original magnification ×400). The tumor cells in mast cell sarcoma show strong staining for KIT (*B*) (original magnification ×40). Conventional cutaneous mastocytosis is seen in the adjacent dermis and is composed of numerous uniform, round mast cells (*C*) (H&E, original magnification ×400), highlighted by a KIT immunostain (*D*) (original magnification ×400). By contrast, the tumor cells of the mast cell sarcoma do not resemble normal mast cells and instead show marked cytologic atypia, nuclear pleomorphism, and frequent multinucleated cells (*E*) (H&E, original magnification ×400). Mast cell lineage is supported by expression of KIT (*F*) (original magnification ×400), as well as tryptase and chymase (not shown).

distinguished from mast cell sarcoma by demonstrating keratin expression; similarly, melanoma typically expresses S100 protein, and often HMB-45 or MART-1. Similar to mast cell sarcoma, a dense infiltrate of eosinophils is usually present in Langerhans cell histiocytosis. However, Langerhans cell histiocytosis is composed of tumor cells with characteristic longitudinal nuclear grooves, which are not seen in mast cell sarcoma, as well as abundant pink cytoplasm and indistinct cell borders. Langerhans cell sarcoma shows considerable cytologic pleomorphism and features that may overlap with mast cell sarcoma. Tumor cells of Langerhans cell histiocytosis and Langerhans cell sarcoma express S100 protein, CD1a, and langerin. ALCL is composed of large epithelioid cells, often with bilobed or multilobed nuclei, similar to mast cell sarcoma. Eosinophilic infiltrates are uncommon in ALCL. ALCL consistently expresses CD30, as well as CD3, CD5, EMA, or cytotoxic granule markers in most cases. ALK expression is present in around half of ALCL cases. Detection of a clonal T-cell receptor gene rearrangement by polymerase chain reaction studies may be helpful in some cases. Variable KIT expression may occasionally be seen in T-cell lymphomas, but the uniformly strong expression seen in mast cell sarcoma is not a feature of lymphomas.

Two cases of mast cell sarcoma arising in association with long-standing cutaneous mastocytosis have been described. One occurred in a patient who had a history of infantile cutaneous mastocytosis 17 years before presenting with a mass on the lip (see **Fig. 5**). A residual lesion of UP was identified adjacent to the mast cell sarcoma.[65] Similarly, the development of mast cell sarcoma has been described in an adult patient with persistent localized cutaneous mastocytosis.[72] These 2 cases appear to represent malignant transformation of a previously indolent form of mastocytosis, implying that at least some cases of mast cell sarcoma may be biologically closely related to pediatric cutaneous mastocytosis.

SUMMARY

The histopathologic findings of mastocytosis have distinguishing features at different anatomic locations, but mast cell infiltrates may be subtle, because of either their sparse nature (eg, in some cases of cutaneous mastocytosis) or focality of involvement (eg, in gastrointestinal mucosa). Advances in immunohistochemical detection of mast cell lineage, along with the identification of aberrant CD25 expression as a marker of neoplasia in mast cell infiltrates, have been extremely useful in the evaluation of mast cell disorders, and broader application of these markers in surgical pathology practice will likely improve the recognition of mastocytosis. Finally, endoscopic GI biopsies are emerging as a useful method of detecting systemic disease in some patients with cutaneous mastocytosis and GI symptoms.

REFERENCES

1. Mihm MC, Clark WH, Reed RJ, et al. Mast cell infiltrates of the skin and the mastocytosis syndrome. Hum Pathol 1973;4(2):231–9.
2. Longley J, Duffy TP, Kohn S. The mast cell and mast cell disease. J Am Acad Dermatol 1995;32(4):545–61.
3. Markey AC, Churchill LJ, MacDonald DM. Human cutaneous mast cells—a study of fixative and staining reactions in normal skin. Br J Dermatol 1989; 120(5):625–31.
4. Horny HP, Sillaber C, Menke D, et al. Diagnostic value of immunostaining for tryptase in patients with mastocytosis. Am J Surg Pathol 1998;22(9):1132–40.
5. Maeda H, Yamagata A, Nishikawa S, et al. Requirement of c-kit for development of intestinal pacemaker system. Development 1992;116(2):369–75.
6. Garcia-Montero AC, Jara-Acevedo M, Teodosio C, et al. KIT mutation in mast cells and other bone marrow hematopoietic cell lineages in systemic mast cell disorders: a prospective study of the Spanish network on mastocytosis (REMA) in a series of 113 patients. Blood 2006;108(7):2366–72.

7. Swerdlow SH, Campo E, Harris NL, et al. WHO classification of tumors of hae-matopoietic and lymphoid tissues. Lyon (France): IARC; 2008.

8. Longley BJ Jr, Metcalfe DD, Tharp M, et al. Activating and dominant inactivating c-KIT catalytic domain mutations in distinct clinical forms of human mastocyto-sis. Proc Natl Acad Sci U S A 1999;96(4):1609–14.

9. Longley BJ, Tyrrell L, Lu SZ, et al. Somatic c-KIT activating mutation in urticaria pigmentosa and aggressive mastocytosis: establishment of clonality in a human mast cell neoplasm. Nat Genet 1996;12(3):312–4.

10. Bodemer C, Hermine O, Palmerini F, et al. Pediatric mastocytosis is a clonal dis-ease associated with D816V and other activating c-KIT mutations. J Invest Der-matol 2010;130(3):804–15.

11. Ma Y, Zeng S, Metcalfe DD, et al. The c-KIT mutation causing human mastocy-tosis is resistant to STI571 and other KIT kinase inhibitors; kinases with enzy-matic site mutations show different inhibitor sensitivity profiles than wild-type kinases and those with regulatory-type mutations. Blood 2002;99(5):1741–4.

12. Zermati Y, De Sepulveda P, Feger F, et al. Effect of tyrosine kinase inhibitor STI571 on the kinase activity of wild-type and various mutated c-kit receptors found in mast cell neoplasms. Oncogene 2003;22(5):660–4.

13. Castells MC, Irani AM, Schwartz LB. Evaluation of human peripheral blood leu-kocytes for mast cell tryptase. J Immunol 1987;138(7):2184–9.

14. Valent P. Mast cell differentiation antigens: expression in normal and malignant cells and use for diagnostic purposes. Eur J Clin Invest 1995;25(10):715–20.

15. Doyle LA, Sepehr GJ, Hamilton MJ, et al. A clinicopathologic study of 24 cases of systemic mastocytosis involving the gastrointestinal tract and assessment of mucosal mast cell density in irritable bowel syndrome and asymptomatic pa-tients. Am J Surg Pathol 2014, in press.

16. Escribano L, Orfao A, Villarrubia J, et al. Immunophenotypic characterization of human bone marrow mast cells. A flow cytometric study of normal and patholog-ical bone marrow samples. Anal Cell Pathol 1998;16(3):151–9.

17. Krauth MT, Majlesi Y, Florian S, et al. Cell surface membrane antigen phenotype of human gastrointestinal mast cells. Int Arch Allergy Immunol 2005;138(2):111–20.

18. Krokowski M, Sotlar K, Krauth MT, et al. Delineation of patterns of bone marrow mast cell infiltration in systemic mastocytosis: value of CD25, correlation with subvariants of the disease, and separation from mast cell hyperplasia. Am J Clin Pathol 2005;124(4):560–8.

19. Sotlar K, Horny HP, Simonitsch I, et al. CD25 indicates the neoplastic phenotype of mast cells: a novel immunohistochemical marker for the diagnosis of systemic mastocytosis (SM) in routinely processed bone marrow biopsy specimens. Am J Surg Pathol 2004;28(10):1319–25.

20. Morgado JM, Sanchez-Munoz L, Teodosio CG, et al. Immunophenotyping in systemic mastocytosis diagnosis: 'CD25 positive' alone is more informative than the 'CD25 and/or CD2' WHO criterion. Mod Pathol 2012;25(4):516–21.

21. Hahn HP, Hornick JL. Immunoreactivity for CD25 in gastrointestinal mucosal mast cells is specific for systemic mastocytosis. Am J Surg Pathol 2007; 31(11):1669–76.

22. Escribano L, Orfao A, Villarrubia J, et al. Expression of lymphoid-associated an-tigens in mast cells: report of a case of systemic mast cell disease. Br J Haema-tol 1995;91(4):941–3.

23. Jordan JH, Walchshofer S, Jurecka W, et al. Immunohistochemical properties of bone marrow mast cells in systemic mastocytosis: evidence for expression of CD2, CD117/Kit, and bcl-x(L). Hum Pathol 2001;32(5):545–52.

24. Sotlar K, Cerny-Reiterer S, Petat-Dutter K, et al. Aberrant expression of CD30 in neoplastic mast cells in high-grade mastocytosis. Mod Pathol 2011;24(4):585–95.
25. Fine J. Mastocytosis. Int J Dermatol 1980;19(3):117–23.
26. Allison MA, Schmidt CP. Urticaria pigmentosa. Int J Dermatol 1997;36(5):321–5.
27. Azana JM, Torrelo A, Mediero IG, et al. Urticaria pigmentosa: a review of 67 pediatric cases. Pediatr Dermatol 1994;11(2):102–6.
28. Berezowska S, Flaig MJ, Rueff F, et al. Adult-onset mastocytosis in the skin is highly suggestive of systemic mastocytosis. Mod Pathol 2013;27(1):19–29.
29. Topar G, Staudacher C, Geisen F, et al. Urticaria pigmentosa: a clinical, hematopathologic, and serologic study of 30 adults. Am J Clin Pathol 1998;109(3):279–85.
30. Olafsson JH, Roupe G, Enerback L. Dermal mast cells in mastocytosis: fixation, distribution and quantitation. Acta Derm Venereol 1986;66(1):16–22.
31. Leder LD. Intraepidermal mast cells and their origin. Am J Dermatopathol 1981; 3(3):247–50.
32. Wolff K, Komar M, Petzelbauer P. Clinical and histopathological aspects of cutaneous mastocytosis. Leuk Res 2001;25(7):519–28.
33. Orkin M, Good RA, Clawson CC, et al. Bullous mastocytosis. Arch Dermatol 1970;101(5):547–64.
34. Hollmann TJ, Brenn T, Hornick JL. CD25 expression on cutaneous mast cells from adult patients presenting with urticaria pigmentosa is predictive of systemic mastocytosis. Am J Surg Pathol 2008;32(1):139–45.
35. Parks A, Camisa C. Reddish-brown macules with telangiectasia and pruritus. Urticaria pigmentosa-telangiectasia macularis eruptiva perstans (TMEP) variant, with systemic mastocytosis. Arch Dermatol 1988;124(3):429–30, 432–433.
36. Sarkany RP, Monk BE, Handfield-Jones SE. Telangiectasia macularis eruptiva perstans: a case report and review of the literature. Clin Exp Dermatol 1998; 23(1):38–9.
37. Gibbs NF, Friedlander SF, Harpster EF. Telangiectasia macularis eruptiva perstans. Pediatr Dermatol 2000;17(3):194–7.
38. Lee HW, Jeong YI, Choi JC, et al. Two cases of telangiectasia macularis eruptiva perstans demonstrated by immunohistochemistry for c-kit (CD 117). J Dermatol 2005;32(10):817–20.
39. Kiszewski AE, Alvarez-Mendoza A, Rios-Barrera VA, et al. Mastocytosis in children: clinicopathological study based on 35 cases. Histol Histopathol 2007; 22(5):535–9.
40. Caplan RM. The natural course of urticaria pigmentosa. Analysis and follow-up of 112 cases. Arch Dermatol 1963;87:146–57.
41. Lee HP, Yoon DH, Kim CW, et al. Solitary mastocytoma on the palm. Pediatr Dermatol 1998;15(5):386–7.
42. Kamysz JJ, Fretzin DF. Necrobiosis in solitary mastocytoma: coincidence or pathogenesis? J Cutan Pathol 1994;21(2):179–82.
43. Wood C, Sina B, Webster CG, et al. Fibrous mastocytoma in a patient with generalized cutaneous mastocytosis. J Cutan Pathol 1992;19(2):128–33.
44. Willemze R, Ruiter DJ, Scheffer E, et al. Diffuse cutaneous mastocytosis with multiple cutaneous mastocytomas. Report of a case with clinical, histopathological and ultrastructural aspects. Br J Dermatol 1980;102(5):601–7.
45. Wawrzycki B, Pietrzak A, Chodorowska G, et al. Diffuse cutaneous bullous mastocytosis in a newborn. Dermatol Ther 2013;26(2):176–9.
46. Golitz LE, Weston WL, Lane AT. Bullous mastocytosis: diffuse cutaneous mastocytosis with extensive blisters mimicking scalded skin syndrome or erythema multiforme. Pediatr Dermatol 1984;1(4):288–94.

47. Oku T, Hashizume H, Yokote R, et al. The familial occurrence of bullous mastocytosis (diffuse cutaneous mastocytosis). Arch Dermatol 1990;126(11):1478–84.

48. Oranje AP, Soekanto W, Sukardi A, et al. Diffuse cutaneous mastocytosis mimicking staphylococcal scalded-skin syndrome: report of three cases. Pediatr Dermatol 1991;8(2):147–51.

49. Bankova LG, Walter JE, Iyengar SR, et al. Generalized bullous eruption after routine vaccination in a child with diffuse cutaneous mastocytosis. J Allergy Clin Immunol Pract 2013;1(1):94–6.

50. Jensen RT. Gastrointestinal abnormalities and involvement in systemic mastocytosis. Hematol Oncol Clin North Am 2000;14(3):579–623.

51. Kirsch R, Geboes K, Shepherd NA, et al. Systemic mastocytosis involving the gastrointestinal tract: clinicopathologic and molecular study of five cases. Mod Pathol 2008;21(12):1508–16.

52. Lee JK, Whittaker SJ, Enns RA, et al. Gastrointestinal manifestations of systemic mastocytosis. World J Gastroenterol 2008;14(45):7005–8.

53. Scolapio JS, Wolfe J 3rd, Malavet P, et al. Endoscopic findings in systemic mastocytosis. Gastrointest Endosc 1996;44(5):608–10.

54. Ammann RW, Vetter D, Deyhle P, et al. Gastrointestinal involvement in systemic mastocytosis. Gut 1976;17(2):107–12.

55. Arguedas MR, Ferrante D. Systemic mastocytosis and giant gastroduodenal ulcer. Gastrointest Endosc 2001;54(4):530–3.

56. Bedeir A, Jukic DM, Wang L, et al. Systemic mastocytosis mimicking inflammatory bowel disease: a case report and discussion of gastrointestinal pathology in systemic mastocytosis. Am J Surg Pathol 2006;30(11):1478–82.

57. Behdad A, Owens SR. Systemic mastocytosis involving the gastrointestinal tract: case report and review. Arch Pathol Lab Med 2013;137(9):1220–3.

58. Tebbe B, Stavropoulos PG, Krasagakis K, et al. Cutaneous mastocytosis in adults. Evaluation of 14 patients with respect to systemic disease manifestations. Dermatology 1998;197(2):101–8.

59. Sokol H, Georgin-Lavialle S, Canioni D, et al. Gastrointestinal manifestations in mastocytosis: a study of 83 patients. J Allergy Clin Immunol 2013;132(4):866–73.

60. Horny HP, Kaiserling E, Campbell M, et al. Liver findings in generalized mastocytosis. A clinicopathologic study. Cancer 1989;63(3):532–8.

61. Metcalfe DD. The liver, spleen, and lymph nodes in mastocytosis. J Invest Dermatol 1991;96(Suppl 3):45S–6S [discussion: 46S, 60S–65S].

62. Horny HP, Ruck MT, Kaiserling E. Spleen findings in generalized mastocytosis. A clinicopathologic study. Cancer 1992;70(2):459–68.

63. Horny HP, Kaiserling E, Parwaresch MR, et al. Lymph node findings in generalized mastocytosis. Histopathology 1992;21(5):439–46.

64. Horny HP, Parwaresch MR, Kaiserling E, et al. Mast cell sarcoma of the larynx. J Clin Pathol 1986;39(6):596–602.

65. Ryan RJ, Akin C, Castells M, et al. Mast cell sarcoma: a rare and potentially under-recognized diagnostic entity with specific therapeutic implications. Mod Pathol 2013;26(4):533–43.

66. Bugalia A, Abraham A, Balasubramanian P, et al. Mast cell sarcoma of the small intestine: a case report. J Clin Pathol 2011;64(11):1035–7.

67. Kojima M, Nakamura S, Itoh H, et al. Mast cell sarcoma with tissue eosinophilia arising in the ascending colon. Mod Pathol 1999;12(7):739–43.

68. Kim YS, Wu H, Pawlowska AB, et al. Pediatric mast cell sarcoma of temporal bone with novel L799F (2395 C>T) KIT mutation, mimicking histiocytic neoplasm. Am J Surg Pathol 2013;37(3):453–8.

69. Brcic L, Vuletic LB, Stepan J, et al. Mast-cell sarcoma of the tibia. J Clin Pathol 2007;60(4):424–5.
70. Georgin-Lavialle S, Aguilar C, Guieze R, et al. Mast cell sarcoma: a rare and aggressive entity–report of two cases and review of the literature. J Clin Oncol 2013;31(6):e90–7.
71. Ma HB, Xu X, Liu WP, et al. Successful treatment of mast cell sarcoma of the uterus with imatinib. Int J Hematol 2011;94(5):491–4.
72. Auquit-Auckbur I, Lazar C, Deneuve S, et al. Malignant transformation of mastocytoma developed on skin mastocytosis into cutaneous mast cell sarcoma. Am J Surg Pathol 2012;36(5):779–82.
73. Bautista-Quach MA, Booth CL, Kheradpour A, et al. Mast cell sarcoma in an infant: a case report and review of the literature. J Pediatr Hematol Oncol 2013; 35(4):315–20.
74. Sperr WR, Escribano L, Jordan JH, et al. Morphologic properties of neoplastic mast cells: delineation of stages of maturation and implication for cytological grading of mastocytosis. Leuk Res 2001;25(7):529–36.

CD30 in Systemic Mastocytosis

Bjorn van Anrooij, BSc[a], Philip M. Kluin, MD, PhD[b],
Joanne N.G. Oude Elberink, MD, PhD[a],
Johanna C. Kluin-Nelemans, MD, PhD[c],*

KEYWORDS

- CD30 • Soluble CD30 • CD30 ligand • CD153 • Systemic mastocytosis

KEY POINTS

- Mast cells from mastocytosis patients frequently aberrantly express CD30, the detection of which can especially aid in establishing the diagnosis of well-differentiated systemic mastocytosis, although other CD30 expressing neoplasms must be considered.
- Expression of CD30 by mast cells is stronger in patients with a high mast cell load; further research is needed to determine whether analysis of CD30 expression can aid identification of advanced subtypes of mastocytosis.
- Mast cell–expressed CD30 and release of soluble CD30 can interfere with normal CD30-CD30L interactions, the effects of which need further investigation.
- Investigations are under way to determine the effects of CD30 expression on mast cell proliferation, hymenoptera venom allergy, and the effectiveness of an anti-CD30 antibody for the treatment of advanced systemic mastocytosis and mast cell leukemia.

INTRODUCTION

The CD30 receptor is similar to mastocytosis itself, in that it constitutes one of the rare bridges between the disciplines of hematology and allergology. Originally CD30 was identified as an antigen expressed by the malignant Reed-Sternberg cells of Hodgkin lymphoma.[1] Expression of CD30 is still widely used in this manner, identifying and prognosticating a variety of hematologic malignancies.[2,3] However, after identifying CD30 as a functional receptor,[4,5] attention has expanded to the role of CD30 in immunity in general and allergic diseases in particular.[6,7] With the discovery of mast cell–expressed CD30 as a marker of systemic mastocytosis, CD30 research has come full circle, further intertwining allergology and hematology.[8] This article aims to

The authors have nothing to disclose.
[a] Department of Allergology, Groningen Research Institute of Asthma and COPD, University Medical Center Groningen, University of Groningen, Groningen, The Netherlands; [b] Department of Pathology and Medical Biology, University Medical Center Groningen, University of Groningen, Groningen, The Netherlands; [c] Department of Hematology, University Medical Center Groningen, University of Groningen, Hanzeplein 1, Groningen 9713 GZ, The Netherlands
* Corresponding author.
E-mail address: j.c.kluin@umcg.nl

summarize the basic science of the CD30 receptor in disease and health, with emphasis on translating bench research to clinical applications relevant for systemic mastocytosis.

THE CD30 RECEPTOR AND ITS LIGAND CD30L

CD30 is encoded for by the tumor necrosis factor receptor superfamily 8 gene (TNFRSF-8).[4] As the name implies, CD30 is sequentially and functionally homologous to the other members of the TNFRSF, such as CD40, RANK, and CD27.[9] The TNFRSF-8 gene is located on chromosome 1p36, and transcription and translation of TNFRSF-8 results in the 105- to 120-kDa transmembrane receptor protein CD30.[9–11]

The same gene can, through alternative splicing, be translated into a 25 kDa cytoplasmic protein called CD30 variant (CD30v), which lacks the transmembrane portion.[12] However, the role of CD30v in health and disease is poorly understood and therefore are not extensively reviewed here. The transmembrane portion of CD30 can strongly bind its ligand CD30L, resulting in downstream signaling in the CD30-expressing cell through tumor necrosis factor (TNF) receptor associated factor (TRAF) 1, 2, 3, and 5, resulting in activation of nuclear factor (NF)-κB and the mitogen-activated protein (MAP) kinase kinases.[13] As is common in the TNF family, binding of CD30L by CD30 results in downstream signaling in the CD30L-expressing cell through reverse signaling as well.[14] The result of this is that both the CD30-expressing and the CD30L-expressing cells receive a transmembrane signal after ligation.

SOLUBLE CD30 AND SCD30L

The final player known to influence CD30-CD30L interactions is the soluble forms of CD30 (sCD30). The metalloproteinases ADAM10 and ADAM17 proteolytically cleave the extracellular portion of the CD30 receptor, resulting in the 85 kDa protein sCD30.[15,16] There is in vitro evidence that cleaving of CD30 and the subsequent release of sCD30 is enhanced by binding of CD30 to CD30L, raising the possibility that sCD30 levels reflect the amount of CD30-CD30L signaling.[17] Levels of sCD30 are clinically relevant, as sCD30 is biologically active. By high-affinity binding to CD30L, sCD30 reduces CD30 transmembrane signaling through competitive antagonism, acting as a negative feedback loop for CD30 signaling through reduction of available CD30L.[18]

In addition, sCD30 itself stimulates additional cleaving of CD30 by the metalloproteinases.[19] Concurrently a sCD30 homologue has been demonstrated to induce transmembrane signaling in CD30L-expressing cells through reverse signaling.[20] Taken together, these investigations illustrate that sCD30 possesses the unique property of being able to reduce CD30 signaling while stimulating CD30L signaling. An overview of all the players influencing the signaling cascades of CD30 is given in **Fig. 1**. Although soluble CD30L (sCD30L) can be detected in serum, its origin and biological effects have not been thoroughly investigated, and both signal-inducing and antagonistic binding has been reported for sCD30L fusion proteins depending on trimerization and immobilization.[21]

EXPRESSION OF CD30 AND CD30L IN PHYSIOLOGY

Under physiologic conditions, expression of CD30 (CD30+) is restricted to a small population of cells, yet expression has been reported to be inducible in a variety of lymphocytes and leukocytes.[7] Mast cells do not express CD30 under these conditions. During neonatal development, transient expression of CD30 is frequent in a

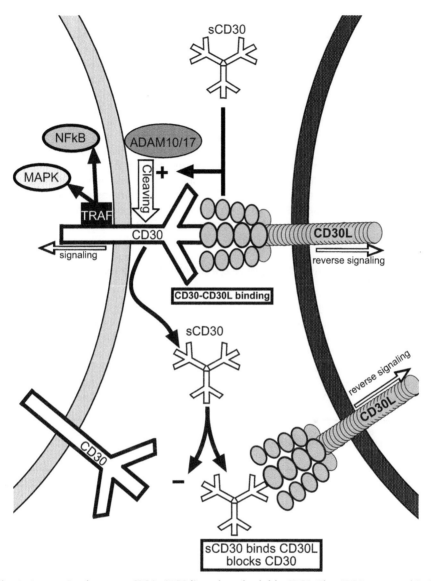

Fig. 1. Interaction between CD30, CD30 ligand, and soluble CD30. The CD30 receptor binds to CD30 ligand (CD30L), initiating transmembrane signaling in both the CD30-expressing cell and the CD30L-expressing cell. CD30 signaling activates the TRAF-MAPK-NFkB signaling cascade. ADAM10/17 cleaves the extracellular portion of CD30, producing sCD30. Cleaving of CD30 by ADAM10/17 is stimulated by ligation of CD30 and circulating sCD30. CD30L is bound by sCD30 with a high affinity, leading to CD30L reverse signaling and reducing CD30 transmembrane signaling. CD30L, CD30 ligand; MAPK, mitogen-activated protein kinases; NFkB, nuclear factor κB; sCD30, soluble CD30; TRAF, tumor necrosis factor receptor–associated factor.

large variety of embryonal tissues.[22] Most CD30+ cells and, subsequently, the greatest sources of circulating sCD30 in adult physiologic conditions are thought to be activated B and T cells.[23] Compared with CD30, expression of CD30L is more prevalent, with CD30L expression in both resting and activated cells of the myeloid and lymphoid lineage, including mast cells.[24,25] There is considerable controversy regarding the expression of CD30 and CD30L on cell types between investigations. This discord in findings presumably reflects differences in methodology. For instance, the initially reported expression of CD30 by macrophages was found to be due to the affinity of an Fc-receptor–like binding site for murine immunoglobulin (Ig)G3 on macrophages binding to the used Ki-1 monoclonal antibody.[26] The anti-CD30 IgG1 antibody Ber-H2 could not detect expression of CD30 on macrophages.[27] Another important consideration is that sCD30 can act as a bridging protein between CD30L and anti-CD30, thereby offering sites for anti-CD30 antibodies to bind, resulting in the possibility of a weak false-positive signal.[15] An overview of cells expressing CD30 and/or CD30L is given in **Table 1**. Increased expression of CD30 and release of sCD30 has been associated with various diseases.

EXPRESSION OF CD30 AND SCD30 IN ALLERGIC AND IMMUNOLOGIC DISEASES

Immunologic diseases associated with increased levels of sCD30 have been extensively reviewed.[41] Traditionally, upregulation of CD30 and increased levels of sCD30 were thought to reflect a T-helper (Th)2-skewed immune system.[6] Accordingly, elevated levels of sCD30 have been found in various Th2-dominated diseases, such as atopic dermatitis,[42] hymenoptera venom allergy,[43] and Graves disease.[44] However, increase in expression and release of sCD30 have also been found in Th1-dominated diseases, such as colitis ulcerosa,[45] and granulomatosis with polyangiitis.[46] The current paradigm is that sCD30 levels in immunologic diseases reflect the activation

Table 1
Expression of CD30 and CD30L in adult physiologic conditions

CD30+			CD30L+		
Cell Type	Characteristics	References	Cell Type	Characteristics	References
T cell	Activated T cells Memory T cells	7,28	T cell	Activated T cells	24
B cell	Activated B cells Epstein-Barr transformed B cells	7,27	B cell	Predominantly lymphoid cells	29,30
Plasma cells	Disputed	31	Neutrophils	—	14,25
Macrophages	Disputed	26,27	Mast cells	—	32
NK cells	Induced	33	Dendritic cells	Mostly immature DCs	34
Extrafollicular lymphoid blasts	Partial coexpression of AID	7,35	Medullary epithelial cells	Hassall corpuscles	36
Eosinophils	Low expression	37	Eosinophils	—	38
Embryonal cells	—	22,39			
Decidual cells	—	39,40			

Abbreviations: AID, activation-induced cytidine deaminase; DC, dendritic cell; NK, natural killer.

states of the B cells and T cells, not necessarily the Th cell differentiation stage.[23] Levels of sCD30 can be also be increased by aberrant expression of CD30 on malignant cells.

EXPRESSION OF CD30 AND SCD30 IN MALIGNANCY

Aberrant expression of CD30 and elevated levels of sCD30 has been reported in a large variety of malignancies. Mastocytosis has recently been added to the list of CD30-expressing neoplasms. Initially, CD30 expression on mast cells was reported to indicate advanced forms of mastocytosis, such as aggressive systemic mastocytosis and smoldering systemic mastocytosis.[8] Follow-up studies report more widespread expression of CD30, with CD30-expressing mast cells being frequently found in cutaneous mastocytosis (CM) and indolent systemic mastocytosis (ISM) as well.[47–49] Moreover, the authors have found mastocytosis to be associated with marked elevations of sCD30 in serum for both patients with advanced systemic mastocytosis and those with ISM, correlating with the mast cell load (article in preparation). For further details, see the section "Soluble CD30 and mastocytosis." Determination of CD30 expression and levels of sCD30 have proved to be clinically relevant for other malignancies as both diagnostic and prognostic tools. For instance, CD30 expression is used for establishing the diagnosis of Hodgkin lymphoma and anaplastic large-cell lymphoma.[50,51] In addition, CD30 identifies a subcategory of diffuse large B-cell lymphoma, with a better disease-free and overall survival.[51] In contrast to CD30, aberrant expression of CD30L is not used as a marker for malignancy and has not been associated with a clinical phenotype. Expression of CD30L in malignancy is therefore not reviewed here.

The soluble form of CD30 has been successfully used as a parameter of tumor burden in Hodgkin lymphoma, and a high level of serum sCD30 is an independent predictor for lower survival in Hodgkin lymphoma and CD30+ cutaneous lymphomas.[52–54] **Table 2** shows malignancies associated with frequent expression of

Table 2
Malignancies frequently expressing CD30

	CD30 Clinical Relevance		CD30 of Unknown Relevance	
Tumor Type	Clinical Importance	References	Tumor Type	References
Classic Hodgkin lymphoma	Diagnosis sCD30 predicts survival	54,55	Enteropathy-associated T-cell lymphoma	56
Anaplastic large cell lymphoma	Diagnosis	50	Follicular lymphoma	57
Lymphomatoid papulosis	Diagnosis	58	Primary mediastinal B-cell lymphoma	59
Embryonal carcinoma	Diagnosis	60	Primary effusion lymphoma	61
Mastocytosis	Diagnosis	48,49,62	Acute myeloid leukemia	63
Diffuse large B-cell lymphoma	Prognosis	51		
NK/T-cell lymphoma	Prognosis	64		
Mycosis fungoides	Prognosis	65		
Adult T-cell lymphoma/ leukemia	sCD30 predicts prognosis	66,67		

CD30 and the clinical significance of CD30. The expression of CD30 can provide information on the etiology of malignant cells. The Epstein-Barr virus (EBV) and human T-cell leukemia virus types 1 and 2 are capable of transforming and inducing CD30 expression on human lymphocytes. Both are implicated in the pathogenesis of CD30+ neoplasms, and the EBV genome is preferentially found in CD30+ non-Hodgkin lymphoma.[68–70]

FUNCTIONAL ROLE OF CD30 IN PROLIFERATION AND APOPTOSIS

The role of CD30 in neoplastic and immunologic diseases is not limited to CD30 as a marker of malignancy or activation. The signals provided by interaction between CD30 and CD30L have been mechanistically implicated in several physiologic and pathologic processes. Initially it was discovered that ligation of CD30 expressed on Hodgkin lymphoma cell lines resulted in increased proliferation and survival of the malignant cells,[71,72] although results varied depending on the cell line used.[72,73] Dissimilarly, in anaplastic large-cell lymphoma cell lines, CD30 signaling resulted in inhibition of proliferation and increased apoptosis.[73,74] Signaling through CD30 has a potent effect on eosinophils, inducing rapid apoptosis.[37] Antagonistic binding of CD30L by Hodgkin lymphoma–derived sCD30 has been speculated to be responsible for the correlation between sCD30 and eosinophilia in Hodgkin lymphoma.[37,75] Eosinophilia is common in mastocytosis as well, and it is tempting to speculate on a possible inverse association between mast cell–derived sCD30 and concomitant eosinophilia. The observation that mastocytosis-associated mast cells express both CD30 and CD30L raises the question whether autocrine signaling plays a part in the pathogenesis of mastocytosis.[8] At present, an investigation by Valent at the Medical University of Vienna is under way to address this question, using CD30-expressing human mastocytosis cell models to determine the effect of CD30 signaling on proliferation and apoptosis.

FUNCTION OF CD30 IN THE ADAPTIVE IMMUNE SYSTEM

In murine and human studies, CD30 and CD30L signaling between B and T lymphocytes has been found to be an important signaling event in the maintenance of the adaptive immune system by regulating memory antibody responses and Ig class switching to IgE and IgG.[76–78] In mice, abrogation of CD30-CD30L signaling using knockout models or antagonistic antibodies for CD30L reduced allergic lung inflammation, allergic rhinitis, and specific IgE levels.[79–81] In vitro experiments with human cells found a similar effect for CD30-CD30L signaling on isotype switching.[82] Studies with natural killer cells found an increase in the production of interferon-γ and TNF-α.[32]

FUNCTIONAL ROLE FOR CD30L SIGNALING IN MASTOCYTOSIS

When interpreting the literature it is important to consider the difficulty of differentiating between effects of CD30 and CD30L transmembrane signaling. For instance, some previous reports should be interpreted with care, as the human mast cell line HMC-1 was used as CD30L+ cells to stimulate CD30+ cells, whereas it is now known that this cell line also expresses CD30, opening up the possibility of CD30L reverse signaling in the cells under investigation.[15,34] Reverse CD30L signaling has been found to stimulate dendritic cell cytokine secretion and maturation.[34] Important for mastocytosis is the report that reverse signaling through human mast cell–expressed CD30L stimulates degranulation-independent release of chemokines, raising the question as to whether these signals are responsible for part of the mediator release symptoms of mastocytosis.[83] The authors have found no correlation between sCD30, a possible inducer of CD30L reverse signaling, and mediator release symptoms such as flushing, pruritus, and diarrhea in a pilot investigation in 79 patients with systemic mastocytosis (van Anrooij and colleagues, unpublished data, 2013).

EFFECTS OF MASTOCYTOSIS-EXPRESSED CD30 ON IMMUNE HOMEOSTASIS

The effect of CD30 expression in mastocytosis on its environment, such as CD30- and CD30L-expressing B/T cells, could be profound. Expression of CD30 by Hodgkin lymphoma cells has been shown to suppress T-cell proliferation, contributing to an ineffective antitumor response.[84] A similar immune escape mechanism could be present in mastocytosis. Antibody production and IgE biology specifically may be profoundly affected, the latter being of importance considering the frequent IgE-mediated anaphylactic reactions in ISM patients. The induced expression of CD30 on T cells found in (B-cell) chronic lymphocytic leukemia impairs isotope switching through reverse signaling in CD30L-expressing B cells.[85] Furthermore, sCD30 derived from CD30-expressing malignancies reduces the availability of CD30L by antagonistic binding.[18] These antagonistic properties of sCD30 may mimic the earlier mentioned specific IgE-suppressing effects of antagonistic anti-CD30L antibodies.[81,86] The authors have found that levels of sCD30 inversely correlate with hymenoptera venom–specific IgE levels (article in preparation). For further details, see the section "Soluble CD30 and mastocytosis." Antagonistic binding of CD30L by mastocytosis-derived sCD30 downregulating CD30-CD30L interactions may partially explain the lower levels of specific IgE found in allergic mastocytosis patients compared with allergic nonmastocytosis patients.[87]

THE DIAGNOSTIC APPLICABILITY OF CD30 IN MASTOCYTOSIS

The limited expression profile of CD30 makes it attractive both as a marker of disease and as a therapeutic target. Using flow cytometry, identification of CD30 expression on mast cells has sensitivity of 80% and specificity of 95% for diagnosing systemic mastocytosis.[62] In addition, the CD30 marker improves on the performance of the standard flow-cytometric mast cell markers for mastocytosis, CD2 and CD25, by reliably identifying the well-differentiated subcategory of mastocytosis.[62] For the identification of CD30 expression in mastocytosis, flow cytometry has proved to be more sensitive than immunohistochemistry.[62] Nevertheless, immunohistochemical staining for CD30 can aid in supporting the diagnosis of mastocytosis. As discussed previously, CD30+ cells in bone marrow or skin tissue are rare, and CD30 expression is not seen in related diseases such as monoclonal mast cell activation syndrome.[49]

CD30 AS A MARKER OF ADVANCED SYSTEMIC MASTOCYTOSIS

At present the classification of systemic mastocytosis relies on evidence of organ dysfunction, as markers identifying the advanced and potentially life-threatening forms of systemic mastocytosis are unavailable.[88] As the authors have previously described, the applicability of CD30 as a marker of advanced forms of systemic mastocytosis is not yet clear. Initially CD30 expression was reported in 85% of patients with advanced systemic mastocytosis, compared with 27% with indolent systemic mastocytosis.[8] Follow-up investigations found CD30 expression in 50% of patients with cutaneous mastocytosis and in 23% to 100% of ISM patients using immunohistochemistry.[48,49,49–69,68–81] Differences in grading criteria and methodology explain these conflicting results and make comparison of data difficult. For instance, the initial investigation revealing expression of CD30 in 12 of 45 ISM patient samples used expression of CD30 on more than 10% of mast cells as a cutoff point,[8] whereas in a small follow-up study using expression of CD30 on greater than 5% of mast cells it appeared that all (3 of 3) ISM patients expressed CD30.[49] Similarly, the original investigation revealed no expression of CD30 in bone marrow for CM patients,[8] whereas a follow-up investigation found CD30 expression in 6 of 12 CM patients when investigating skin biopsy samples.[49] **Table 3** displays the results of CD30 immunohistochemistry per category of mastocytosis. Taken together, these preliminary results suggest that CD30 is not a reliable marker for advanced systemic mastocytosis. One common finding in these reports is that CD30 expression seems to be higher in patients with greater mast cell burden, which is in accordance with the authors' own findings with sCD30.

SOLUBLE CD30 AND MASTOCYTOSIS

The authors have found that levels of sCD30 in serum are elevated in all categories of systemic mastocytosis and correlate with the mast cell burden as evidenced by baseline serum tryptase, irrespective of grading (article in preparation). Because elevated levels of sCD30 can be found in a large variety of diseases, measurement of sCD30 cannot substitute for baseline serum tryptase as a screening tool for systemic mastocytosis. Although the authors have found sCD30 levels to be significantly higher in advanced forms of systemic mastocytosis in comparison with ISM, levels of sCD30 did not predict for survival in patients with advanced systemic mastocytosis (article in preparation). Clinical significance for sCD30 may be found in the relationship with hymenoptera venom allergy. The authors previously noted that a higher mast cell load reduces the risk of hymenoptera venom anaphylaxis in systemic mastocytosis.[89] As a possible cause, aberrant expression of CD30 was noted. It was hypothesized that mast cell–derived CD30 and sCD30 interfering with constitutional CD30-CD30L interactions might lower the risk of hymenoptera venom anaphylaxis. The authors have found sCD30 levels to be significantly lower in ISM patients with a history of hymenoptera venom anaphylaxis than in ISM patients without such history. Furthermore, sCD30 levels were found to predict for a lower risk of hymenoptera venom anaphylaxis and to be associated with lower levels of wasp venom–specific IgE (article in preparation). The applicability of sCD30 as an identifier for patients at risk of hymenoptera anaphylaxis needs to be further investigated before clinical recommendations can be made.

CD30 AS A TARGET FOR CYTOREDUCTIVE THERAPY

The infrequent expression of CD30 in physiologic conditions assures a high specificity for targeted treatment. In line with this, investigations using monoclonal antibodies directed at the CD30 antigen have resulted in an overall benign safety and tolerability profile.[90,91] However, the efficacy of these antibodies in CD30+ lymphomas was lacking.[91] The finding that the CD30 receptor is internalized makes it an attractive target for antibody-drug conjugates. Recently, the antibody-drug conjugate SNG-35/brentuximab vedotin has proved to be both tolerable and effective in inducing tumor regression.[92] These findings have resulted in the Food and Drug Administration granting accelerated approval of SGN35/brentuximab vedotin for the treatment of relapsed Hodgkin lymphoma and relapsed anaplastic large-cell lymphoma.[93] SNG-35/brentuximab vedotin consists of an anti-CD30 chimeric monoclonal antibody coupled to monomethyl-auristatin E, a microtubule toxin that inhibits cell division on internalization. These reports raise the question as to whether similar results for anti-CD30 monoclonal antibodies can be achieved in mastocytosis. To answer this question,

Table 3
Expression profile of CD30 in mastocytosis

Classification	Sotlar et al,[8] 2011 IHC — CD30 >10% Mast Cells	Arredondo et al,[49] 2011 IHC — CD30 >5% Mast Cells	Moonim et al, 2012 IHC — NR	Chiu et al,[48] 2013 IHC — NR	Morgado et al,[62] 2013 IHC — CD30 >10% Mast Cells	Morgado et al,[62] 2013 FCM — CD30 MFI >2 rSD Background MFI
CM	0/3 (0%)	6/12 (50%)	—	—	—	—
ISM	12/45 (27%)	3/3 (100%)	10/26 (38%)	0/11 (0%)	13/57 (23%)	89/123 (80%)
SSM	2/2 (100%)	0/2 (0%)	2/2 (100%)	—	—	—
SM-AHNMD	—	6/11 (55%)	6/12 (50%)	6/19 (32%)	—	—
ASM	5/5 (100%)	3/3 (100%)	2/3 (67%)	6/11 (55%)	5/7 (71%)	8/8 (100%)
MCL	5/7 (71%)	4/4 (100%)	—	1/2 (50%)	—	0/2 (0%)

Abbreviations: ASM, aggressive systemic mastocytosis; CM, cutaneous mastocytosis; FCM, flow cytometry; IHC, immunohistochemistry; ISM, indolent systemic mastocytosis; MCL, mast cell leukemia; MFI, median fluorescence intensity; NR, not reported; rSD, robust standard deviation; SM-AHNMD, systemic mastocytosis with an associated hematologic non–mast cell lineage disorder; SSM, smoldering systemic mastocytosis.

a single-arm open-label trial for SGN-35 in aggressive systemic mastocytosis and mast cell leukemia is under way (ClinicalTrials.gov number NCT01807598).

SUMMARY

In physiologic conditions, CD30 is a receptor with an expression profile limited to activated B and T cells, and is implicated in the regulation of proliferation and antibody production. The expression of CD30 by mastocytosis mast cells may influence the clinical phenotype and (future) management of mastocytosis.

REFERENCES

1. Schwab U, Stein H, Gerdes J, et al. Production of a monoclonal antibody specific for Hodgkin and Sternberg-Reed cells of Hodgkin's disease and a subset of normal lymphoid cells. Nature 1982;299(5878):65–7.
2. Savage KJ, Harris NL, Vose JM, et al. ALK- anaplastic large-cell lymphoma is clinically and immunophenotypically different from both ALK+ ALCL and peripheral T-cell lymphoma, not otherwise specified: report from the international peripheral T-cell lymphoma project. Blood 2008;111(12):5496–504.
3. Swerdlow SH. 4th edition. International Agency for Research on Cancer. WHO classification of tumours of haematopoietic and lymphoid tissues, vol. 15. Lyon (France): International Agency for Research on Cancer IARC; 2008. p. 439.
4. Durkop H, Latza U, Hummel M, et al. Molecular cloning and expression of a new member of the nerve growth factor receptor family that is characteristic for Hodgkin's disease. Cell 1992;68(3):421–7.
5. Smith CA, Gruss HJ, Davis T, et al. CD30 antigen, a marker for Hodgkin's lymphoma, is a receptor whose ligand defines an emerging family of cytokines with homology to TNF. Cell 1993;73(7):1349–60.
6. Romagnani S, Del Prete G, Maggi E, et al. CD30 and type 2 T helper (Th2) responses. J Leukoc Biol 1995;57(5):726–30.
7. Falini B, Pileri S, Pizzolo G, et al. CD30 (ki-1) molecule: a new cytokine receptor of the tumor necrosis factor receptor superfamily as a tool for diagnosis and immunotherapy. Blood 1995;85(1):1–14.
8. Sotlar K, Cerny-Reiterer S, Petat-Dutter K, et al. Aberrant expression of CD30 in neoplastic mast cells in high-grade mastocytosis. Mod Pathol 2011;24(4): 585–95.
9. Aizawa S, Satoh H, Horie R, et al. Cloning and characterization of a cDNA for rat CD30 homolog and chromosomal assignment of the genomic gene. Gene 1996; 182(1–2):155–62.
10. Fonatsch C, Latza U, Durkop H, et al. Assignment of the human CD30 (ki-1) gene to 1p36. Genomics 1992;14(3):825–6.
11. Froese P, Lemke H, Gerdes J, et al. Biochemical characterization and biosynthesis of the ki-1 antigen in Hodgkin-derived and virus-transformed human B and T lymphoid cell lines. J Immunol 1987;139(6):2081–7.
12. Horie R, Ito K, Tatewaki M, et al. A variant CD30 protein lacking extracellular and transmembrane domains is induced in HL-60 by tetradecanoylphorbol acetate and is expressed in alveolar macrophages. Blood 1996;88(7):2422–32.
13. Schneider C, Hubinger G. Pleiotropic signal transduction mediated by human CD30: a member of the tumor necrosis factor receptor (TNFR) family. Leuk Lymphoma 2002;43(7):1355–66.
14. Wiley SR, Goodwin RG, Smith CA. Reverse signaling via CD30 ligand. J Immunol 1996;157(8):3635–9.

15. Eichenauer DA, Simhadri VL, von Strandmann EP, et al. ADAM10 inhibition of human CD30 shedding increases specificity of targeted immunotherapy in vitro. Cancer Res 2007;67(1):332–8.
16. Hansen HP, Dietrich S, Kisseleva T, et al. CD30 shedding from karpas 299 lymphoma cells is mediated by TNF-alpha-converting enzyme. J Immunol 2000; 165(12):6703–9.
17. Rossi FM, Degan M, Mazzocut-Zecchin L, et al. CD30L up-regulates CD30 and IL-4 expression by T cells. FEBS Lett 2001;508(3):418–22.
18. Hargreaves PG, Al-Shamkhani A. Soluble CD30 binds to CD153 with high affinity and blocks transmembrane signaling by CD30. Eur J Immunol 2002;32(1): 163–73.
19. Hansen HP, Recke A, Reineke U, et al. The ectodomain shedding of CD30 is specifically regulated by peptide motifs in its cysteine-rich domains 2 and 5. FASEB J 2004;18(7):893–5.
20. Saraiva M, Smith P, Fallon PG, et al. Inhibition of type 1 cytokine-mediated inflammation by a soluble CD30 homologue encoded by ectromelia (mousepox) virus. J Exp Med 2002;196(6):829–39.
21. Powell IF, Li T, Jack HM, et al. Construction and expression of a soluble form of human CD30 ligand with functional activity. J Leukoc Biol 1998;63(6):752–7.
22. Tamiolakis D, Maroulis G, Simopoulos C, et al. Human embryonal tissues of all three germ layers can express the CD30 antigen. an immunohistochemical study of 30 fetuses coming after therapeutic abortions from week 8th to week 16th of gestation. Cesk Patol 2006;42(1):9–15.
23. Kennedy MK, Willis CR, Armitage RJ. Deciphering CD30 ligand biology and its role in humoral immunity. Immunology 2006;118(2):143–52.
24. Lane PJ, Gaspal FM, Kim MY. Two sides of a cellular coin: CD4(+)CD3- cells regulate memory responses and lymph-node organization. Nat Rev Immunol 2005;5(8):655–60.
25. Gruss HJ, Pinto A, Gloghini A, et al. CD30 ligand expression in nonmalignant and Hodgkin's disease-involved lymphoid tissues. Am J Pathol 1996;149(2): 469–81.
26. Andreesen R, Brugger W, Lohr GW, et al. Human macrophages can express the Hodgkin's cell-associated antigen ki-1 (CD30). Am J Pathol 1989;134(1):187–92.
27. Durkop H, Foss HD, Eitelbach F, et al. Expression of the CD30 antigen in non-lymphoid tissues and cells. J Pathol 2000;190(5):613–8.
28. Ellis TM, Simms PE, Slivnick DJ, et al. CD30 is a signal-transducing molecule that defines a subset of human activated CD45RO+ T cells. J Immunol 1993; 151(5):2380–9.
29. Klein U, Tu Y, Stolovitzky GA, et al. Transcriptional analysis of the B cell germinal center reaction. Proc Natl Acad Sci U S A 2003;100(5):2639–44.
30. Feldhahn N, Schwering I, Lee S, et al. Silencing of B cell receptor signals in human naive B cells. J Exp Med 2002;196(10):1291–305.
31. Schwarting R, Gerdes J, Durkop H, et al. BER-H2: A new anti-ki-1 (CD30) monoclonal antibody directed at a formol-resistant epitope. Blood 1989;74(5): 1678–89.
32. Cerutti A, Schaffer A, Goodwin RG, et al. Engagement of CD153 (CD30 ligand) by CD30+ T cells inhibits class switch DNA recombination and antibody production in human IgD+ IgM+ B cells. J Immunol 2000;165(2):786–94.
33. Bekiaris V, Gaspal F, McConnell FM, et al. NK cells protect secondary lymphoid tissue from cytomegalovirus via a CD30-dependent mechanism. Eur J Immunol 2009;39(10):2800–8.

34. Simhadri VL, Hansen HP, Simhadri VR, et al. A novel role for reciprocal CD30-CD30L signaling in the cross-talk between natural killer and dendritic cells. Biol Chem 2012;393(1–2):101–6.

35. Cattoretti G, Buttner M, Shaknovich R, et al. Nuclear and cytoplasmic AID in extrafollicular and germinal center B cells. Blood 2006;107(10):3967–75.

36. Romagnani P, Annunziato F, Manetti R, et al. High CD30 ligand expression by epithelial cells and Hassal's corpuscles in the medulla of human thymus. Blood 1998;91(9):3323–32.

37. Matsumoto K, Terakawa M, Miura K, et al. Extremely rapid and intense induction of apoptosis in human eosinophils by anti-CD30 antibody treatment in vitro. J Immunol 2004;172(4):2186–93.

38. Pinto A, Aldinucci D, Gloghini A, et al. Human eosinophils express functional CD30 ligand and stimulate proliferation of a Hodgkin's disease cell line. Blood 1996;88(9):3299–305.

39. Tamiolakis D, Papadoupoulos N, Venizelos I, et al. CD30 (ki-1) molecule expression in human embryonal epithelial cells of the basal layer of the developing epidermis and epidermal buds and its potential significance for embryogenesis. Acta Dermatovenerol Alp Panonica Adriat 2005;14(3):85–90, 92.

40. Ito K, Watanabe T, Horie R, et al. High expression of the CD30 molecule in human decidual cells. Am J Pathol 1994;145(2):276–80.

41. Oflazoglu E, Grewal IS, Gerber H. Targeting CD30/CD30L in oncology and auto-immune and inflammatory diseases. Adv Exp Med Biol 2009;647:174–85.

42. Di Lorenzo G, Gangemi S, Merendino RA, et al. Serum levels of soluble CD30 in adult patients affected by atopic dermatitis and its relation to age, duration of disease and scoring atopic dermatitis index. Mediators Inflamm 2003;12(2):123–5.

43. Foschi FG, Emiliani F, Savini S, et al. CD30 serum levels and response to hymenoptera venom immunotherapy. J Investig Allergol Clin Immunol 2008;18(4):279–83.

44. Phenekos C, Vryonidou A, Gritzapis AD, et al. Th1 and Th2 serum cytokine profiles characterize patients with Hashimoto's thyroiditis (Th1) and graves' disease (Th2). Neuroimmunomodulation 2004;11(4):209–13.

45. Somada S, Muta H, Nakamura K, et al. CD30 ligand/CD30 interaction is involved in pathogenesis of inflammatory bowel disease. Dig Dis Sci 2012;57(8):2031–7.

46. Wang G, Hansen H, Tatsis E, et al. High plasma levels of the soluble form of CD30 activation molecule reflect disease activity in patients with Wegener's granulomatosis. Am J Med 1997;102(6):517–23.

47. Moonim M, Kossier T, van Der Walt J, et al. CD30/CD123 expression in systemic mastocytosis does not correlate with aggressive disease. Poster presented at: 54th Annual Meeting of the American Society of Hematology. Atlanta, GA, December 8, 2012.

48. Chiu A, Czader MB, Ochs RC, et al. Subtypes of systemic mastocytosis exhibit distinct immunomorphologic features in bone marrow biopsies. Lab Invest 2013;93:324A.

49. Arredondo AR, Jennings CD, Shier L, et al. CD30 expression in mastocytosis. Lab Invest 2011;91:285A–6A.

50. Delsol G, Jaffe E, Falini B. Anaplastic large cell lymphoma (ALCL), ALK-positive. In: Swerdlow S, Campo E, Harris N, editors. WHO classification of tumours of haematopoietic and lymphoid tissues. 4th edition. Lyon (France): IARC; 2008. p. 312–6.

51. Hu S, Xu-Monette ZY, Balasubramanyam A, et al. CD30 expression defines a novel subgroup of diffuse large B-cell lymphoma with favorable prognosis and distinct gene expression signature: a report from the international DLBCL rituximab-CHOP consortium program study. Blood 2013;121(14):2715–24.

52. Kadin ME, Pavlov IY, Delgado JC, et al. High soluble CD30, CD25, and IL-6 may identify patients with worse survival in CD30+ cutaneous lymphomas and early mycosis fungoides. J Invest Dermatol 2012;132(3 Pt 1):703–10.

53. Nadali G, Tavecchia L, Zanolin E, et al. Serum level of the soluble form of the CD30 molecule identifies patients with Hodgkin's disease at high risk of unfavorable outcome. Blood 1998;91(8):3011–6.

54. Visco C, Nadali G, Vassilakopoulos TP, et al. Very high levels of soluble CD30 recognize the patients with classical Hodgkin's lymphoma retaining a very poor prognosis. Eur J Haematol 2006;77(5):387–94.

55. von Wasielewski R, Mengel M, Fischer R, et al. Classical Hodgkin's disease. clinical impact of the immunophenotype. Am J Pathol 1997;151(4):1123–30.

56. Delabie J, Holte H, Vose JM, et al. Enteropathy-associated T-cell lymphoma: clinical and histological findings from the international peripheral T-cell lymphoma project. Blood 2011;118(1):148–55.

57. Gardner LJ, Polski JM, Evans HL, et al. CD30 expression in follicular lymphoma. Arch Pathol Lab Med 2001;125(8):1036–41.

58. Kempf W, Pfaltz K, Vermeer MH, et al. EORTC, ISCL, and USCLC consensus recommendations for the treatment of primary cutaneous CD30-positive lymphoproliferative disorders: Lymphomatoid papulosis and primary cutaneous anaplastic large-cell lymphoma. Blood 2011;118(15):4024–35.

59. Pileri SA, Gaidano G, Zinzani PL, et al. Primary mediastinal B-cell lymphoma: High frequency of BCL-6 mutations and consistent expression of the transcription factors OCT-2, BOB.1, and PU.1 in the absence of immunoglobulins. Am J Pathol 2003;162(1):243–53.

60. Leroy X, Augusto D, Leteurtre E, et al. CD30 and CD117 (c-kit) used in combination are useful for distinguishing embryonal carcinoma from seminoma. J Histochem Cytochem 2002;50(2):283–5.

61. Ansari MQ, Dawson DB, Nador R, et al. Primary body cavity-based AIDS-related lymphomas. Am J Clin Pathol 1996;105(2):221–9.

62. Morgado JM, Perbellini O, Johnson RC, et al. CD30 expression by bone marrow mast cells from different diagnostic variants of systemic mastocytosis. Histopathology 2013;63(6):780–7.

63. Zheng W, Medeiros LJ, Hu Y, et al. CD30 expression in high-risk acute myeloid leukemia and myelodysplastic syndromes. Clin Lymphoma Myeloma Leuk 2013;13(3):307–14.

64. Hong J, Park S, Baek HL, et al. Tumor cell nuclear diameter and CD30 expression as potential prognostic parameter in patients with extranodal NK/T-cell lymphoma, nasal type. Int J Clin Exp Pathol 2012;5(9):939–47.

65. Benner MF, Jansen PM, Vermeer MH, et al. Prognostic factors in transformed mycosis fungoides: a retrospective analysis of 100 cases. Blood 2012;119(7):1643–9.

66. Takeshita M, Akamatsu M, Ohshima K, et al. CD30 (ki-1) expression in adult T-cell leukaemia/lymphoma is associated with distinctive immunohistological and clinical characteristics. Histopathology 1995;26(6):539–46.

67. Nishioka C, Takemoto S, Kataoka S, et al. Serum level of soluble CD30 correlates with the aggressiveness of adult T-cell leukemia/lymphoma. Cancer Sci 2005;96(11):810–5.

68. Kanavaros P, Jiwa NM, de Bruin PC, et al. High incidence of EBV genome in CD30-positive non-Hodgkin's lymphomas. J Pathol 1992;168(3):307–15.
69. Herbst H, Stein H. Tumor viruses in CD30-positive anaplastic large cell lymphomas. Leuk Lymphoma 1993;9(4–5):321–8.
70. Niedobitek G. The role of Epstein-Barr virus in the pathogenesis of Hodgkin's disease. Ann Oncol 1996;7(Suppl 4):11–7.
71. Zheng B, Fiumara P, Li YV, et al. MEK/ERK pathway is aberrantly active in Hodgkin disease: a signaling pathway shared by CD30, CD40, and RANK that regulates cell proliferation and survival. Blood 2003;102(3):1019–27.
72. Guo F, Sun A, Wang W, et al. TRAF1 is involved in the classical NF-kappaB activation and CD30-induced alternative activity in Hodgkin's lymphoma cells. Mol Immunol 2009;46(13):2441–8.
73. Hirsch B, Hummel M, Bentink S, et al. CD30-induced signaling is absent in Hodgkin's cells but present in anaplastic large cell lymphoma cells. Am J Pathol 2008;172(2):510–20.
74. Staber PB, Noehammer C, Durkop H, et al. mRNA expression patterns indicate CD30 mediated activation of different apoptosis pathways in anaplastic large cell lymphoma but not in Hodgkin's lymphoma. Leuk Res 2006;30(3):343–8.
75. Horn-Lohrens O, Tiemann M, Lange H, et al. Shedding of the soluble form of CD30 from the Hodgkin-analogous cell line L540 is strongly inhibited by a new CD30-specific antibody (ki-4). Int J Cancer 1995;60(4):539–44.
76. Withers DR, Gaspal FM, Bekiaris V, et al. OX40 and CD30 signals in CD4(+) T-cell effector and memory function: a distinct role for lymphoid tissue inducer cells in maintaining CD4(+) T-cell memory but not effector function. Immunol Rev 2011;244(1):134–48.
77. Gaspal FM, Kim MY, McConnell FM, et al. Mice deficient in OX40 and CD30 signals lack memory antibody responses because of deficient CD4 T cell memory. J Immunol 2005;174(7):3891–6.
78. Shanebeck KD, Maliszewski CR, Kennedy MK, et al. Regulation of murine B cell growth and differentiation by CD30 ligand. Eur J Immunol 1995;25(8):2147–53.
79. Polte T, Fuchs L, Behrendt AK, et al. Different role of CD30 in the development of acute and chronic airway inflammation in a murine asthma model. Eur J Immunol 2009;39(7):1736–42.
80. Nam SY, Kim YH, Do JS, et al. CD30 supports lung inflammation. Int Immunol 2008;20(2):177–84.
81. Fuchiwaki T, Sun X, Fujimura K, et al. The central role of CD30L/CD30 interactions in allergic rhinitis pathogenesis in mice. Eur J Immunol 2011;41(10):2947–54.
82. Molin D, Fischer M, Xiang Z, et al. Mast cells express functional CD30 ligand and are the predominant CD30L-positive cells in Hodgkin's disease. Br J Haematol 2001;114(3):616–23.
83. Fischer M, Harvima IT, Carvalho RF, et al. Mast cell CD30 ligand is upregulated in cutaneous inflammation and mediates degranulation-independent chemokine secretion. J Clin Invest 2006;116(10):2748–56.
84. Su CC, Chiu HH, Chang CC, et al. CD30 is involved in inhibition of T-cell proliferation by Hodgkin's Reed-Sternberg cells. Cancer Res 2004;64(6):2148–52.
85. Cerutti A, Kim EC, Shah S, et al. Dysregulation of CD30+ T cells by leukemia impairs isotype switching in normal B cells. Nat Immunol 2001;2(2):150–6.
86. Polte T, Behrendt AK, Hansen G. Direct evidence for a critical role of CD30 in the development of allergic asthma. J Allergy Clin Immunol 2006;118(4):942–8.

87. Muller U, Helbling A, Hunziker T, et al. Mastocytosis and atopy: a study of 33 patients with urticaria pigmentosa. Allergy 1990;45(8):597–603.

88. Horny HP, Metcalfe DD, Bennett JM, et al. Mastocytosis. In: Swerdlow SH, Campo E, Harris NL, et al, editors. WHO classification of tumours of haemato-poietic and lymphoid tissues. Lyon (France): IARC Press; 2008. p. 54–63.

89. van Anrooij B, van der Veer E, de Monchy JG, et al. Higher mast cell load de-creases the risk of hymenoptera venom-induced anaphylaxis in patients with mastocytosis. J Allergy Clin Immunol 2013;132(1):125–30.

90. Bartlett NL, Younes A, Carabasi MH, et al. A phase 1 multidose study of SGN-30 immunotherapy in patients with refractory or recurrent CD30+ hematologic malignancies. Blood 2008;111(4):1848–54.

91. Ansell SM, Horwitz SM, Engert A, et al. Phase I/II study of an anti-CD30 mono-clonal antibody (MDX-060) in Hodgkin's lymphoma and anaplastic large-cell lymphoma. J Clin Oncol 2007;25(19):2764–9.

92. Younes A, Bartlett NL, Leonard JP, et al. Brentuximab vedotin (SGN-35) for relapsed CD30-positive lymphomas. N Engl J Med 2010;363(19):1812–21.

93. de Claro RA, McGinn K, Kwitkowski V, et al. U.S. food and drug administration approval summary: brentuximab vedotin for the treatment of relapsed Hodgkin lymphoma or relapsed systemic anaplastic large-cell lymphoma. Clin Cancer Res 2012;18(21):5845–9.

Eosinophilia in Mast Cell Disease

Anna Kovalszki, MD[a,*], Peter F. Weller, MD[b,c]

KEYWORDS

- Eosinophilia • Chronic eosinophilic leukemia (CEL) • Hypereosinophilic syndrome
- Systemic mastocytosis • Tryptase • FIP1L1-PDGFRA fusion • Imatinib

KEY POINTS

- The interplay between mast cells and eosinophils is complicated and those interactions are currently being studied.
- Certain clonal and nonclonal entities exist in which these 2 cell types are increased in tissues and other sites, and in which they play a role in pathogenesis.
- The specific type of clonal disorder is important to diagnose correctly, because treatment needs to be carefully tailored to the specific entity.

INTRODUCTION

Eosinophils and mast cells coexist in tissues in some benign conditions, and also in bone marrow biopsies of patients affected by clonal diseases. Some clonal and non-clonal disorders in which mast cells are affected are also associated with peripheral eosinophilia. These disorders include such varied presentations as allergic and asthmatic disorders, eosinophilic esophagitis (EoE), and both clonal and probably nonclonally expanded lines within the category of malignancies.

Discussed are the complex interplay of eosinophils and mast cells in these disorders. Also what is known about these disorders is described, a schematic in thinking about these disorders in one rubric is offered, and treatment options, which are usually tailored specifically to the patient presentation and underlying disorder, if it can be elucidated, are discussed.

MAST CELL AND EOSINOPHIL BIOLOGY
Mast Cells

Mast cells derive from the pluripotent precursor cell (CD34+, CD117+(Kit)). They develop and mature with the influence of stem cell factor (SCF) via Kit, the

The authors have nothing to disclose.
[a] Division of Allergy and Inflammation, Department of Medicine, Beth Israel Deaconess Medical Center, Harvard Medical School, 330 Brookline Avenue, Boston, MA 02215, USA; [b] Division of Allergy and Inflammation, Department of Medicine, Beth Israel Deaconess Medical Center, Harvard Medical School, 330 Brookline Avenue CLS943, Boston, MA 02215, USA; [c] Division of Infectious Diseases, Department of Medicine, Beth Israel Deaconess Medical Center, Harvard Medical School, 330 Brookline Avenue CLS943, Boston, MA 02215, USA
* Corresponding author.
E-mail address: akovalsz@bidmc.harvard.edu

Immunol Allergy Clin N Am 34 (2014) 357–364
http://dx.doi.org/10.1016/j.iac.2014.01.013
0889-8561/14/$ – see front matter © 2014 Elsevier Inc. All rights reserved.

transmembrane tyrosine kinase receptor for SCF.[1] Many other cytokines, including interleukins (IL) IL-3, IL-4, IL-5, IL-6, IL-9, and IL-15, can potentiate the growth and maturation of mast cells.

Mast cells are a rich source of inflammatory mediators which include histamine, prostaglandin D_2, cysteinyl leukotrienes (LTC_4), platelet activating factor, IL-3, IL-5, IL-6, IL-16, and SCF. Mast cell products that likely provide some interaction with eosinophils include IL-5, which is a potent growth and survival factor, CCL5 (RANTES), which is a chemotactic molecule, chymase (eosinophil apoptosis suppressor), tumor necrosis factor (survival and chemotaxis), heparin (stabilize eotaxins), and Kit, which interacts with eosinophil-derived SCF to induce differentiation, proliferation, and activation of mast cells.[2]

Eosinophils

Eosinophils also derive from the pluripotent CD34[+] cell line. Granulocyte-macrophage colony-stimulating factor, IL-3, and IL-5 are all growth factors for eosinophils. IL-5 is the major cytokine that influences eosinophilopoiesis, as well as eliciting their activation and chemotaxis.[3] As discussed above, mast cells do produce both IL-3 and IL-5. Eosinophil mediators include many chemokines and cytokines. A notable feature of eosinophils as a source of cytokines is that they store these cytokines preformed within eosinophil granules and secretory vesicles. Some of these mediators that have potential for mast cell interactions include IL-3, IL-5, IL-6, IL-16, and LTC_4. More recently IL-9 was found to be produced by eosinophils in the context of mast cell interactions in EoE.[4] Platelet activating factor is a known chemoattractant for eosinophils. IL-16, prostaglandin D_2, and LTC_4 are produced by eosinophils and eosinophils express receptors for these agents, enhancing the interaction between mast cells and eosinophils.[5]

Therefore, in addition to interacting with each other, these 2 cells have the capacity to influence the tissue microenvironment, which self-promotes their own existence and attracts cells that help activate and stimulate them into the area (such as TH2 CD4+ T cells, macrophages).

The Mast Cell-Eosinophil Pair

One interesting concept regarding the interaction between them is the existence of the eosinophil and mast cell couplets or pairs, reported in papers from 2011 and 2013.[6,7] The research was mainly done on tissues with allergic inflammation, and the authors found several colocalized pairs of mast cells and eosinophils in human nasal polyps, asthmatic bronchi, as well as in mouse atopic dermatitis tissues. In vitro, they found that the 2 cells form stable conjugates and there is clear membrane contact established between them. Eosinophils were more viable when mast cells were present, dependent on soluble mediators and on physical cell contact (interestingly more so in the presence of SCF-enriched media than in granulocyte-macrophage colony-stimulating factor–enriched media). Mast cells were not as clearly affected or made more viable by eosinophil coculture. They were found to influence each other in a paracrine/physical pathway, using human and murine cells in vitro.[7] This concept is discussed later when discussing the role of anti-IL-5 in EoE.

NONCLONAL DISORDERS IN WHICH BOTH CELLS ARE PRESENT AND LIKELY DRIVE DISEASE PATHOGENESIS
Asthma and Allergic Rhinitis

In allergic disorders, mast cells degranulate in response to immunoglobulin E–mediated allergic stimulation. Mediators released locally recruit eosinophils to cause further damage. Previous work has shown that both cells are present in asthmatic airways more often than in patients without allergic asthma.[8] They are also present in the nasal fluid of patients with allergic rhinitis.[9] Bronchoalveolar lavage (BAL) tryptase level, albeit elevated, however, did not correlate with worse lung function in asthmatic patients. In the same way, in a study done to evaluate tryptase/mast cell burden in eosinophilic pneumonia patients, while tryptase was elevated in BAL of these patients versus normal controls, the actual level of elevation between those patients did not correlate with lung function parameters.[10]

EoE

Both mast cells and eosinophils are present in biopsy specimens of patients with EoE. There is a great mast cell signature in EoE,[11] and the presence of mast cells has been found to be useful in distinguishing between EoE and gastroesophageal reflux disease in biopsy specimens.[12] The relative contribution of both cell types to disease pathogenesis is under investigation. Some patients with EoE respond to anti-IL-5 therapy. In those who respond, mast cells were found to be decreased along with eosinophils after therapy in biopsy specimens.[4] Interestingly, these cells existed as couplets in EoE as with other disorders mentioned above within biopsy specimens. The mechanism under which this occurred was thought to be due to mutual cross-talk as others previously had shown, as well as through the role of IL-9-producing cells (70% of which were eosinophils per their evaluation). IL-9 produced by mostly eosinophils served as a potent mast cell growth factor.

Idiopathic Hypereosinophilic Syndrome

In the general workup of uncharacterized eosinophilia, sometimes one reaches the conclusion that a patient has idiopathic hypereosinophilic syndrome (HES) (no myeloproliferative criteria or lymphoproliferative criteria are met, no allergic cause is found, no vasculitis or features of it are elucidated such as in eosinophilic polyangiitis with granulomatous formerly known as Churg-Strauss syndrome) (**Box 1**, **Fig. 1**). In the paper with the largest database of published HES patients from 2009, 20% of patients without myeloproliferative variant HES or chronic eosinophilic leukemia (CEL) had elevated tryptase levels (66% of the patients total had tryptase levels checked during

---

Box 1
World Health Organization criteria for systemic mastocytosis

One major and one minor criterion or 3 minor criteria must be met for diagnosis.

Major Criterion

Multifocal, dense aggregates of mast cells (15 or more) detected in sections of bone marrow and confirmed by tryptase immunohistochemistry or other special stains

Minor Criteria

- In biopsy section, more than 25% of the mast cells in the infiltrate have atypical morphology, or, of all the mast cells in the aspirate smear, more than 25% are immature or atypical

- Mast cells coexpress CD117 with CD2 and/or CD25

- Detection of *KIT* point mutation at codon 816 in bone marrow, blood, or other extracutaneous organs

- Serum total tryptase persistently >20 ng/mL (not a valid criteria in cases of systemic mastocytosis with associated clonal hematologic non-mast-cell lineage disease)

Adapted from Valent P, Horny HP, Escribano L, et al. Diagnostic criteria and classification of mastocytosis: a consensus proposal. Leuk Res 2001;25:603–25.

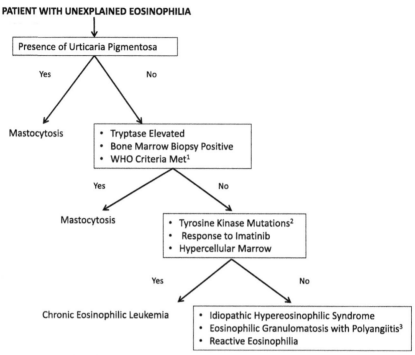

PATIENT WITH UNEXPLAINED EOSINOPHILIA

Presence of Urticaria Pigmentosa

Yes / No

Mastocytosis

- Tryptase Elevated
- Bone Marrow Biopsy Positive
- WHO Criteria Met[1]

Yes / No

Mastocytosis

- Tyrosine Kinase Mutations[2]
- Response to Imatinib
- Hypercellular Marrow

Yes / No

Chronic Eosinophilic Leukemia

- Idiopathic Hypereosinophilic Syndrome
- Eosinophilic Granulomatosis with Polyangiitis[3]
- Reactive Eosinophilia

Fig. 1. Workup of uncharacterized eosinophilia. 1. World Health Organization criteria for systemic mastocytosis (see **Box 1**). 2. Tyrosine kinase mutations in chronic eosinophilic leukemia. Including but not limited to *FIP1L1-PDGFRA* fusion, fusion of *PDGFRA* with other partner genes, fusions involving *PDGFRB*. 3. Formerly known as Churg-Strauss syndrome.

workup in this population).[13] Idiopathic HES can be α-interferon-responsive,[14] something that is also used to control systemic mastocytosis in more severe cases.[15]

CLONAL DISORDERS AFFECTING MAST CELLS AND EOSINOPHILS
Chronic Eosinophilic Leukemia

FIP1L1/PDFGRA-positive HES, described in 2003, also variably called myeloproliferative HES versus CEL, is the most significant entity in which an aberrant population of eosinophils is found with increased numbers of mast cells. These eosinophils are activated to cause end-organ damage, and there are elevated numbers of mast cells as well as serum tryptase levels. However, the mast cells do not carry the c-kit D816V mutation typically associated with mastocytosis nor do they cause any clinical symptoms of systemic mastocytosis.[16] Eleven percent of HES patients have this mutation.[13] The mutation is found in eosinophils, neutrophils, mast cells, T lymphocytes, B lymphocytes, and monocytes; hence, a pluripotent hematopoietic progenitor cell is affected. However, it seems to preferentially cause expansion of the eosinophil and mast cell populations.[17] Dysplastic eosinophils and spindle-shaped mast cells are present, along with a hypercellular marrow, and usually elevated B12 and tryptase levels (**Fig. 2**). The mast cells also have CD25 positivity, yet they do not usually have the CD2 positivity often seen in systemic mastocytosis.[18] Tryptase levels seem to at least partially normalize in response to imatinib treatment, like the eosinophilia does.[19]

CEL associated with F/P mutation can be confused with systemic mastocytosis due to the histopathologic and immunohistochemical features of mast cells shared among

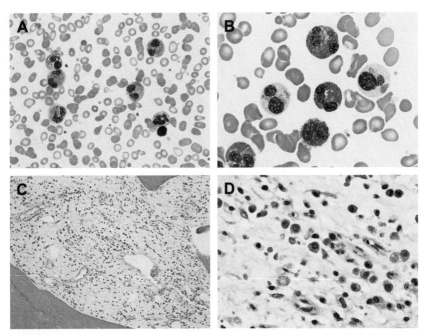

Fig. 2. Bone marrow biopsy and aspirate in a patient with chronic eosinophilic leukemia carrying the FIP1L1-PDGFRA rearrangement. Increased numbers of hypogranulated neoplastic eosinophils are observed in the aspirate (*A, B*) (Wright-Giemsa, original magnification ×100). The infiltrate predominantly consists of eosinophils in a background of fibrosis in the biopsy (*C, D*) (Hematoxylin and Eosin, original magnification ×400) as opposed to mastocytosis whereby the predominant infiltrate is that of mast cells. (*Courtesy of* German A. Pihan, MD, Beth Israel Deaconess Medical Center, Harvard Medical School, Boston, MA.)

the 2 disorders. As mentioned above, mast cells in both of these disorders are spindle-shaped and express CD25+, which is an abnormal marker. However, they do not form compact aggregates, express CD2, or carry c-Kit D816V mutation in CEL. This confusion has contributed to the suggestion of imatinib as a therapy for mast cell disease in earlier reports, whereas an overwhelming majority of mastocytosis cases do not respond to imatinib due to the presence of D816V c-Kit mutation rendering resistance to this drug.[20] Therefore, establishing the correct diagnosis is crucial for selecting the appropriate therapy. One paper suggests an algorithm based on the extent of eosinophilia and tryptase levels (see discussion below).[16]

Mastocytosis

Most patients with mastocytosis carry a D816V gain-of-function mutation in KIT, the gene encoding the c-kit receptor. There are limited data that SCF overexpression may play a role in some cases.[21,22]

Up to 28% of patients with systemic mastocytosis have peripheral eosinophilia, greater than 650 cells/mm[3], although the frequency increases in advanced forms of mastocytosis.[16,23] Eosinophilia is frequently noted in bone marrow biopsies and aspirates even in patients without significant peripheral eosinophilia (**Fig. 3**). Histopathology on these patients is usually positive for aberrant expression of CD2+ and CD25+. CKIT D816V mutation is positive in bone marrow or peripheral blood by sensitive PCR techniques[24]; no mutation for the FIP1L1-PDGFRA fusion is present. The CKIT

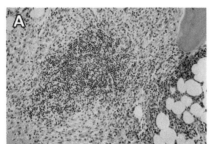 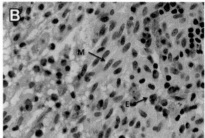

Fig. 3. (A) Bone marrow biopsy in systemic mastocytosis, intermediate magnification (Hematoxylin and Eosin, 100×) featuring atypical, spindle-shaped mast cells and intermingled eosinophils surrounding a lymphoid aggregate. (B) Bone marrow biopsy in systemic mastocytosis, high magnification (Hematoxylin and Eosin, 400×) showing atypical, spindle-shaped mast cells (M) with numerous intermingled eosinophils (E). (*Courtesy of* Charles W. Ross, MD, University of Michigan, Ann Arbor, MI.)

mutation in mastocytosis is also interestingly multilineage yet preferentially affects mast cell expansion.[25,26] The eosinophilia in mastocytosis is often not pathologic and does not necessitate treatment. The presentation is that of systemic mastocytosis, rather than that of clonal eosinophilia with end-organ damage.

In a paper from 2007 comparing the 2 entities (D816V-positive systemic mastocytosis vs FIP1L1/PDGFRA-positive CEL), distinguishing features for CEL included the degree of eosinophilia in relation to tryptase level, the absence of dense mast cell aggregates, the degree of B12 elevation, pulmonary symptoms, and cardiac symptoms.[16] Mastocytosis rather than CEL was more likely in those with elevated tryptase to absolute eosinophil count ratio, dense mast cell aggregates on bone marrow biopsy, gastrointestinal symptoms, urticaria pigmentosa, female sex, and thrombocytosis. The 2 disorders can occasionally coexist, although it is very unusual to exhibit both D816V c-Kit mutation and PDGFRA fusion concurrently.[27]

FUTURE DIRECTIONS
Therapies

Although some therapies are known to target both mast cell disease and eosinophilia (systemic steroids, α-interferon), others are potentially used in one versus the other disorder[13,28,29]; hence, distinguishing between entities is of vital importance with careful evaluation. Imatinib is useful in FIP1L1-PDGFRA fusion disease but has no effect and theoretically can worsen c-Kit D816V-positive mastocytosis, by selectively inhibiting the cells carrying the wild-type c-Kit.[19,30,31] Conversely, anti-IL5 therapy, although promising in HES,[32] EoE,[4] eosinophilic asthma[33] (diseases which all have a mast cell signature), remains to be studied in the treatment of mastocytosis, which has associated eosinophilia. Omalizumab (anti-immunoglobulin E therapy), although useful in allergic asthma,[34,35] has not been carefully studied in mastocytosis, although case reports have shown it to be useful in recurrent anaphylaxis associated with mastocytosis.[36] Finally, up and coming therapies, such as midostaurin (PKC412), one of the tyrosine kinase inhibitors currently under study, have reportedly been shown to help with both systemic mastocytosis and associated eosinophilia.[2]

Bone marrow transplantation is a last-resort therapy in the more aggressive and malignant forms of both mastocytosis and eosinophilic disorders. Further papers on experience with bone marrow transplant in these disorders (often written as case studies) will shed some light on both the cure rate and the complications related to treating these disorders.

REFERENCES

1. Metcalfe DD. Mastocytosis. In: Adkinson NF Jr, editor. Middleton's allergy principles and practice, vol. 2, 8th edition. Philadelphia: Saunders Elsevier; 2014. p. 1224–36.
2. Gotlib J, Akin C. Mast cells and eosinophils in mastocytosis, chronic eosinophilic leukemia, and non-clonal disorders. Semin Hematol 2012;49(2):128–37.
3. Klion AD, Weller PF. Eosinophilia and eosinophil related disorders. In: Adkinson NF Jr, editor. Middleton's allergy principles and practice, vol. 2, 8th edition. Philadelphia: Saunders Elsevier; 2014. p. 1205–23.
4. Otani IM, Anilkumar AA, Newbury RO, et al. Anti-IL-5 therapy reduces mast cell and IL-9 cell numbers in pediatric patients with eosinophilic esophagitis. J Allergy Clin Immunol 2013;131(6):1576–82.
5. Kovalszki A, Sheikh J, Weller PF. Eosinophils and eosinophilia. In: Rich RR, editor. Clinical immunology principles and practice, vol. 1, 4th edition. Philadelphia: Elsevier Saunders; 2013. p. 298–309.
6. Elishmereni M, Alenius HT, Bradding P, et al. Physical interactions between mast cells and eosinophils: a novel mechanism enhancing eosinophil survival in vitro. Allergy 2011;66(3):376–85.
7. Elishmereni M, Bachelet I, Nissim Ben-Efraim AH, et al. Interacting mast cells and eosinophils acquire an enhanced activation state in vitro. Allergy 2013;68(2):171–9.
8. Jarjour NN, Calhoun WJ, Schwartz LB, et al. Elevated bronchoalveolar lavage fluid histamine levels in allergic asthmatics are associated with increased airway obstruction. Am Rev Respir Dis 1991;144(1):83–7.
9. Rasp G, Hochstrasser K. Tryptase in nasal fluid is a useful marker of allergic rhinitis. Allergy 1993;48(2):72–4.
10. Bargagli E, Bigliazzi C, Leonini A, et al. Tryptase concentrations in bronchoalveolar lavage from patients with chronic eosinophilic pneumonia. Clin Sci 2005; 108(3):273–6.
11. Abonia JP, Blanchard C, Butz BB, et al. Involvement of mast cells in eosinophilic esophagitis. J Allergy Clin Immunol 2010;126(1):140–9.
12. Kirsch R, Bokhary R, Marcon MA, et al. Activated mucosal mast cells differentiate eosinophilic (allergic) esophagitis from gastroesophageal reflux disease. J Pediatr Gastroenterol Nutr 2007;44(1):20–6.
13. Ogbogu PU, Bochner BS, Butterfield JH, et al. Hypereosinophilic syndrome: a multicenter, retrospective analysis of clinical characteristics and response to therapy. J Allergy Clin Immunol 2009;124(6):1319–25.e3.
14. Butterfield JH, Weiler CR. Use of pegylated interferon in hypereosinophilic syndrome. Leuk Res 2012;36(2):192–7.
15. Cardet JC, Akin C, Lee MJ. Mastocytosis: update on pharmacotherapy and future directions. Expert Opin Pharmacother 2013;14(15):2033–45.
16. Maric I, Robyn J, Metcalfe DD, et al. KIT D816V-associated systemic mastocytosis with eosinophilia and FIP1L1/PDGFRA-associated chronic eosinophilic leukemia are distinct entities. J Allergy Clin Immunol 2007;120(3):680–7.
17. Robyn J, Lemery S, McCoy JP, et al. Multilineage involvement of the fusion gene in patients with FIP1L1/PDGFRA-positive hypereosinophilic syndrome. Br J Haematol 2006;132(3):286–92.
18. Klion AD, Noel P, Akin C, et al. Elevated serum tryptase levels identify a subset of patients with a myeloproliferative variant of idiopathic hypereosinophilic

syndrome associated with tissue fibrosis, poor prognosis, and imatinib responsiveness. Blood 2003;101(12):4660–6.

19. Klion AD, Robyn J, Akin C, et al. Molecular remission and reversal of myelofibrosis in response to imatinib mesylate treatment in patients with the myeloproliferative variant of hypereosinophilic syndrome. Blood 2004;103(2):473–8.

20. Akin C, Metcalfe DD. The biology of Kit in disease and the application of pharmacogenetics. J Allergy Clin Immunol 2004;114(1):13–9 [quiz: 20].

21. Valent P, Akin C, Sperr WR, et al. Mastocytosis: pathology, genetics, and current options for therapy. Leuk Lymphoma 2005;46(1):35–48.

22. Valent P, Horny HP, Escribano L, et al. Diagnostic criteria and classification of mastocytosis: a consensus proposal. Leuk Res 2001;25(7):603–25.

23. Pardanani A, Lim KH, Lasho TL, et al. Prognostically relevant breakdown of 123 patients with systemic mastocytosis associated with other myeloid malignancies. Blood 2009;114(18):3769–72.

24. Kristensen T, Vestergaard H, Moller MB. Improved detection of the KIT D816V mutation in patients with systemic mastocytosis using a quantitative and highly sensitive real-time qPCR assay. J Mol Diagn 2011;13(2):180–8.

25. Akin C, Kirshenbaum AS, Semere T, et al. Analysis of the surface expression of c-kit and occurrence of the c-kit Asp816Val activating mutation in T cells, B cells, and myelomonocytic cells in patients with mastocytosis. Exp Hematol 2000;28(2):140–7.

26. Yavuz AS, Lipsky PE, Yavuz S, et al. Evidence for the involvement of a hematopoietic progenitor cell in systemic mastocytosis from single-cell analysis of mutations in the c-kit gene. Blood 2002;100(2):661–5.

27. Florian S, Esterbauer H, Binder T, et al. Systemic mastocytosis (SM) associated with chronic eosinophilic leukemia (SM-CEL): detection of FIP1L1/PDGFRalpha, classification by WHO criteria, and response to therapy with imatinib. Leuk Res 2006;30(9):1201–5.

28. Valent P, Sperr WR, Akin C. How I treat patients with advanced systemic mastocytosis. Blood 2010;116(26):5812–7.

29. Kluin-Nelemans HC, Jansen JH, Breukelman H, et al. Response to interferon alfa-2b in a patient with systemic mastocytosis. N Engl J Med 1992;326(9):619–23.

30. Cools J, DeAngelo DJ, Gotlib J, et al. A tyrosine kinase created by fusion of the PDGFRA and FIP1L1 genes as a therapeutic target of imatinib in idiopathic hypereosinophilic syndrome. N Engl J Med 2003;348(13):1201–14.

31. Akin C, Brockow K, D'Ambrosio C, et al. Effects of tyrosine kinase inhibitor STI571 on human mast cells bearing wild-type or mutated c-kit. Exp Hematol 2003;31(8):686–92.

32. Rothenberg ME, Klion AD, Roufosse FE, et al. Treatment of patients with the hypereosinophilic syndrome with mepolizumab. N Engl J Med 2008;358(12):1215–28.

33. Pavord ID, Korn S, Howarth P, et al. Mepolizumab for severe eosinophilic asthma (DREAM): a multicentre, double-blind, placebo-controlled trial. Lancet 2012;380(9842):651–9.

34. Corren J, Casale T, Deniz Y, et al. Omalizumab, a recombinant humanized anti-IgE antibody, reduces asthma-related emergency room visits and hospitalizations in patients with allergic asthma. J Allergy Clin Immunol 2003;111(1):87–90.

35. Chiang DT, Clark J, Casale TB. Omalizumab in asthma: approval and postapproval experience. Clin Rev Allergy Immunol 2005;29(1):3–16.

36. Carter MC, Robyn JA, Bressler PB, et al. Omalizumab for the treatment of unprovoked anaphylaxis in patients with systemic mastocytosis. J Allergy Clin Immunol 2007;119(6):1550–1.

Epidemiology, Diagnosis, and Treatment of *Hymenoptera* Venom Allergy in Mastocytosis Patients

Marek Niedoszytko, MD, PhD[a],[*],[1], Patrizia Bonadonna, MD[b],[1],
Joanne N.G. Oude Elberink, MD, PhD[c],[1],
David B.K. Golden, MD, PhD[d]

KEYWORDS

- Hymenoptera venom allergy • Venom immunotherapy • Immunoglobulin E serology
- Mastocytosis

KEY POINTS

- Hymenoptera venom allergy (HVA) is a typical immunoglobulin E (IgE)-mediated reaction caused by sensitization to 1 or more allergens of the venom, and accounts for 1.5% to 34% of all cases of anaphylaxis.
- Patients suffering from mastocytosis are more susceptible for the anaphylactic reactions to an insect sting.
- Total avoidance of Hymenoptera is not feasible, and there is no preventive pharmacologic treatment available. HVA patients should carry an emergency kit with autoinjectable epinephrine.
- Venom immunotherapy (VIT) represents a safe and effective treatment decreasing the risk of subsequent systemic reactions.
- In addition to the regular workup for mastocytosis, specific diagnostic examinations for insect venom allergy include specific IgE measurements, such as serologic IgE (sIgE) measurement and skin test with standardized allergen concentrations.
- Skin tests in mastocytosis can be complicated by systemic allergic reactions. Specific IgE might be more often negative in comparison with the insect venom allergic population with no mastocytosis.
- If standard tests are negative, basophil activation test or recombinant sIgE assessment might be helpful in making a correct diagnosis, which was studied in the general population of patients with insect venom allergy (IVA).

Continued

The authors contributed equally to the article.
[a] Department of Allergology, Medical University of Gdansk, Debinki 7, Gdańsk 80-210, Poland;
[b] Allergy Unit, Azienda Ospedaliera Universitaria Integrata of Verona, Piazzale Aristide Stefani 1, 37126, Verona, Italy; [c] Department of Allergology, University Hospital Groningen, Hanzeplein 1, 9700 RB Groningen, Netherlands; [d] Division of Allergy-Immunology, Johns Hopkins Bayview Medical Center, 4940 Eastern Avenue, Baltimore, MD 21224, USA
[1] Members of the European Competence Network on Mastocytosis.
* Corresponding author.
E-mail address: mnied@gumed.edu.pl

Immunol Allergy Clin N Am 34 (2014) 365–381
http://dx.doi.org/10.1016/j.iac.2014.02.004   immunology.theclinics.com

Continued

- The only treatment that is able to reduce the risk of systemic reactions to IVA is allergen immunotherapy.
- Lifelong treatment is recommended in subjects with diagnosed mastocytosis and mast-cell activation syndrome.

INTRODUCTION

Hymenoptera venom allergy (HVA) is a typical immunoglobulin E (IgE)-mediated reaction caused by sensitization to 1 or more allergens of the venom, and accounts for 1.5% to 34% of all cases of anaphylaxis.[1] The severity can vary from large local reactions (a swelling >10 cm lasting up to 24 hours) to systemic anaphylaxis. Systemic reactions are classified with 4° of increasing severity according to Mueller.[2] The diagnostic procedures, which are mandatory for a correct prescription of venom immunotherapy (VIT), include skin-prick or intradermal tests, and serum-specific IgE assays.

The culprit insects of allergic reactions are Hymenoptera belonging to the suborder Aculeate, which includes the families Apidae, Vespidae, and Formicidae. The Apidae family comprises *Apis mellifera* and *Bombus*. The Vespidae family includes the Vespinae subfamilies (*Vespula* and *Dolichovespula* species, and *Vespa crabro*) and Polistinae subfamilies (*Polistes* species).[3,4] The Formicidae family is represented in the United States by the imported fire ants (*Solenopsis* species).

Total avoidance of Hymenoptera is not feasible, and there is no preventive pharmacologic treatment available.[4] HVA patients should carry an emergency kit with autoinjectable epinephrine in addition to antihistamines and oral corticosteroid, although the effect of the latter 2 in acute anaphylaxis is doubtful. VIT represents a safe and effective treatment that decreases the risk of subsequent systemic reactions[4] and improves the quality of life.[5] VIT is prescribed to all subjects with a clear history of systemic reaction and positive skin test or venom-specific IgE in serum.

Over the preceding years, by studying those patients with anaphylaxis, it was progressively realized that there is a preferential association between HVA and mastocytosis, a group of clonal disorders of the mast-cell lineage.[6–13] In addition, the risk of anaphylaxis increased with increasing levels of tryptase.[13] Whereas in the general population the prevalence of HVA is lower than 2%,[8] in patients with mastocytosis the prevalence of IVA is about 25%.[7] Anaphylactic reactions to an insect sting affect a substantial percentage of patients with systemic mastocytosis.[6] The study by van Anrooij and colleagues[7] shows in patients with mastocytosis that the prevalence of HVA differs according to the specific form of mastocytosis and basal tryptase level. The highest prevalence was found in patients with a tryptase level of 20.4 to 29.9 µg/L, in whom prevalence reaches 50%. On the other hand, the prevalence among patients with levels below 6.1 µg/L and above 191 µg/L is lower than 10%.[7] Nevertheless it is higher than the prevalence in the general population, which is lower than 2%.[8] The expected life expectancy of patients with the cutaneous and indolent forms of mastocytosis is similar to that of the general population.[9] Anaphylactic reactions (the most common being to an insect sting) and osteoporotic fractures are the most important risk factors among mastocytosis patients.[9] This article aims to answer the most important clinical questions raised by the diagnosis and treatment of IVA in mastocytosis patients.

EPIDEMIOLOGY

Severe anaphylactic reactions after Hymenoptera stings were initially described in case reports or a small series of patients with cutaneous or systemic mastocytosis.[10–13] Of note, increased baseline serum tryptase is associated with a history of more severe sting reactions also in patients without systemic mastocytosis.[14]

Two large studies reported 19% and 5% of patients who experienced an anaphylactic reaction to Hymenoptera venom among 74 and 163 adults with mastocytosis, mostly systemic,[6,15] demonstrating a higher incidence of HVA in mast-cell disease. More recently, other studies confirmed that the most common triggers for anaphylactic episodes among clonal patients are stings from Hymenoptera such as yellowjacket (Vespula), honey bee (Apis), Polistes, and imported fire ants (Solenopsis).[7,16,17] Reactions to other stings are exceptional in the United States and Europe. To date only 2 cases of anaphylaxis to mosquito bites have been reported, 1 in a Spanish case series[15] and 1 in a case report.[18]

The prevalence of Hymenoptera stings in eliciting anaphylaxis in children with mastocytosis is lower in comparison with adults.[6,15]

The prevalence of mastocytosis in the general population is estimated to be in the range of 3 to 13 per 100,000 inhabitants.[19,20] By contrast, the frequency of clonal mast-cell disease (CMD) in screened subjects with HVA ranges from 1% to 7.9% (**Table 1**). The lower prevalence rate reported in some studies might be explained by the low sensitivity of the test used for screening,[21] or by the lack of a bone marrow evaluation,[14] or the evaluation of CD25/CD2 mast-cell coexpression and/or Kit mutation.[22,24,25] The first report of routine bone marrow evaluation of patients with HVA and raised tryptase, including the detection of minor criteria for mastocytosis, reported a percentage of CMD as high as 7.9%.[23] In this series, 20% of cases of systemic mastocytosis/mast-cell activation syndrome would not have been diagnosed without flow cytometry, Kit mutation analysis, or both. For this reason it is recommended to refer patients with raised tryptase without skin involvement to a tertiary research center with experience in mast-cell disorders.

The relation between HVA and mastocytosis seems to be quite specific, as it has been shown that the prevalence of mast-cell disorder in food or drug hypersensitivity is far lower than in patients with HVA.[23] Urticaria pigmentosa is not a confounder because insects are also the most common trigger for anaphylaxis in patients with

Table 1
Prevalence of clonal mast cell disease (CMD) in patients with systemic reactions to Hymenoptera venom, screened on the basis of elevated tryptase

Authors,[Ref.] Year	No. of Patients	Raised Tryptase (%)	CMD	%
Haeberli et al,[14] 2003[a]	259	19 (7.3)	3 CM	1
Dubois,[21] 2004[b]	2375	32 (1.3)	22 SM	1
Rueff et al,[22] 2006[c]	1102	106 (9.6)	21 CM + 8 SM	2.6
Bonadonna et al,[23] 2009	379	44 (11.6)	21 ISM + 9 MMAS	7.9
Potier et al,[24] 2009[c]	138	22 (15.9)	1 CM + 5 SM	4.4
Guenova et al,[25] 2010[c,d]	274	30 (10.9)	1 CM + 3 ISM	1.5

Abbreviations: CM, cutaneous mastocytosis; ISM, indolent systemic mastocytosis; MMAS, monoclonal mast-cell activation syndrome; SM, systemic mastocytosis.
[a] Bone marrow evaluation not performed.
[b] Screening with urinary histamine metabolite.
[c] Evaluation of CD25/CD2 mast cell coexpression and Kit mutation not performed or reported.
[d] Bone marrow evaluation performed if baseline serum tryptase >15 ng/mL.

indolent systemic mastocytosis without skin involvement. This finding suggests some specificity in the association between mast-cell disorders and HVA, deserving more detailed mechanistic investigation.

Initially the association between HVA and CMD was described mainly in patients with urticaria pigmentosa,[12,22,26] but gradually it became clear that patients with mastocytosis and HVA more frequently have no skin involvement.[7,15,21,23,26–29]

The main characteristics of CMD in patients with a systemic reaction to Hymenoptera venom are reported in **Table 2**. Systemic mastocytosis was the more frequent diagnosis (72%), although in several series bone marrow biopsy was not performed or performed only in a portion of patients. Median age ranges from 34 to 50 years, and most patients are males (ratio 1.61). In 50% of cases, baseline serum tryptase is less than 20 ng/mL.

In most patients with mastocytosis without urticaria pigmentosa, Hymenoptera sting anaphylaxis is characterized by absence of angioedema and erythema and the presence of syncope during reaction.[27–29] In fact, the so-called REMA (Red Española de Mastocitosi) score, proposed by Alvarez-Twose and colleagues,[16] based on male sex, baseline serum tryptase greater than 25 ng/mL, and presence of syncope/presyncope without angioedema and/or urticaria, shows sensitivity of 92% and specificity of 67% in detecting CMD in HVA patients without urticaria pigmentosa.

A recent study found lower median baseline serum tryptase levels in insect venom allergic mastocytosis patients without urticaria pigmentosa when compared with other mastocytosis patients.[28,29] Surprisingly, Hymenoptera venom anaphylaxis seems to be absent in patients with the aggressive subtypes of systemic mastocytosis, who harbor the highest mast-cell load.[7,38] This finding might question the assumption that the risk of Hymenoptera venom anaphylaxis continuously increases with increasing mast-cell load. In fact, the highest prevalence was found in patients with indolent systemic mastocytosis (ISM) with tryptase levels ranging from 20.4 to 29.9 µg/L, with a prevalence of 50%, whereas in mastocytosis patients with levels below 6.1 µg/L and above 191 µg/L the prevalence of HVA is lower than 10%.[7]

In a study by Niedoszytko and colleagues[37] it has been shown that gene-expression profiles in the peripheral blood cells were different between patients with a history of HVA and those without, reflecting a more pronounced mast-cell dysfunction in patients without a history of anaphylaxis. The investigators found in patients with HVA a trend toward lower levels of tryptase in serum and lower urinary excretion of the histamine metabolites methylhistamine and methylimidazole acetic acid, which are also thought to reflect mast-cell burden.[37]

Ultimately, it seems that patients with ISM and without skin involvement with Hymenoptera venom anaphylaxis as main symptom have a lower frequency of symptoms resulting from the release of mast-cell mediators.[27–29]

DIAGNOSIS

The first problem is the indication for the diagnosis of IVA. Current guidelines indicate that additional diagnostic tests should be performed in patients who have suffered historically from an anaphylactic reaction.[1,4] However, the prevalence of positive venom skin tests in the general population is estimated at 20%, and differs according to population and risk of field sting.[8] The current guidelines of the European Academy of Allergy and of the US Joint Task Force on Practice Parameters do not advise VIT for patients with positive skin test or sIgE who were never stung or tolerated stings without systemic reaction. However, because many patients were never stung or were stung before the first symptoms of mastocytosis occurred, there is debate as

Table 2
Characteristics of most reported mast cell clonal diseases (CMD) presenting with systemic reactions to Hymenoptera sting

Authors,[Ref.] Year	No. of Patients	Diagnosis	M/F	Median Age in Years (Range)	Tryptase <20 ng/mL, n (%)	Without Skin Involvement, n (%)
Müller et al,[10] 1983	3	2 CMᵃ + 1 SM	1/2	34 (32–50)	Not reported	3 (0)
Kors et al,[11] 1993	5	5 SM	0/5	49 (29–71)	Not reported	2 (40)
Fricker et al,[30] 1997	10	7 CMᵃ + 3 SM	4/6	39 (29–51)	5 (50)	0 (0)
Oude Elberink et al,[12] 1997	2	2 SM	0/2	44–43	Not reported	2 (0)
Biederman et al,[31] 1999	1	1 CMᵃ	1/0	40	0	0
Ludolph-Hauser et al,[26] 2001	13	13 CM	5/8	42 (30–66)	7 (54)	13 (0)
Dubois,[21] 2004	17	17 SM	—	—	—	8 (53)
Rueff et al,[22] 2006ᵃ	29	21 CM + 8 SM	—	—	—	—
Sonneck et al,[32] 2007	5	4 ISM 1 MMAS	4/0 0/1	40 (33–50) 39	1 (25) 1/1	5 (100)
Akin et al,[33] 2007	1	1 MMAS	1	42	1/1	0 (100)
González de Olano et al,[34] 2008	21	21 ISM	17/4	50 (29–74)	2 (9)	16 (76)
Potier et al,[24] 2009ᵇ	6	1 CM + 5 ISM	5/1	41 (29–59)	1 (17)	1 (16.6)
Bonadonna et al,[23] 2009	30	21 ISM 9 MMAS	13/8 9/0	48 (19–76) 51 (32–69)	6 (29) 6 (67)	26 (81)
Dugas-Breit et al,[35] 2009ᵃ	56	32 CM + 24 SM	—	—	—	—
Müller & Haeberli,[36] 2009	1	1 SM	1	50	0	1
Guenova et al,[25] 2010	4	1 CM + 3 SM	3/1	64 (57–71)	1	Not reported
Niedoszytko et al,[37] 2011	12	12 ISM	2/10	49 (25–70)	3 (25)	Not reported
Alvarez-Twose et al,[28] 2013	143	143 ISM	111/32	44 (16–76)	88 (62)	143 (100)
Total	359	78 CM, 270 ISM, 11 MMAS	177/110 (ratio 1.61)	—	121 (50)	221 (86)

ᵃ Bone marrow evaluation not performed or in a portion of cases.
ᵇ Bone marrow histology without evaluation of CD25/CD2 mast cell expression.

to whether prophylactic treatment could be performed in mastocytosis. This approach is currently not recommended, and therefore only patients who have suffered an anaphylactic reaction to an insect sting are candidates for diagnostic testing.

Second, there is the issue of which diagnostic methods might be used. The safe test that can be performed in most patients is sIgE measurement. When possible, the analysis should be done approximately 4 weeks after the reaction; if negative the test can be easily repeated, and in some cases it becomes positive a few weeks later.[39] On the other hand, if the time period between the sting and the test is longer, the result may be falsely negative. The cutoff level for the venom-specific IgE test is the value of 0.35 IU/L and higher. Recent data indicate that in some patients with clear medical history, even values higher than 0.1 may indicate the presence of an allergy.[40] There is a difference in sensitivity and specificity of the methods. Sensitivity of specific IgE depends on the method used and ranges from 70% to 87%.[41,42] It is possible that the false-positive results may be due to cross-reactive carbohydrate determinants (CCD), which may occur in 35% of the whole population of IVA patients.[39] In cases of IgE negativity a second analysis is recommended, to be performed at least 6 weeks after the first diagnosis. In most cases the diagnosis is performed once.[39] If the sIgE level is in a range 0.1 to 0.35 IU/L, the sIgE analysis should be repeated after few weeks. In most clinically significant cases the increase of the sIgE level can be observed.[39] It should be emphasized that contrary to the food allergy, the level of IgE does not correlate with the severity of the reaction. In general, the sIgE level is lower in mastocytosis patients than in the general population of HVA patients (Oude Elberink, in preparation for publication).

Skin-prick tests are performed with the standard concentration of insect venom ranging from 1 to 100 μg/L. If skin-prick tests are negative, the intradermal tests should be performed with concentrations of 0.001 to 1 μg/mL. Higher concentrations may lead to the false-positive results.[42] As the skin tests with the insect venom diagnose the reactivity of the skin and can be considered an allergen challenge on the skin, the facilities used in the treatment of anaphylaxis should be used (intravenous access, the possibility of immediate administration of epinephrine, fluids, oxygen, steroids, and antihistamine drugs). As mastocytosis patients are at high risk of fatal anaphylaxis, in some cases the diagnosis may be performed in an inpatient ward.[43] The third problem concerns patients who have suffered from an anaphylactic reaction but in whom the standard tests described here are negative.[9,44–46] Such a situation is found more often in mastocytosis patients than in the general population of IVA patients.[45] Thus the tryptase level may indicate a higher risk of fatal reaction in the future and the need for further, repeated skin test and sIgE analysis. In such cases the alternative methods, such as the basophil activation test (BAT) or sIgE using recombinant allergens, may be useful. The data on BAT in patients with a negative skin test and sIgE vary in different centers. The study by Bonadonna and colleagues[42] showed that negative standard tests are reliable because BAT did not add useful information. By contrast, the groups of Gonzales de Olano,[47] Korosec[41] and Bidad[48] showed the usefulness of the method in false-negative patients, with sensitivity reaching 81% to 87% in patients with mastocytosis. The analysis of IgE to recombinant allergen Api m1, Ves v1, and Ves v5 can be helpful in doubly sensitized patients, and increase the detection of yellowjacket venom allergy. In the general population the sensitivity of recombinant allergen diagnosis in yellowjacket allergy is excellent, reaching 95%, while in bee-allergic patients it is estimated at 78%.[49] The additional value of this is not yet known in the mastocytosis population. Sting challenges with living insects used in the assessment of the effectiveness of insect VIT are normally contraindicated in patients not receiving VIT, particularly in high-risk patients such as those with mastocytosis.[39,43]

The fourth problem concerns patients with double sensitivity, which may be found in 50% of the general IVA population. In patients who have had only one reaction to an insect in their medical history but in whom the tests indicate a positive reaction to multiple venoms, the aforementioned diagnostics methods can be used. In addition, inhibition tests using the analysis of sIgE levels in serum mixed with venom may be helpful.[50] In true-positive cases the addition of venom to the serum containing sIgE leads to the negative results of subsequent sIgE. In some cases the double-positive results may be caused by CCD. The true double-positive results may be diagnosed in cases where at least 2 anaphylactic reactions have occurred in the medical history. Using new methods such as BAT and recombinant allergen may be helpful in doubly sensitized patients. A positive result of sIgE using recombinant allergens to bee venom while negative to yellowjacket venom may indicate true bee-venom allergy. However, a positive result to yellowjacket alone does not exclude bee-venom allergy, owing to the low sensitivity of the test already described. In such cases, additional tests such as BAT should be performed.[49] If the tests to both recombinant allergens are positive, IVA testing should be performed with both venoms.[49]

The fifth problem concerns patients with IVA who may suffer from mastocytosis. The epidemiologic data show that approximately 5% (range 1%–7.9%) of IVA patients suffer from mastocytosis.[23,39] The tryptase level should be measured before and at the end of immunotherapy, as the development of mastocytosis may be preceded by an anaphylactic reaction. In addition, patients should also consult a dermatologist. New diagnostic methods such as highly sensitive D816V mutation analysis[51] and gene expression studies[52] may be helpful; however, further studies are needed to establish the diagnostic value of these methods.

TREATMENT

Because of the severity of the reactions,[28] patients are advised to carry at least 2 epinephrine autoinjectors.

Treatment of Hymenoptera venom anaphylaxis has been and still is a matter of debate. Although VIT is an established, safe, and effective treatment for the prevention of anaphylaxis in patients with previous systemic reactions after Hymenoptera stings without mastocytosis,[4] there are concerns about both the safety and efficacy of this treatment in mastocytosis patients.[12,21] Moreover, the indication for this treatment is a matter of debate, as specific IgE is low, or even absent, in mastocytosis patients, and anaphylactic reactions in patients with mastocytosis might be non–IgE-mediated,[45] therefore the question is whether VIT would be of benefit.

Data available thus far concerning immunotherapy in mastocytosis come from case reports and observational studies, most of which are retrospective with a high risk of selection bias. There are no randomized trials.

The efficacy of VIT in mastocytosis has been reviewed previously,[43] evaluating 7 publications (**Table 3**).[13–15,21–23,30,53] Recently Bonadonna and colleagues[54] combined data from Italy and Spain, which confirmed the safety and efficacy of the treatment. Overall, the efficacy of VIT can be evaluated in a total of 132 patients with mastocytosis receiving VIT by sting challenges or field stings (see **Table 3**).

There is a large variation in the protection rate, varying from 14% to 85%. In the larger and more recent studies, protection rates are lowest. The question is whether this is due to selection bias, as in the past the awareness of mastocytosis was lower, tryptase measurements were only widely available for routine practice from the beginning of this millennium, and more specific markers such as CD25 and c-kit mutation were less available. It is reasonable to suppose that screening for mastocytosis was

Table 3
Effectiveness of venom immunotherapy (VIT) in mastocytosis

Authors,[Ref.] Year	Time of Sting Challenge	No. (%) of Patients with Systemic Reaction in Sting Challenge	No. (%) of Patients with Systemic Reaction on Field Sting	Cumulative No. of Reactions to Re-Sting
Rueff et al,[22] 2006	6–12 mo after reaching maintenance dose	7/33 (21.6)	—	7/33 (21.6)
Dubois,[21] 2004	ND	—	6/7 (85)	6/7 (85)
Bonadonna et al,[23] 2009	ND	—	2/13 (15)	2/13 (15)
Haeberli et al,[14] 2003	3–5 y of VIT	4/10 (40)	—	4/10 (40)
Fricker et al,[30] 1997	Maintenance dose	0/3	1/3 (33)	1/6 (16)
González de Olano et al,[15] 2007	ND	—	3/12 (25)	3/12 (25)
Engler & Davis,[53] 1994	ND	—	0/1	0/1
Bonadonna et al,[54] in press	ND	—	7/50 (14)	7/50 (14)
Total	—	11/46 (23.9)	19/132 (20.0)	30/132 (22.7)

Abbreviation: ND, not done.

initiated in the past only in cases with severe adverse effects. However, this was not the case in a small study from Groningen (the Netherlands) with a high percentage of side effects,[21] where from the 1980s all patients with HVA were screened routinely for mastocytosis by urine methylhistamine (with sensitivity comparable to that of tryptase).[55] By contrast, recent data from this hospital also show a far lower percentage of side effects (H. Oude Elberink, personal observation, 2013).

The efficacy of VIT has been evaluated by sting challenges and field stings. In general, sting challenges were only performed in Munich and Bern.

In total, systemic reactions were observed in 11 of 46 (23.9%) sting challenges described, whereas a systemic reaction to a field sting occurred in 19 of 86 (20.0%) patients during VIT. The most severe reaction described (requiring resuscitation and intubation) was found in a patient who was not yet on a maintenance phase of VIT.[15] Overall, the protection rate in these studies is lower than 80%, which is lower than that in patients without mastocytosis, where the protection is about 80% in honey bee–allergic patients and about 95% in yellowjacket-allergic patients during the maintenance phase of VIT.[56] Of note, the efficacy of VIT in these patients might even be overstated because of the relatively low predictive value of a single negative sting reaction in a patient.[57]

Side effects during VIT might be an indication of treatment failure, as has also been demonstrated for the general population.[58] In the study by González de Olano and colleagues,[15] all patients with a reaction to a later sting had side effects during the build-up phase of VIT, which may suggest that at least these patients should be warned that VIT might be less efficacious.

In the general IVA population, it has been suggested that by increasing the dose of venom, protection can be increased or achieved.[58] In mastocytosis, the effect of a higher maintenance dose was demonstrated in 2 mastocytosis patients reacting to a field sting who tolerated subsequent stings after increasing the maintenance dose.[59] In a study by Rueff and colleagues[60] of 8 patients with an elevated tryptase level (>13.5 ng/mL) and a positive challenge, 7 were protected at a subsequent sting challenge after increasing the dose up to the one providing the protection to an insect sting, which was 150, 200, or 250 µg, whereas in the other patient the sting challenge was not repeated.[10,60,61]

No data are available to date evaluating the long-term efficacy of VIT in mastocytosis patients. However, 2 fatalities have been described in 2 patients who were stung after stopping VIT: one 4 years after a 5-year course of VIT, and the other 6 months after a 2.5-year course of VIT.[11] Although the guidelines of the European Academy of Allergology and Clinical Immunology advise lifelong treatment of this group of patients,[4] it is presently unclear as to whether continuation of VIT will be able to prevent fatal anaphylactic reactions.

Overall it can be concluded that although the efficacy of VIT in mastocytosis might be less in comparison with the general IVA population treated with VIT, the number of systemic reactions in patients with mastocytosis seems to be reduced.

Side Effects of VIT in Mastocytosis

Table 4 summarizes the evaluation of the safety of VIT in mastocytosis in a total of 201 patients.

Overall, side effects during VIT were documented in 38 (23.9%) patients, most of which are systemic (73.7%). In the study by Bonadonna and colleagues,[23] side effects were specifically related to the honey bee, which is in accordance with the general IVA population whereby side effects caused by honey bee venom occur more frequently in comparison with patients allergic to yellowjacket venom, varying from 26.6% (12%–30%) in honey bee venom–treated patients to 11.2% (range 2%–20.9%) of the yellowjacket venom–treated patients.[4,8,43] In the review by Niedoszytko and colleagues,[43] no differences in side effects between treatments for yellowjacket and honey bee venom were found in patients with mastocytosis.

Overall, compared with the general IVA population, side effects are more frequent, especially in yellowjacket-allergic patients.

Pretreatment during the build-up phase of VIT in mastocytosis patients was described in 2 articles.[15,53] Engler and Davis[53] used prednisone, hydroxyzine, ranitidine and astemizole during the 5 days of rush therapy. González de Olano and colleagues[15] considered VIT in mastocytosis patients as a risky procedure, and therefore used premedication (oral disodium cromoglycate) and intensive care unit or monitored setting with management for resuscitation in all patients. However, in a recent study by Bonadonna and colleagues,[54] the use of pretreatment regimens is not mentioned. Concerning the maintenance phase of VIT, systemic reactions also have been reported.[12,21] Therefore, pretreatment may also be considered in this phase of treatment.

Patients with mastocytosis who have experienced systemic reactions should carry 2 or more epinephrine self-injectors. This practice is also advised for all VIT-treated mastocytosis patients despite having reached the maintenance dose, because of the persistent risk of a systemic reaction and the possibility that systemic reactions may also occur after a sting of an insect whose venom was not used for VIT.[62]

Overall, the following conclusions can be drawn in relation to treatment[43]:

1. Mastocytosis patients have a high risk of severe sting reactions
2. VIT is also recommended for mastocytosis patients
3. VIT probably should be performed lifelong

Table 4
Side effects of venom immunotherapy (VIT) in mastocytosis patients

Authors,[Ref.] Year	VIT	No. (%) of Mastocytosis Patients		
			Side Effects	
		Total	Systemic	Adrenaline[1] was Used or Caused Discontinuation of Treatment[2]
Rueff et al,[22] 2006	48 mastocytosis	9 (18.8) build-up phase of VIT	9 (18.8) build-up phase of VIT	2[a]
Dubois,[21] 2004	7 ISM	6 (85)	6 (85)	4
Bonadonna et al,[23] 2009	16 ISM (2 UP+, 14 UP−)	2 (12.5)	0	0
Haeberli et al,[14] 2003	10 patients with tryptase >13.5 µg/L and sting challenge performed	1 (10)	1 (10)	0
Fricker et al,[30] 1997	3 ISM UP+ 3 ISM UP− 4 UP, no bone marrow diagnosis	2 (20)	1 (10)	0
González de Olano et al,[15] 2007	21 ISM (5 UP+, 16 UP−)	6 (29) 3 build-up, 3 maintenance phase of VIT	5 (24)	1
Engler & Davis,[53] 1994 Mueller,[2] 1996 Oude Elberink et al,[12] 1997	4 UP, 1 ISM	2 (33)	2 (33)	2
Bonadonna et al,[54] in press	77 ISM (12 UP+, 65 UP−) MMAS 7	10 (8.4)	4 (build-up) (4.8)	1
Total	201	38 (18.9)	28 (13.9)	10 (5.0)

Abbreviation: UP, urticaria pigmentosa.
[a] Unpublished data.

4. VIT in mastocytosis might be accompanied by a slightly higher frequency of side effects
5. Special precautions might be taken into account, notably during the build-up phase of the therapy
6. VIT is able to reduce systemic reactions, but to a lesser extent in comparison with the general IVA population
7. Patients should be warned that the efficacy of VIT might be less than optimal, and they should continue carrying at least 2 epinephrine autoinjectors.

The United States Perspective

The mutual relationship between mastocytosis and IVA has been the subject of increasing attention and research over the past 10 to 15 years. On participation in both the European and American Academy activities during these years, one recognizes 2 very different perceptions of this area by allergy specialists in these 2 different regions. A review of the literature suggests that the United States may be vaguely aware that venom allergy can play a role in mastocytosis, but Europe is increasingly aware that mastocytosis plays an important role in venom allergy.

The United States perspective about the role of mastocytosis in venom allergy has long held that the only reason to consider the possibility is when a patient with a clear history of sting anaphylaxis has negative venom skin tests and specific sIgE tests; this was viewed as the coincidence of 2 rare conditions, and therefore extremely rare. Many allergists in the United States are likely to consider that they will never see such a case in their careers.

Review of investigational activity in the United States in the area of mastocytosis helps to explain this view. Mastocytosis has been intensively and successfully characterized in United States studies, but the published reports make no mention of venom allergy in patients with mastocytosis. There has also been outstanding research on serum tryptase expression and the meaning of elevated serum levels.[63] Serum tryptase has been studied for its role as a marker of acute anaphylaxis, and has been viewed as a marker of mastocytosis when it exceeds 20 ng/mL, but throughout the United States published literature on serum tryptase there is no mention of any relation between baseline levels and the risk of venom allergy. Unless the total serum tryptase level is consistently higher than 20 ng/mL it has not been considered abnormal by many allergists, so the frequency and significance of baseline serum tryptase of 12 to 18 ng/mL in patients with insect-sting anaphylaxis has been largely ignored.

Review of the published literature on mast cells and venom allergy is also revealing. In 1983, Müller[10] reported an association of urticaria pigmentosa with insect sting reactions; there were no United States publications on the subject at the time. In 1993, Kors and colleagues[11] reported on mastocytosis and sting reactions. In 1994, Engler and Davis[53] published the first United States report on the subject (rush VIT in a patient with mastocytosis). In 1997, Fricker and colleagues[30] reported the association of urticaria pigmentosa with sting reactions and elevated tryptase, as well as the safety of VIT in such patients. Also in 1997, Oude Elberink and colleagues[12] published their case reports of fatal sting reactions in patients with mastocytosis. There had been no further publications at that time in the United States. In 2001, Ludolph-Hauser and colleagues[26] published a study of tryptase levels and sting reactions, and in 2003 Haeberli and colleagues[14] reported the relation of tryptase level to severity of sting reaction, as well as the safety of VIT in such patients. Again were no further reports on the subject in the United States at that time. Since 2005 there have been almost 20 European publications on this subject, with no academic studies and only one case report in the United States.

It is also very telling to examine the US Joint Task Force Practice Parameters on Hymenoptera Venom Allergy that have been published in the past decade.[64,65] One of the co-authors of this article (D.G.) was a contributing author to the 2004 document and the Work Group Chair (and lead author) of the 2011 update. The 2004 Practice Parameters stated that "rarely, patients can have an anaphylactic reaction with a subsequent sting despite negative skin and in vitro test responses, possibly because of a non–IgE-mediated mechanism."[64] There is no mention of tryptase or mastocytosis anywhere in the document. In the 2011 update, there are several statements made in various sections of the document, as follows. "Baseline serum tryptase levels have been found to be increased, particularly in patients who had severe anaphylactic shock reactions to insect stings." "Such patients might require evaluation for mastocytosis or disorders of mast cell function." "Patients with mastocytosis, or an increased baseline serum tryptase level, are also at higher risk for severe reactions to future stings." There is no mention anywhere in the document of the frequency and demographics of mastocytosis or elevated tryptase, or of indications for measurement of baseline serum tryptase.[65]

To illustrate the United States perspective on mastocytosis and venom allergy, 3 sentinel cases drawn from the authors' files are reviewed here. The first case is the only case report in the United States literature, and was published as a prelude to a review article on insect allergy and cardiac disease by Professor Muller[66] (*Current Opinion in Allergy and Immunology*, 2007). This 53-year-old man was stung on the neck by a yellowjacket, and after 10 minutes felt nausea and dizziness. He drove to a gas station, where he collapsed on the pavement. Emergency responders found him in ventricular fibrillation, with no hives or other signs. He was cardioverted 4 times and intubated, and no epinephrine was given. In the emergency room he had a heavy chest and dyspnea, and ST changes on electrocardiogram. He underwent cardiac catheterization, but no significant abnormality was found. There is a family history that his father died suddenly at age 34. His medications include metoprolol, losartan, celecoxib, atorvastatin, Glucophage, glyburide, metformin, rosiglitazone, lansoprazole, and lithium. The discharge diagnosis was familial idiopathic ventricular tachycardia, with no mention of insect sting. He received an implanted defibrillator. Venom skin tests were performed 6 weeks later and were negative, but serum IgE was positive (1 ng/mL) for yellowjacket, hornet, and *Polistes* venoms. The baseline serum tryptase was 30 ng/mL. Bone marrow biopsy was reported with clusters of abnormal mast cells. The debate centered on whether this was cardiac anaphylaxis in a patient with mastocytosis (and absent hives, as is so often the case), or familial idiopathic ventricular fibrillation. The cardiologist insisted it could not be anaphylaxis because there were no hives. There was debate as to whether it was efficacious and safe for the patient to undergo VIT, and also whether he should stop the β1-selective blocker and/or the angiotensin receptor blocker. At the time this case was published, there was virtually no awareness in the United States of any relationship between insect sting anaphylaxis, mastocytosis, and baseline serum tryptase.

The second case illustrates many of the typical clinical features of patients with IVA and mastocytosis. The patient was first evaluated in 2010, but his history begins in the 1970s and 1980s with multiple near-fatal reactions to insect stings characterized by rapid-onset shock and unconsciousness with no hives. He received VIT from 1986 to 1992 with no reactions to VIT or stings during those years. In 1992 he had a severe anaphylactic reaction to a VIT injection. Although he underwent uneventful rush VIT, he chose to discontinue treatment. In 1993 he had an unexplained anaphylactic reaction (with no sting), but he had many stings without reaction between 1994 and 2010. In 2010 he had a near-fatal sting reaction. He now admits many episodes over many years of flushing and dizziness. Baseline serum tryptase was 23.5. He underwent rush VIT (with omalizumab pretreatment) with no problems, and remains on VIT. Bone marrow biopsy in 2011 confirmed the diagnosis of mastocytosis.

The third case illustrates the United States perspective on mastocytosis and insect allergy. In an email query to one of the authors (D.G.), a practicing allergist described a 40-year-old woman who had 10 yellowjacket stings that caused rapid-onset collapse with no hives. Her blood pressure was 70/40 mm Hg, and she responded well to epinephrine and intravenous fluids. The allergist suspects that the severe reaction was due to the toxic effect of multiple stings. He questions the need for testing, but is concerned that skin tests may cause severe reaction. The authors recommended checking the baseline serum tryptase and to perform venom skin tests. The allergist later reported with great surprise that the tryptase was 16.7 ng/mL. He stated that "I never do it unless venom IgE and skin tests are negative," and went on to question "what is the meaning of this 'random' tryptase level without rashes or other symptoms?"

In summary, mastocytosis and venom allergy is not merely a European problem, but is recognized as a problem only in Europe. Allergists in the United States have been generally unaware of the frequency of mastocytosis in insect allergy patients, or the clinical significance of baseline serum tryptase measurement in patients with insect-sting anaphylaxis. Baseline serum tryptase is not normally measured in the United States (unless skin tests and serum IgE tests are negative). The work group for the United States practice parameters continues to review the current status of our knowledge, and has advanced several other questions. Should baseline serum tryptase be measured in every patient who is evaluated for insect sting allergy, or just those with severe or hypotensive reactions? Should venom IgE or skin tests be done in every patient with mastocytosis (and should they receive VIT if the tests are positive)? Should patients with severe sting anaphylaxis be routinely tested in the future for abnormal levels of other mediators of anaphylaxis, such as platelet-activating factor (PAF) (or PAF acetylyhydrolase), prostaglandin D_2, leukotriene C_4, chymase, and carboxypeptidase?

SUMMARY

The occurrence of CMDs (particularly ISM without skin lesions or monoclonal mast-cell activation syndrome) in patients with HVA is now well ascertained, but probably underestimated.

In particular, HVA represents one of the most frequent clinical presentations in ISM without skin lesions.

The strong association between CMD and HVA is of particular interest, because it suggests a specific pathogenetic link between CMD and anaphylaxis from Hymenoptera venom, which probably differs from that of anaphylaxis attributable to drugs and foods.

The diagnosis of CMD is of clinical relevance to establish proper VIT, which can protect the patient from other serious or even fatal reactions.

The critical points in the association of HVA and CMD are the patients with systemic reactions to Hymenoptera venom with negative skin and serologic tests, the appropriate management of sensitized patients without previous systemic reactions, and, most importantly, the selection criteria for bone marrow biopsy.

The diagnosis of IVA is obligatory in patients with mastocytosis who have suffered from IVA. If the results are negative, the procedures such as skin tests and sIgE analysis should be repeated. If the result is still negative, BAT and recombinant allergens increase the sensitivity and lead to the correct diagnosis in most cases.

The only causative treatment of IVA is allergen immunotherapy. The effectiveness of the treatment in mastocytosis patients with standard dosage is slightly lower than in the general population. The safety of the treatment is also lower, thus the inpatient administration of the drug should be considered. Lifelong treatment is recommended in subjects with diagnosed mastocytosis and mast-cell activation syndrome, owing to the lack of long-term protection achievement caused by the presence of atypical mast cells.

REFERENCES

1. Bilò BM, Bonifazi F. Epidemiology of insect-venom anaphylaxis. Curr Opin Allergy Clin Immunol 2008;8:330–7.
2. Mueller H. Diagnosis and treatment of insect sensitivity. J Asthma Res 1966;3: 331.
3. Severino MG, Campi P, Macchia D, et al. European Polistes venom allergy. Allergy 2006;61(7):860–3.
4. Bonifazi F, Jutel M, Bilò BM, et al. EAACI Interest Group on insect venom hypersensitivity. Prevention and treatment of hymenoptera venom allergy: guidelines for clinical practice. Allergy 2005;60:1459–70.
5. Oude Elberink JN, De Monchy JG, Van Der Heide S, et al. Venom immunotherapy improves health-related quality of life in patients allergic to yellow jacket venom. J Allergy Clin Immunol 2002;110(1):174–82.
6. Brockow K, Jofer C, Behrendt H, et al. Anaphylaxis in patients with mastocytosis: a study on history, clinical features and risk factors in 120 patients. Allergy 2008;63(2):226–32.
7. van Anrooij B, van der Veer E, de Monchy JG, et al. Higher mast cell load decreases the risk of Hymenoptera venom-induced anaphylaxis in patients with mastocytosis. J Allergy Clin Immunol 2013;132(1):125–30.
8. Golden DB, Marsh DG, Freidhoff LR, et al. Natural history of Hymenoptera venom sensitivity in adults. J Allergy Clin Immunol 1997;100:760–6.
9. Sperr WR, Valent P. Diagnosis, progression patterns and prognostication in mastocytosis. Expert Rev Hematol 2012;5:261–74.
10. Müller UR, Horat W, Wüthrich B, et al. Anaphylaxis after Hymenoptera sting in three patients with urticaria pigmentosa. J Allergy Clin Immunol 1983;72:685–9.
11. Kors JW, van Doormaal JJ, de Monchy JG. Anaphylactoid shock following Hymenoptera sting as a presenting symptom of systemic mastocytosis. J Intern Med 1993;233:255–8.
12. Oude Elberink JN, de Moncky JG, Kors JW, et al. Fatal anaphylaxis after a yellow jacket sting, despite venom immunotherapy, in two patients with mastocytosis. J Allergy Clin Immunol 1997;99:153–4.
13. Florian S, Krauth MT, Simonitsch-Klupp I, et al. Indolent systemic mastocytosis with elevated serum tryptase, absence of skin lesions, and recurrent severe anaphylactoid episodes. Int Arch Allergy Immunol 2005;136:273–80.
14. Haeberli G, Bronnimann M, Hunziker T, et al. Elevated basal serum tryptase and hymenoptera venom allergy: relation to severity of sting reactions and to safety and efficacy of venom immunotherapy. Clin Exp Allergy 2003;33:1216–20.
15. González de Olano D, de la Hoz Caballer B, Núñez López R, et al. Prevalence of allergy and anaphylactic symptoms in 210 adult and pediatric patients with mastocytosis in Spain: a study of the Spanish network on mastocytosis (REMA). Clin Exp Allergy 2007;37:1547–55.
16. Alvarez-Twose I, González de Olano D, Sánchez-Muñoz L, et al. Clinical, biological, and molecular characteristics of clonal mast cell disorders presenting with

systemic mast cell activation symptoms. J Allergy Clin Immunol 2010;125: 1269–78.

17. Wein M. Sting anaphylaxis and urticaria pigmentosa. J Allergy Clin Immunol 1998;101:432.

18. Reiter N, Reiter M, Altrichter S, et al. Anaphylaxis caused by mosquito allergy in systemic mastocytosis. Lancet 2013;19:382.

19. Rosbotham JL, Malik NM, Syrris P, et al. Lack of c-kit mutation in familial urticaria pigmentosa. Br J Dermatol 1999;140:849–52.

20. van Doormaal JJ, Arends S, Brunekreeft KL, et al. Prevalence of indolent systemic mastocytosis in a Dutch region. J Allergy Clin Immunol 2013;131:1429–31.

21. Dubois AE. Mastocytosis and Hymenoptera allergy. Curr Opin Allergy Clin Immunol 2004;4:291–5.

22. Rueff F, Placzek M, Przybilla B. Mastocytosis and Hymenoptera venom allergy. Curr Opin Allergy Clin Immunol 2006;6:284–8.

23. Bonadonna P, Perbellini O, Passalacqua G, et al. Clonal mast cell disorders in patients with systemic reactions to Hymenoptera stings and increased serum tryptase levels. J Allergy Clin Immunol 2009;123:680–6.

24. Potier A, Lavigne C, Chappard D, et al. Cutaneous manifestations in Hymenoptera and Diptera anaphylaxis: relationship with basal serum tryptase. Clin Exp Allergy 2009;39:717–25.

25. Guenova E, Volz T, Eichner M, et al. Basal serum tryptase as risk assessment for severe Hymenoptera sting reactions in elderly. Allergy 2010;65:919–23.

26. Ludolph-Hauser D, Rueff F, Fries C, et al. Constitutively raised serum concentrations of mast-cell tryptase and severe anaphylactic reactions to Hymenoptera stings. Lancet 2001;357:361–2.

27. Zanotti R, Bonadonna P, Bonifacio M, et al. Isolated bone marrow mastocytosis: an underestimated subvariant of indolent systemic mastocytosis. Haematologica 2011;96:482–4.

28. Alvarez-Twose I, Bonadonna P, Matito A, et al. Systemic mastocytosis as a risk factor for severe Hymenoptera sting-induced anaphylaxis. J Allergy Clin Immunol 2013;131:614–5.

29. Alvarez-Twose I, Zanotti R, González-de-Olano D, et al, on behalf of the Spanish Network on Mastocytosis (REMA) and the Italian Network on Mastocytosis (RIMA). Nonaggressive systemic mastocytosis (SM) without skin lesions associated with insect-induced anaphylaxis shows unique features versus other indolent SM. J Allergy Clin Immunol 2013. [Epub ahead of print].

30. Fricker M, Helbling A, Schwartz L, et al. Hymenoptera sting anaphylaxis and urticaria pigmentosa: clinical findings and results of venom immunotherapy in ten patients. J Allergy Clin Immunol 1997;100:11–5.

31. Biedermann T, Ruëff F, Sander CA, et al. Mastocytosis associated with severe wasp sting anaphylaxis detected by elevated serum mast cell tryptase levels. Br J Dermatol 1999;141:1110–2.

32. Sonneck K, Florian S, Müllauer L, et al. Diagnostic and subdiagnostic accumulation of mast cells in the bone marrow of patients with anaphylaxis: monoclonal mast cell activation syndrome. Int Arch Allergy Immunol 2007;142: 158–64.

33. Akin C, Scott LM, Kocabas CN, et al. Demonstration of an aberrant mast-cell population with clonal markers in a subset of patients with "idiopathic" anaphylaxis. Blood 2007;110:2331–3.

34. González de Olano D, Alvarez-Twose I, Esteban-López MI, et al. Safety and effectiveness of immunotherapy in patients with indolent systemic mastocytosis

presenting with Hymenoptera venom anaphylaxis. J Allergy Clin Immunol 2008; 121:519–26.

35. Dugas-Breit S, Przybilla B, Dugas M, et al. Serum concentration of baseline mast cell tryptase: evidence for a decline during long-term immunotherapy for Hymenoptera venom allergy. Clin Exp Allergy 2010;40:643–9.

36. Müller UR, Haeberli G. The problem of anaphylaxis and mastocytosis. Curr Allergy Asthma Rep 2009;9:64–70.

37. Niedoszytko M, Oude Elberink JN, Bruinenberg M, et al. Gene expression profile, pathways, and transcriptional system regulation in indolent systemic mastocytosis. Allergy 2011;66:229–37.

38. Wimazal F, Geisser O, Shnawa P, et al. Severe life-threating or disabling anaphylaxis in patients with systemic mastocytosis: a single-center experience. Int Arch Allergy Immunol 2011;157:399–405.

39. Przybilla B, Rueff F. Insect stings: clinical features and management. Dtsch Arztebl Int 2012;109:238–48.

40. Biagini RE, MacKenzie BA, Sammons DL, et al. Latex specific IgE: performance characteristics of the IMMULITE 2000 3gAllergy assay compared with skin testing. Ann Allergy Asthma Immunol 2006;97:196–202.

41. Korošec P, Šilar M, Eržen R, et al. Clinical routine utility of basophil activation testing for diagnosis of hymenoptera-allergic patients with emphasis on individuals with negative venom-specific IgE antibodies. Int Arch Allergy Immunol 2013;161:363–8.

42. Bonadonna P, Zanotti R, Melioli G, et al. The role of basophil activation test in special populations with mastocytosis and reactions to hymenoptera sting. Allergy 2012;67:962–5.

43. Niedoszytko M, de Monchy J, van Doormaal JJ, et al. Mastocytosis and insect venom allergy: diagnosis, safety and efficacy of venom immunotherapy. Allergy 2009;64:1237–45.

44. Golden DB, Tracy JM, Freeman TM, et al. Negative venom skin test results in patients with histories of systemic reaction to a sting. Insect Committee of the American Academy of Allergy, Asthma and Immunology. J Allergy Clin Immunol 2003;112:495–8.

45. Kranke B, Sturm G, Aberer W. Negative venom skin test results and mastocytosis. J Allergy Clin Immunol 2004;113:180–1.

46. Golden DB, Kagey-Sobotka A, Norman PS, et al. Insect sting allergy with negative venom skin test responses. J Allergy Clin Immunol 2001;107:897–901.

47. Gonzalez-de-Olano D, Alvarez-Twose I, Morgado JM, et al. Evaluation of basophil activation in mastocytosis with Hymenoptera venom anaphylaxis. Cytometry B Clin Cytom 2011;80:167–75.

48. Bidad K, Nawijn MC, van Oosterhout AJ, et al. Basophil Activation Test in the diagnosis and monitoring of mastocytosis patients with wasp venom allergy. Cytometry B Clin Cytom 2013. [Epub ahead of print].

49. Muller U, Schmid-Grendelmeier P, Hausmann O, et al. IgE to recombinant allergens Api m 1, Ves v 1, and Ves v 5 distinguish double sensitization from cross-reaction in venom allergy. Allergy 2012;67:1069–73.

50. Holzweber F, Svehla E, Fellner W, et al. Inhibition of IgE binding to cross-reactive carbohydrate determinants enhances diagnostic selectivity. Allergy 2013;68:1269–77.

51. Kristensen T, Broesby-Olsen S, Vestergaard H, et al. Mastocytosis Centre Odense University Hospital (MastOUH) Circulating KIT D816V mutation-positive

non-mast cells in peripheral blood are characteristic of indolent systemic masto-cytosis. Eur J Haematol 2012;89:42–6.

52. Niedoszytko M, Bruinenberg M, de Monchy J, et al. Changes in gene expression caused by insect venom immunotherapy responsible for the long-term protection of insect venom-allergic patients. Ann Allergy Asthma Immunol 2011; 106:502–10.

53. Engler RJ, Davis WS. Rush Hymenoptera venom immunotherapy: successful treatment in a patient with systemic mast cell disease. J Allergy Clin Immunol 1994;94:556–9.

54. Bonadonna P, et al. Venom immunotherapy in patients with clonal mast cell disorders: efficacy, safety, and practical considerations. J Allergy Clin Immunol Pract 2013;1:474–8.

55. van Doormaal JJ, van der Veer E, van Voorst Vader PC, et al. Tryptase and histamine metabolites as diagnostic indicators of indolent systemic mastocytosis without skin lesions. Allergy 2012;67(5):683–90.

56. Golden DB. Insect sting anaphylaxis. Immunol Allergy Clin North Am 2007;27: 261–72.

57. Franken HH, Dubois AE, Minkema HJ, et al. Lack of reproducibility of a single negative sting challenge response in the assessment of anaphylactic risk in patients with suspected yellow jacket hypersensitivity. J Allergy Clin Immunol 1994; 93:431–6.

58. Golden D, Kwiterovich K, Kagey-Sobotka A, et al. Discontinuing venom immunotherapy: extended observations. J Allergy Clin Immunol 1998;101:298–305.

59. Bonadonna P, Zanotti R, Caruso B, et al. Allergen specific immunotherapy is safe and effective in patients with systemic mastocytosis and Hymenoptera allergy. J Allergy Clin Immunol 2008;121:256–7.

60. Ruëff F, Wenderoth A, Przybilla B. Patients still reacting to a sting challenge while receiving conventional Hymenoptera venom immunotherapy are protected by increased venom doses. J Allergy Clin Immunol 2001;108:1027–32.

61. Price LA, Safko M. Bee venom allergy in a patient with urticaria pigmentosa. J Allergy Clin Immunol 1987;79:407–9.

62. Reimers A, Müller U. Fatal outcome of a vespula sting in a patient with mastocytosis after specific immunotherapy with honey bee venom. Allergy Clin Immunol Int J WAO Org 2005;17(Suppl 1):69–70.

63. Schwartz LB, Metcalfe DD, Miller JS, et al. Tryptase levels as an indicator of mast-cell activation in systemic anaphylaxis and mastocytosis. N Engl J Med 1987;316(26):1622–6.

64. Moffitt JE, Golden DB, Reisman RE, et al. Stinging insect hypersensitivity: a practice parameter update. J Allergy Clin Immunol 2004;114:869–86.

65. Golden DB, Moffitt J, Nicklas RA, et al, Joint Task Force on Practice Parameters, American Academy of Allergy, Asthma & Immunology (AAAAI), American College of Allergy, Asthma & Immunology (ACAAI), Joint Council of Allergy, Asthma and Immunology. Stinging insect hypersensitivity: a practice parameter update 2011. J Allergy Clin Immunol 2011;127:852–4.

66. Müller UR, Golden DB, Demarco PJ, et al. Immunotherapy for hymenoptera venom and biting insect hypersensitivity. Clin Allergy Immunol 2007;7:337–41.

Bone Involvement and Osteoporosis in Mastocytosis

Maurizio Rossini, MD*, Roberta Zanotti, MD,
Ombretta Viapiana, MD, Gaia Tripi, MD, Giovanni Orsolini, MD,
Luca Idolazzi, MD, Patrizia Bonadonna, MD,
Donatella Schena, MD, Luis Escribano, MD, PhD, Silvano Adami, MD,
Davide Gatti, MD

KEYWORDS

- Mastocytosis • Osteoporosis • Osteosclerosis • Fracture • Bone mineral density
- Bone turnover markers

KEY POINTS

- Bone involvement is frequent in patients with systemic mastocytosis.
- Osteoporosis is the most prevalent bone manifestation, but diffuse osteosclerosis or focal osteolytic or osteosclerotic lesions are not infrequent.
- The risk of osteoporotic fractures is high, especially at the spine and in men.
- Routine measurements of bone mineral density and vertebral morphometry are warranted.
- The bone turnover markers indicate involvement of complex bone metabolism in mastocytosis-related manifestations.
- Bisphosphonates represent the first-line treatment for mastocytosis-related osteoporosis.

EPIDEMIOLOGY

Bone manifestations are one of the frequent symptoms of systemic mastocytosis (SM), particularly in adults. Patients may present with poorly localized bone pain, diffuse osteopenia or osteoporosis with fragility or pathologic fractures, diffuse osteosclerosis, or both focal osteolytic and osteosclerotic bone lesions.

SM has long been identified as a potential cause of osteoporosis. Nevertheless, until recently the bone involvement frequently has been described only in case reports or in small groups of patients.[1–14] In recent years studies on larger numbers of patients[15–18] and use of the dual X-ray absorptiometry (DXA) technique, which is universally accepted as the gold standard for assessing bone mass, have become available.[19]

The authors have nothing to disclose.
University of Verona, Policlinico Borgo Roma, Piazzale Scuro, 10, Verona 37134, Italy
* Corresponding author.
E-mail address: maurizio.rossini@univr.it

Immunol Allergy Clin N Am 34 (2014) 383–396
http://dx.doi.org/10.1016/j.iac.2014.01.011   immunology.theclinics.com

According to the traditional World Health Organization (WHO) criteria (T score, standard deviation [SD] below the mean of young healthy adults <−2.5),[19] osteoporosis ranged from 18% to 31% (**Fig. 1**). However, in these studies the reports also included elderly patients, so the real incidence of mastocytosis-related osteoporosis remains unclear. In previous published experience[17] the authors decided, in accord with guidelines of the International Society for Clinical Bone Densitometry,[20] to use the Z score (SD below the age- and gender-matched mean reference value) in addition to the WHO osteoporosis definition based on the T score. The threshold for that value to diagnose mastocytosis-related low bone mineral density (BMD) was set at less than −2, similar, for example, to what has been done for bone mineral classification in cystic fibrosis.[21] Adopting the traditional WHO criteria, osteoporosis was found in 20% of patients with indolent SM (ISM), whereas with the more accurate criteria, mastocytosis-related low BMD was found in 9% of women and 28% of men.[17]

The higher prevalence of osteoporosis in men compared with women, recently confirmed by others,[18] is somewhat consistent with the 9% prevalence of mastocytosis observed in bone biopsies in men with idiopathic osteoporosis.[22]

The percentage of bone involvement in 'the authors' series of ISM was 36%, lower than that reported by Barete and colleagues[16] (46%), who included a higher number of SM variants associated with a poorer prognosis.

Also observed was that patients without skin involvement, 55% versus only 5% in the study of Barete and colleagues,[16] have the same risk of osteoporosis as patients with skin lesions[17]: this is an important issue because in the absence of trigger factors for anaphylaxis, osteoporosis might be the only manifestation of a latent ISM. ISM without mastocytosis in the skin might be a challenge for the physician,[23] and the prevalence is possibly underestimated.[24] The authors' study indicates that osteoporosis of unknown etiology should lead to the suspicion of bone marrow mastocytosis. Moreover, the Z score at the total hip was significantly lower in those patients who did not have previous anaphylaxis when compared with those who did. This finding might simply reflect an earlier diagnosis in the latter group of patients.[25]

A recent update of data from this ISM cohort confirmed the results of the previous analysis carried out on a smaller group. The authors have records from 199 patients (81 women, mean age 53 years, age range 23–84 years; 118 men, mean age 49 years, age range 20–82 years). Among these subjects 65% had anaphylactic reaction to hymenoptera bite or drugs, and skin involvement was evident in 51%. Serum tryptase level higher than 20 μg/L was observed in 70% of cases, whereas in 9 patients it was below the more restrictive threshold of 11.4 μg/L. Osteoporosis, defined by OMS criteria (T score <−2.5), was documented more frequently in women (**Fig. 2**), but on average they were older than the men and most of them were already postmenopausal. Indeed, lower lumbar or femoral BMD, in comparison with age-matched and

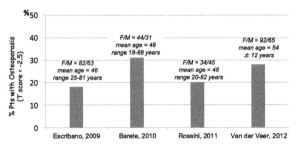

Fig. 1. Prevalence of osteoporosis in the largest available studies.

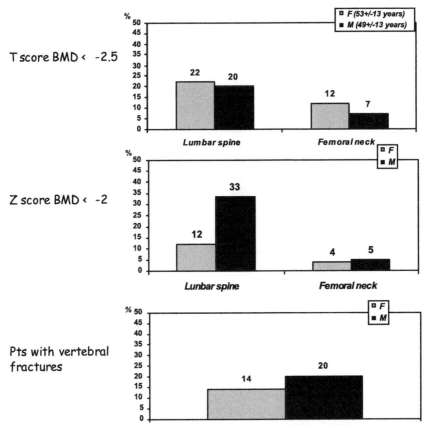

Fig. 2. Prevalence of osteoporosis, mastocytosis-related low bone mineral density (BMD), and vertebral fractures in the authors' 199 patients (81 women, 118 men) with indolent systemic mastocytosis.

sex-matched healthy controls (Z score <−2), were found more frequently in male than in female patients, especially at the lumbar site (33% vs 12%, respectively) (see **Fig. 2**). Moreover, the prevalence of at least 1 vertebral fracture was 20% in men and 14% in women (see **Fig. 2**), as already reported by the authors and other investigators.[17,18]

In the authors' experience about 1 male patient out of 5 had multiple vertebral fractures at the time of SM diagnosis, similar to what is seen in glucocorticoid-induced osteoporosis (**Fig. 3**), and this indicates the need for an earlier diagnosis. All vertebral sites, including the cervical spine, can be involved. There was no difference in the prevalence of low BMD between patients with or without skin involvement, whereas it was greater in the subgroup with no personal history of anaphylaxis.

In a recent study,[18] fracture prevalence was assessed in 157 patients (65 men, 92 women) affected by ISM with mean age 54 ± 12 years. A total of 235 fractures were reported, 140 of which were secondary to low-energy trauma. Of these 62% were vertebral, 1% pelvic, and 36% other nonvertebral. The prevalence of osteoporosis as diagnosed by DXA or osteoporotic fractures was 28% and 37% of patients, respectively. Prevalence of osteoporotic manifestation in men (46% <50 years, 73% ≥50 years) was much greater than in women (18% <50 years, 58% ≥50 years), as

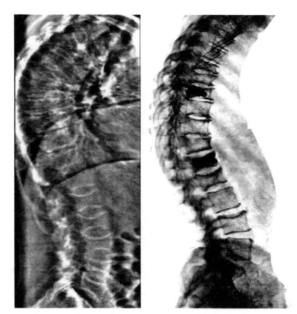

Fig. 3. Vertebral fracture assessment by dual X-ray absorptiometry; on the right, imaging outcomes of vertebroplasty are visible.

observed in a previous study.[17] Old age, male gender, and high urinary methylhistamine levels were independently correlated with bone porotic manifestations.[18] In the study of van der Veer and colleagues,[18] consistent with another study,[26] ISM patients without urticaria pigmentosa had a higher prevalence of osteoporotic fractures or osteoporosis at DXA, which could be due to an earlier diagnosis in patients with more evident clinical manifestations.

Diffuse osteosclerosis was described in 2% to 8% of patients with SM,[15–17,27] with a female/male ratio of 3:1.[26] Of importance, fragility fractures were not reported in the patients with ISM-related osteosclerosis. Overall, the reported percentages of focal or diffuse osteosclerosis ranged from 8% to 19% in series of patients with various forms of SM.[15,16,28] It should be borne in mind that, at variance with osteoporosis, this condition is apparently asymptomatic and, therefore, it is likely that a large proportion of the affected patients remains undiagnosed.

In SM either focal osteolytic or osteosclerotic bone lesions have been reported,[15,16] and the coexistence of these lesions is frequent: in a study of 75 adult mastocytosis patients, 37 had bone involvement, 23 had osteoporosis, 6 had axial osteosclerosis, 1 had an osteolytic lesion, and 3 had a mixed pattern.[16] Probably the prevalence of these focal bone lesions is not well known because in most of the studies a full skeletal radiographic examination in all patients is lacking.

The main limitation of the available studies is their cross-sectional nature, which does not allow establishment of the relationship between actual bone involvement and progression of the disease. Longitudinal studies are needed to understand the evolution of skeletal involvement in patients with SM.

PATHOPHYSIOLOGY

Osteoporosis was more frequently identified at the spine than at the hip, with fragility fractures most often involving the vertebral bodies. This finding suggests a prevalent involvement of trabecular bone tissue, although the reasons for this selective involvement remain unclear. Possible reasons include the higher propensity of clonal mast cells to colonize the bone marrow, or a rapid progression of the bone loss, with a prevalent involvement of the most metabolically active bone tissue. However, one cannot exclude that purely cortical bone loss may occur in mastocytosis, as previously suggested,[29] or based on the recently observed high incidence of nonvertebral fractures.[18]

Osteoporosis in SM has been attributed to either neoplastic infiltration or the local release of mediators (histamine, heparin, tryptase, lipid mediators, and cytokines). In particular, cytokines such as tumor necrosis factor α (TNF-α), interleukin (IL)-1, and IL-6, promotion of osteoclast activity, or inhibition of osteoblast function have been suggested to play a role.[30–35] Histamine is the most abundant product and acts directly on both osteoclasts and their precursors through autocrine/paracrine mechanisms.[33,34] Some mast cell products, such as histamine, have complex effects on bone remodeling. In the knock-out mice for histamine decarboxylase, the enzyme responsible for the production of histamine, osteoclast number is decreased and bone formation is increased.[36] A positive correlation between histamine metabolites and the risk of osteoporotic manifestation has been reported.[18]

Men with ISM are more prone than women with ISM to osteoporotic involvement,[17,18] suggesting a possibility that the influence of mast cell mediators on bone metabolism and the release of these mediators are different between the sexes.

Focusing on the bone histomorphometric analysis, in a few patients with osteoporosis in whom a bone biopsy was obtained, an increased[1,2,26,37] or normal[27] number of osteoclasts was reported. Regarding the histologic aspect,[26] an important article has been recently published about a quantitative histomorphometric technique applied to a large number of patients. Because 66% of patients were affected by ISM without the typical skin lesions, an analysis has been carried out comparing forms with or without cutaneous involvement. Histomorphometric analysis revealed that both forms of ISM are characterized by deterioration of bone structure (decrease in bone trabeculae) and increased amount of osteoid and bone cell (both osteoclasts and osteoblasts), without significant differences between patients with or without cutaneous involvement.

Thus, even if some morphologic and histologic features, such as reduction in trabeculae number and thickness, are similar to those observed in glucocorticoid-induced osteoporosis, others are completely different, especially the presence of osteoblasts that are typically decreased by glucocorticoids. ISM is associated with high bone turnover, and the extent of bone cell activity depends on mast cell number rather than cutaneous involvement.

Surprisingly, in mastocytosis osteoporosis the increase in osteoclast and osteoblast number was greater when mast cells were gathered to form granulomas, rather than scattered. Therefore, severity of bone involvement depended more on mast cell number and distribution in the bone marrow than on the presence or absence of skin manifestations.

Systemic bone-remodeling activity can be quantified using biochemical bone turnover markers (BTM), such as bone-specific alkaline phosphatase (bALP) or C-telopeptides of type I collagen (CTX). However, as previously reported,[17] in the patients with osteoporotic manifestations serum BTM often were found to be normal, sometimes above (and in such cases associated with increased uptake on bone scintiscan) or even below the normal range; unlike other forms of osteoporosis, such as postmenopausal, they did not correlate with BMD (**Fig. 4**). Moreover, in the authors' experience, as recently confirmed by others,[26] none of these serum markers were predictive for vertebral fractures in patients with ISM. These results might suggest that

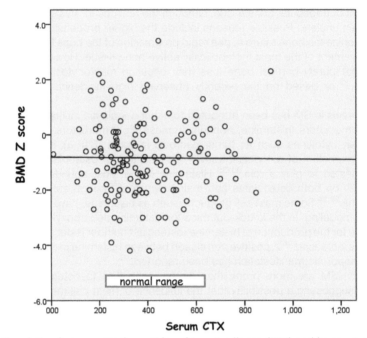

Fig. 4. Correlation between C-telopeptides of type I collagen (CTX) and bone mineral density (BMD) Z score in the authors' ISM patients.

mastocytosis-related osteoporosis could be characterized both by absolute and relative prevalence of osteoclastic activity, consistent with the positive results reported with bisphosphonate treatment.[16,29]

In a recent study[38] the behavior of serum BTM has been investigated in 45 adult patients with different categories of mastocytosis. Serum BTM assessing resorption (CTX, deoxypyridinoline), neoformation (bALP), or a serum osteoclast function–modulating cytokine (osteoprotegerin [OPG]) were significantly increased in patients compared with controls, although they showed a wide variability. CTX and OPG levels were higher in patients with aggressive SM than with cutaneous or indolent systemic forms; moreover, they significantly correlated with serum tryptase level. The correlations between serum tryptase and BTM levels, as well as among BTM levels and disease aggressiveness, support the existence of a link between the bone-remodeling process and the number of mast cells.

Similar to previous reports that elevated tryptase levels can be associated with greater bone density in patients with SM,[8] in the subgroup of ISM patients with osteoporosis there was a significant positive correlation between tryptase serum levels and Z-score BMD (**Fig. 5**). Of note, in these patients serum tryptase levels also significantly correlated with bALP serum levels (**Fig. 6**), a marker of bone formation, but not with CTX.

In the patients with diffuse osteosclerosis secondary to SM, serum tryptase levels were particularly high.[17] Moreover, in these patients the markers of bone turnover were particularly elevated, consistent with an increased and diffuse uptake at the scintiscan[17]: this was the first complete documentation that the diffuse osteosclerosis associated with SM is not an "osteopetrosis-like osteopathy," as previously reported,[39] but a skeletal disease characterized by increased bone turnover.

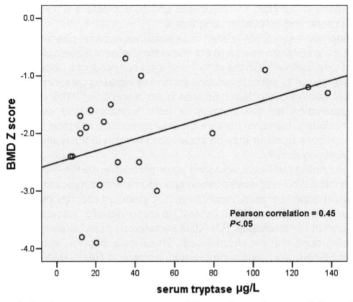

Fig. 5. Correlation between serum tryptase and Z score in a subgroup of the authors' ISM patients with osteoporosis.

This finding has been recently histologically confirmed on biopsies of patients with osteosclerosis in which, in addition to an increase in trabecular bone volume, there was an elevation of histologic bone turnover features,[26] according to what was revealed by the measurement of serum BTM or scintiscan.[17] Therefore, it appears

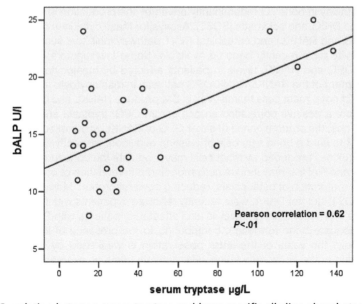

Fig. 6. Correlation between serum tryptase and bone-specific alkaline phosphatase (bALP) levels in a subgroup of the authors' ISM patients with osteoporosis.

that an increase in numbers of osteoclasts and osteoblasts is a common feature of both osteoporotic and osteosclerosing forms.

The pathophysiology of SM-related osteosclerosis remains obscure, although it is known that mast cells can exert a direct stimulatory effect on osteoblast proliferation, recruitment, and activity.[40] On the other hand mast cell products, possibly via tryptase release, were shown to activate osteoblasts and to increase osteoprotegerin production, thereby limiting osteoclast-mediated bone resorption.[40] The authors have no obvious explanation for the findings of both increased and decreased bone-formation markers in the same disease. One may surmise that in this condition, opposite effects on bone turnover may be observed in relation to the number of mast cells and their secreting activity.

The main signaling pathways regulating bone remodeling are the RANKL/OPG/RANK and the canonical WNT pathways promoting predominantly osteoclast bone resorption and osteoblast bone formation, respectively.[41] Osteoclast precursors express RANK, and the ligand that activates RANK (RANKL) is responsible for the recruitment, activation, and survival of osteoclasts. RANKL is secreted by osteoblasts but also by other cells including bone marrow stromal cells. These cells express also OPG, a decoy receptor for RANKL, and thus a physiologic inhibitor of RANK-RANKL signaling. Of interest, the same cell, the osteoblast, is able to express both the stimulator (RANKL) and the suppressor (OPG) of RANK and consequently to affect osteoclast differentiation and activity. Osteoblast differentiation is predominantly regulated by the canonical WNT pathway, which acts as the master regulator of osteogenesis together with bone morphogenetic proteins. The WNT pathway plays a key role in determining the fate of mesenchymal stem cells. In the absence of β-catenin, these cells do not differentiate into mature osteocalcin-expressing osteoblasts but only into chondrocytes. This pathway also promotes osteoblastogenesis by suppressing adipogenesis, through peroxisome proliferator activated receptor γ (PPARγ) inhibition. Increased WNT signaling might also, in some circumstances, result in a reduced osteoclastogenesis and bone resorption by promoting the osteoblast expression of OPG. The regulation of WNT pathway in bone is predominantly driven by the production of receptor inhibitors such as DKK1 and sclerostin (SOST). Assays for these cytokines controlling osteoclast (OPG and RANKL) and osteoblast (WNT pathway inhibitors such as SOST and DKK1) activity have recently become available. Some investigators reported an increase in OPG and RANKL levels in patients affected by mastocytosis, suggesting the involvement of the RANKL/RANK/OPG pathway in mastocytosis-related osteoporosis.[38,42] Of note, mast cells themselves in SM produce RANKL and OPG.[42]

In addition, a positive correlation among serum OPG, tryptase, and BTM was reported.[38] Thus, the predominance of either OPG or RANKL would direct bone involvement in SM toward a bone sclerosis or wasting evolution, respectively.

Bone cytokines produced by mast cells may modulate the bone turnover in various ways. IL-6 and RANKL may induce activation and differentiation of osteoclasts. OPG may inhibit maturation of osteoclasts, reducing bone resorption. Moreover, enhanced levels of SOST, but not DKK1, were recently reported in patients with ISM,[42] suggesting that the WNT/β-catenin pathway is also affected in patients with SM, with consequent inadequate bone formation, contributing to the presence of low bone mass. Unfortunately, the value of the latter observation is weakened by the inadequate age matching of the study population, with patients being on average 15 years older than controls, and it has been described in many studies that SOST increases in tandem with age. In their cohort of ISM patients with osteopenia or osteoporosis, the authors have been unable to detect differences in a comparison with perfectly matched healthy subjects, and have confirmed a positive significant correlation between age and SOST.[43] The authors observed in the data of Rabenhorst and colleagues[42] that the serum levels of SOST and 25-hydroxyvitamin D were negatively correlated, which might suggest that vitamin D levels are determinants of SOST levels, at least in ISM patients.[43]

CLINICAL FEATURES

The principal clinical manifestation of bone involvement in SM is the fragility fracture, in particular at the vertebral bodies. According to experience, at the time of diagnosis 20% of male patients had multiple deformities, with medial collapses resembling those typically seen in glucocorticoid-induced osteoporosis (see **Fig. 3**).

Recently it has been observed in ISM patients that 36% of fragility fractures occurs at nonvertebral sites,[18] suggesting a relevant involvement of cortical bone also.

Patients frequently (54%) report bone pain, described as severe or intolerable in 18% of cases.[44]

Nearly nothing is known regarding the clinical evolution of focal lesions, especially of sclerosing lesions, in SM patients. Forms of diffuse osteosclerosis usually are asymptomatic, even if in the authors' experience they seem to be at risk of developing early osteoarthritic features.

DIAGNOSIS

Vertebral osteoporosis and fractures are frequent in patients with SM, particularly in young males and also in patients without skin involvement. All patients with idiopathic osteoporosis, particularly males, should be evaluated for mast cell disease. Both total spine radiography and densitometric examination are warranted in all patients with SM, as is evaluation by DXA according to T scores and Z scores. Indeed, in patients with vertebral fractures the authors observed on average a lower T score and Z score. Although there is great variability, in about half of the patients these values were not pathologic (**Fig. 7**), or not valuable because of inaccuracy caused by fracture or

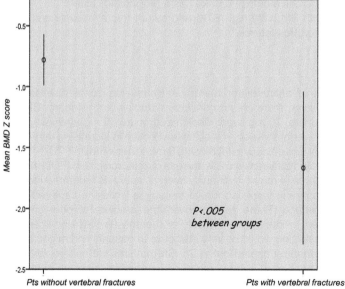

Fig. 7. Mean bone mineral density (BMD) Z score in ISM patients with or without fractures.

osteoarthritis deformities. Therefore, DXA sensitivity and specificity to predict vertebral fracture is limited. In SM the association between fracture and DXA diagnosis
of osteoporosis is inconstant, likely because of the patchy distribution of neoplastic
mast cells, or because there are other bone features, in addition to BMD, affected;
these should be evaluated with a different approach. In the absence of other diagnostic tools for bone assessment, the authors recommend obtaining a total spine
radiograph for vertebral morphometry in all SM patients. Vertebral fractures are
assessed visually. The semiquantitative system of Genant is commonly used.[45] A
vertebral deformity of at least 20% loss in height is typically considered a fracture.
This system grades the deformities from I to III, with grade I representing a 20% to
24% reduction in vertebral height and ranging up to grade III, which is a 40% or greater
reduction in height. Vertebral fracture assessment by DXA (see **Fig. 3**) can be useful in
the evaluation of vertebral fractures in these patients, especially in the follow-up. The
authors typically perform a DXA scan once every year until stability is achieved, with
less frequent monitoring thereafter.

The observation that less than 5% of patients with ISM had a normal serum tryptase
level suggests that this assay can be used confidently for screening in selected cases
of unexplained osteoporosis, even if the serum tryptase level in the normal range
cannot exclude SM diagnosis. On the other hand, high levels of serum tryptase can
be found in other diseases such as chronic urticaria, renal insufficiency, other hematologic diseases, onchocercosis, ischemic myocardial disease, or in the presence of
heterophilic antibodies. In the authors' experience, serum tryptase levels cannot be
used as a predictor of osteoporosis involvement in patients with SM. It has been reported that the urinary histamine metabolites, in particular methylhistamine, are associated with a higher risk of osteoporotic manifestations.[18]

In SM, tryptase levels, which reflect mast cell burden, correlate significantly with
BTM.[38] The role of BTM in clinical practice remains uncertain. However, high serum
levels of BTM are suspicious for mastocytosis bone involvement, and in this condition
a scintigraphy bone scan is recommended. Increased uptake at the scintiscan can
detect focal and asymptomatic bone lesions, to be subjected to targeted radiographic
assessment, whereas a diffuse uptake has a prognostic value.[46]

In patients with SM, very high BTM and serum tryptase levels are suspicious for
diffuse osteosclerotic features.[17]

MANAGEMENT

Early institution of antimediator therapy may reverse some disease-related bone
changes[47]; however, there are no conclusive studies in this regard. Bisphosphonate
therapy (alendronate, 70 mg every week; risedronate 35 mg every week; pamidronic
acid, 90 mg intravenously every 4 weeks) is effective in increasing vertebral BMD, but
has considerably less efficacy in increasing femoral neck BMD.[16,29,48,49] In the absence
of a specific study in patients with SM, the use of zoledronic acid (ZOL) at the dose used
in multiple myeloma (4 mg intravenously every 4 weeks) is recommended.[50]

Evidence supporting bisphosphonate therapy is limited to case reports or studies
of very small groups (**Table 1**). Moreover, the problem of poor compliance with
bisphosphonates, whether given weekly or monthly, is well documented, and less
frequent administration would be very attractive to patients and might further increase
compliance. In therapy carried out in 25 ISM patients with osteoporosis, one 5-mg
intravenous infusion of ZOL guaranteed a therapeutic effect on surrogate markers
(BMD and BTM) of antifracture efficacy for at least 1 year (Rossini, unpublished
data, 2013). Mean BMD gain was at least twice as great as those reported in previous

Table 1
Evidence supporting bisphosphonate therapy

Authors,[Ref.] Year	Treatment	Cases (N)
Cundy et al,[29] 1987	Oral clodronate	1
Marshall et al,[49] 1997	IV pamidronate	3
Brumsen et al,[48] 2002	IV + oral pamidronate	1
Lim et al,[7] 2005	IV pamidronate + oral alendronate	6
Laroche et al,[54] 2007	Interferon-α + IV pamidronate	4
Laroche et al,[55] 2011	IV pamidronate $\pm$ interferon-α	10

Abbreviation: IV, intravenous.

small series with daily oral treatment with alendronate or with monthly pamidronate infusions, both in lumbar and femoral sites. Moreover, at 1 year after the only ZOL infusion the BTM were still suppressed, suggesting that there may be a safe time window during which subsequent infusions may be administered.

In severe and bisphosphonate-refractory cases and in mastocytosis-related bone pain, interferon-α can be useful.[50–55]

REFERENCES

1. Fallon MD, Whyte MP, Teitelbaum SL. Systemic mastocytosis associated with generalized osteopenia. Histopathological characterization of the skeletal lesion using undecalcified bone from two patients. Hum Pathol 1981;12:813–20.
2. Chines A, Pacifici R, Avioli LV, et al. Systemic mastocytosis presenting as osteoporosis: a clinical and histomorphometric study. J Clin Endocrinol Metab 1991; 72:140–4.
3. Schoenaers P, De Clerck LS, Timmermans U, et al. Systemic mastocytosis, an unusual cause of osteoporosis. Clin Rheumatol 1987;6:458–62.
4. Harvey JA, Anderson HC, Borek D, et al. Osteoporosis associated with mastocytosis confined to bone: report of two cases. Bone 1989;10:237–41.
5. Lidor C, Frisch B, Gazit D, et al. Osteoporosis as the sole presentation of bone marrow mastocytosis. J Bone Miner Res 1990;5:871–6.
6. Floman Y, Amir G. Systemic mastocytosis presenting with severe spinal osteopenia and multiple compression fractures. J Spinal Disord 1991;4:369–73.
7. Lim AY, Ostor AJ, Love S, et al. Systemic mastocytosis: a rare cause of osteoporosis and its response to bisphosphonate treatment. Ann Rheum Dis 2005;64:965–6.
8. Kushnir-Sukhov NM, Brittain E, Reynolds JC, et al. Elevated tryptase levels are associated with greater bone density in a cohort of patients with mastocytosis. Int Arch Allergy Immunol 2006;139:265–70.
9. Salles M, Holgado S, Navarro JT, et al. Osteoporosis as a first manifestation of systemic mastocytosis. Study of 6 cases. Med Clin (Barc) 2007;128:216–8.
10. King JJ, Crawford EA, Iwenofu OH, et al. Pathologic long bone fracture in a patient with systemic mastocytosis. Clin Orthop Relat Res 2007;459:263–9.
11. Donker ML, Bakker NA, Jaspers WJ, et al. Two patients with osteoporosis: initial presentation of systemic mastocytosis. J Bone Miner Metab 2008;26:199–202.
12. Stein JA, Kamino H, Walters RF, et al. Mastocytosis with urticaria pigmentosa and osteoporosis. Dermatol Online J 2008;14:2.
13. Mathew R, Dhillon V, Shepherd P. Systemic mastocytosis presenting as osteoporosis-a case report. Clin Rheumatol 2009;28:865–6.

14. Manara M, Varenna M, Cantoni S, et al. Osteoporosis with vertebral fractures in young males, due to bone marrow mastocytosis: a report of two cases. Clin Exp Rheumatol 2010;28:97–100.

15. Escribano L, Alvarez-Twose I, Sánchez-Muñoz L, et al. Prognosis in adult indolent systemic mastocytosis: a long-term study of the Spanish Network on Mastocytosis in a series of 145 patients. J Allergy Clin Immunol 2009;124:514–21.

16. Barete S, Assous N, de Gennes C, et al. Systemic mastocytosis and bone involvement in a cohort of 75 patients. Ann Rheum Dis 2010;69:1838–41.

17. Rossini M, Zanotti R, Bonadonna P, et al. Bone mineral density, bone turnover markers and fractures in patients with indolent systemic mastocytosis. Bone 2011;49:880–5.

18. van der Veer E, van der Goot W, de Monchy JG, et al. High prevalence of fractures and osteoporosis in patients with indolent systemic mastocytosis. Allergy 2012;67:431–8.

19. Kanis JA. Assessment of fracture risk and its application to screening for postmenopausal osteoporosis: synopsis of a WHO report. WHO study Group. Osteoporos Int 1994;4:368–81.

20. Lewiecki EM, Gordon CM, Baim S, et al. International society for clinical densitometry 2007 adult and pediatric official positions. Bone 2008;43:1115–21.

21. Report of the UK Cystic Fibrosis Trust Bone Mineralisation Working Group. Bone mineralisation in cystic fibrosis. Cystic Fibrosis Trust 2007. Available at: www.cftrust.org.uk. Accessed February 20, 2014.

22. Brumsen C, Papapoulos SE, Lentjes EG, et al. A potential role for the mast cell in the pathogenesis of idiopathic osteoporosis in men. Bone 2002;31:556–61.

23. Valent P, Akin C, Escribano L, et al. Standards and standardization in mastocytosis: consensus statements on diagnostics, treatment recommendations and response criteria. Eur J Clin Invest 2007;37:435–53.

24. Zanotti R, Bonadonna P, Bonifacio M, et al. Isolated bone marrow mastocytosis: an underestimated subvariant of indolent systemic mastocytosis. Haematologica 2011;96:482–4.

25. Bonadonna P, Perbellini O, Passalacqua G, et al. Clonal mast cell disorders in patients with systemic reactions to hymenoptera stings and raised serum tryptase. J Allergy Clin Immunol 2009;123:680–6.

26. Seitz S, Barvencik F, Koehne T, et al. Increased osteoblast and osteoclast indices in individuals with systemic mastocytosis. Osteoporos Int 2013;24:2325–34.

27. Delling G, Ritzel H, Werner M. Histological characteristics and prevalence of secondary osteoporosis in systemic mastocytosis. A retrospective analysis of 158 cases. Pathologe 2001;22:132–40.

28. Travis WD, Li CY, Bergstralh EJ, et al. Systemic mast cell disease. Analysis of 58 cases and literature review. Medicine (Baltimore) 1988;67:345–68.

29. Cundy T, Beneton MN, Darby AJ, et al. Osteopenia in systemic mastocytosis: natural history and responses to treatment with inhibitors of bone resorption. Bone 1987;8:149–55.

30. Metcalfe DD. Mast cells and mastocytosis. Blood 2008;112:946–55.

31. Theoharides TC, Boucher W, Spear K. Serum interleukin-6 reflects disease severity and osteoporosis in mastocytosis patients. Int Arch Allergy Immunol 2002;128:344–50.

32. Brockow K, Akin C, Huber M, et al. IL-6 levels predict disease variant and extent of organ involvement in patients with mastocytosis. Clin Immunol 2005;115:216–23.

33. Dobigny C, Saffar JL. H1 and H2 histamine receptors modulate osteoclastic resorption by different pathways: evidence obtained by using receptor antagonists in a rat synchronized resorption model. J Cell Physiol 1997;173:10–8.
34. Biosse-Duplan M, Baroukh B, Dy M, et al. Histamine promotes osteoclastogenesis through the differential expression of histamine receptors on osteoclasts and osteoblasts. Am J Pathol 2009;174:1426–34.
35. Kanzaki S, Takahashi T, Kanno T, et al. Heparin inhibits BMP-2 osteogenic bioactivity by binding to both BMP-2 and BMP receptor. J Cell Physiol 2008;216: 844–50.
36. Fitzpatrick LA, Buzas E, Gagne TJ, et al. Targeted deletion of histamine decarboxylase gene in mice increases bone formation and protects against ovariectomy-induced bone loss. Proc Natl Acad Sci U S A 2003;100:6027–32.
37. De Gennes C, Kuntz D, de Vernejoul MC. Bone mastocytosis. A report of nine cases with a bone histomorphometric study. Clin Orthop Relat Res 1992;279:281–91.
38. Guillaume N, Desoutter J, Chandesris O, et al. Bone complications of mastocytosis: a link between clinical and biological characteristics. Am J Med 2013;126: 75.e1–7.
39. Reinacher-Schick A, Petrasch S, Longley BJ, et al. c-Kit mutation and osteopetrosis-like osteopathy in a patient with systemic mast cell disease. Ann Hematol 1998;77:131–4.
40. Chiappetta N, Gruber B. The role of mast cells in osteoporosis. Semin Arthritis Rheum 2006;36:32–6.
41. Rossini M, Gatti D, Adami S. Involvement of WNT/β-catenin signaling in the treatment of osteoporosis. Calcif Tissue Int 2013;93:121–32.
42. Rabenhorst A, Christopeit B, Leja S, et al. Serum levels of bone cytokines are increased in indolent systemic mastocytosis associated with osteopenia or osteoporosis. J Allergy Clin Immunol 2013;132:1234–7.
43. Rossini M, Adami S, Zanotti R, et al. Serum levels of bone cytokines in indolent systemic mastocytosis associated with osteopenia or osteoporosis. J Allergy Clin Immunol 2013. [Epub ahead of print]. http://dx.doi.org/10.1016/j.jaci. 2013.12.007.
44. Hermine O, Lortholary O, Leventhal PS, et al. Case-control cohort study of patients' perceptions of disability in mastocytosis. PLoS One 2008;3(5):e2266.
45. Genant HK, Wu CY, van Kuijk C, et al. Vertebral fracture assessment using a semiquantitative technique. J Bone Miner Res 1993;8:1137–48.
46. Chen CC, Andrich MP, Mican JM, et al. A retrospective analysis of bone scan abnormalities in mastocytosis: correlation with disease category and prognosis. J Nucl Med 1994;35:1471–5.
47. Graves L III, Stechschulte DJ, Morris DC, et al. Inhibition of mediator release in systemic mastocytosis is associated with reversal of bone changes. J Bone Miner Res 1990;5:1113–9.
48. Brumsen C, Hamdy NA, Papapoulos SE. Osteoporosis and bone marrow mastocytosis: dissociation of skeletal responses and mast cell activity during long-term bisphosphonate therapy. J Bone Miner Res 2002;17:567–9.
49. Marshall A, Kavanagh RT, Crisp AJ. The effect of pamidronate on lumbar spine bone density and pain in osteoporosis secondary to systemic mastocytosis. Br J Rheumatol 1997;36:393–6.
50. Pardanani A. How I treat patients with indolent and smoldering mastocytosis (rare conditions but difficult to manage). Blood 2013;121:3085–94.
51. Weide R, Ehlenz K, Lorenz W, et al. Successful treatment of osteoporosis in systemic mastocytosis with interferon alpha-2b. Ann Hematol 1996;72:41–3.

52. Lehmann T, Beyeler C, Lammle B, et al. Severe osteoporosis due to systemic mast cell disease: successful treatment with interferon alpha-2B. Br J Rheumatol 1996;35:898–900.

53. Butterfield JH. Interferon treatment for hypereosinophilic syndromes and systemic mastocytosis. Acta Haematol 2005;114:26–40.

54. Laroche M, Bret J, Brouchet A, et al. Clinical and densitometric efficacy of the association of interferon alpha and pamidronate in the treatment of osteoporosis in patients with systemic mastocytosis. Clin Rheumatol 2007;26:242–3.

55. Laroche M, Livideanu C, Paul C, et al. Interferon alpha and pamidronate in osteoporosis with fracture secondary to mastocytosis. Am J Med 2011;124:776–8.

Drug Allergy in Mastocytosis

Patrizia Bonadonna, MD*, Carla Lombardo, MD

KEYWORDS

- Mastocytosis • Mast cell diseases • Clonal mast cell disorders • Drug allergy
- Drug hypersensitivity • Anaphylaxis

KEY POINTS

- Mastocytosis in adults is associated with a history of anaphylaxis in 22% to 49%.
- Drugs are known to elicit anaphylaxis in patients with mastocytosis, but data on patients with drug hypersensitivity and mast cell diseases are scarce.
- In unselected patients with drug hypersensitivity, only a few patients with unrecognized mast cell disease have been described.
- In patients with drug anaphylaxis, basal serum tryptase determination and careful skin inspection are recommended to exclude mast cell disease.
- The risk of systemic reactions during general anesthesia can be reduced by an assessment of a patient's personal risks (previous reaction to a drug or during surgery) and by avoiding specific trigger factors (patient's temperature changes, infusion of cold solution, tissue trauma, friction and other mechanical factors).

INTRODUCTION

Patients with mastocytosis have an increased risk of anaphylaxis with a prevalence reported between 22% and 49% in adults and between 6% and 9% in children.[1,2] Fatal anaphylaxis has been described after Hymenoptera sting; anesthesia; the intake of drugs, such as nonsteroidal anti-inflammatory drugs (NSAIDs), codeine, and perioperative drugs; foods and unknown causes.[2–4]

Immunologic drug hypersensitivity reactions may commonly be divided into immediate (<1 h) and nonimmediate (>1 h) reactions depending on the time of onset of symptoms.[4] Immediate reactions, possibly IgE-mediated, appear within 1 to 6 hours after drug intake and usually include urticaria, angioedema, conjunctivitis, rhinitis, bronchospasm, gastrointestinal symptoms (nausea, vomiting, diarrhea), and anaphylaxis.[5] However, the frequency of underlying mast cell diseases (MCD) in patients with drug hypersensitivity is still unknown.

Conflict of Interest: None.
Allergy Unit, Azienda Ospedaliera Universitaria Integrata of Verona, Piazzale Aristide Stefani 1, Verona 37126, Italy
* Corresponding author.
E-mail address: patrizia.bonadonna@ospedaleuniverona.it

Drug Anaphylaxis in Patients with Mastocytosis

Drugs are among the listed trigger factors for anaphylaxis in patients with mastocytosis. There are no data on drug-induced urticaria alone. Nevertheless, published data are based on case reports and a few small case series that do not lead to clear indications.

NSAIDs, β-lactam antibiotics, radiocontrast media (RCM), aminoglycosides, streptomycin, phenylephrine, codeine, and local and general anesthesia have been listed as trigger factors in patient histories.[1,2] However, there are no formal confirmations by positive skin test or provocation test described in the literature.

MCD in Patients with Drug Hypersensitivity

In patients with anaphylaxis, a few recently published case reports have indicated an association between severe systemic reactions during general anesthesia and persistent high tryptase values, but bone marrow biopsy was performed only in some cases.[6–8] In addition to reactions to general anesthesia or antibiotics, anaphylaxis to iodinated contrast media has been described in a patient who was subsequently diagnosed with systemic mastocytosis (SM).[9] Another paper reports a case of an acetylsalicylic acid–dependent anaphylaxis to carrot in a young patient with SM, and oral allergy syndrome to raw carrots was confirmed by oral provocation test.

Only selected studies have tried to investigate undetected MCD. In contrast to studies in patients with Hymenoptera venom allergy, where 88% of patients with anaphylaxis and raised tryptase values had a clonal MCD (SM or monoclonal mast cell activation syndrome), the association between severe systemic reactions to drug and MCD is far lower.[10] An Italian study determined the frequency of MCD in patients with food- or drug-induced anaphylaxis: out of 86 patients with drug hypersensitivity only 7 patients (8.1%) had increased serum tryptase levels greater than 11.4 ng/mL.[11] However, only one out of five bone marrow–tested patients was finally diagnosed with SM. No case of monoclonal mast cell activation syndrome was documented. Moreover, the study authors observed that the severity of reactions was significantly greater in patients with drug hypersensitivity.

These data were confirmed in another publication where the clinical, biologic, and molecular characteristics of 83 patients with anaphylaxis and other symptoms attributable to MCD without skin involvement were analyzed. In patients with clonal MCD the most common trigger for anaphylactic episodes was Hymenoptera sting, whereas drugs were mostly involved as a trigger in nonclonal MCD.[12]

In other studies on drug hypersensitivity, which included serum tryptase measurements after reactions, bone marrow biopsy to diagnose MCD was not performed.[13–16]

MCDS AND GENERAL ANESTHESIA

The literature on perioperative drug safety in patients with mastocytosis is very limited, and is taken from a few case reports and some small case series that often give conflicting information on single drugs and drug groups tolerated or not by these patients. Large cohort studies looking at the prevalence of reactions during general anesthesia in patients with SM have not been published. Thus, it is not possible to provide general recommendations regarding drugs or groups of drugs that are either well tolerated or not tolerated. A recent review of the available literature on surgical procedures in patients with mastocytosis tries to provide indications on how to manage perioperative courses and avoid known trigger factors.[17]

Given the improvement of anesthetic procedures in the last few decades, those drugs reported as potential trigger factors in early case reports are no longer considered to be valid in most countries. Particular attention to physical potential trigger factors should be observed: sudden temperature changes in patients and the operating room, infusion of cold solutions, wide tissue trauma, frictions, and other mechanical factors should all be avoided. Because mast cell degranulation can be triggered by anxiety, premedication with sedatives, such as benzodiazepines, should be considered in selected patients.

Risk Factors

The current literature does not make it possible to quantify the risk of systemic reaction during general anesthesia in patients with mastocytosis. Anaphylaxis in children with pediatric-onset mastocytosis is rare and limited to patients with extensive skin disease (>40% of body surface) and higher serum tryptase levels.[2] In a retrospective study of patients with pediatric mastocytosis that includes 24 general anesthesias and five cases of sedation and local anesthesia in 22 patients, adverse reactions were limited to flushing in 9% and gastrointestinal reactions with nausea, vomiting, and/ or diarrhea in 18% of patients.[18] Patients did not follow any prophylactic treatment with H_1 and H_2 blockers or steroids, but they continued their chronic antimediator therapy; no special anesthetic recommendations were reported. Moreover, a review of pediatric cases of anesthesia in children with mastocytosis has suggested that the risk for most pediatric patients is probably overstated by mastocytosis Web sites.[19]

Risk for adults seems higher and occurs mainly in systemic forms of mastocytosis, such as indolent SM, regardless of skin involvement.[2] The risk is probably lower in patients that never have experienced anaphylaxis and/or have tolerated previous general anesthesia. Instead, patients who have reported anaphylaxis, especially those that have experienced systemic reactions after drug administration or during anesthesia, should be considered at higher risk and an allergy evaluation should be strongly considered for these patients before elective procedures.

Value of Premedication

Currently, there is no evidence of the efficacy of premedication with antihistamine (anti-H_1 and anti-H_2) and corticosteroids to prevent systemic reactions in patients with mastocytosis. However, there is no evidence to the contrary either: some groups of specialists suggest premedication only in selected cases, whereas other groups recommend pretreatment in all patients in addition to their chronic antimediator therapy.[20]

A reasonable, but unproved approach is to consider premedication with an intravenous antihistamine (eg, chlorphenamine, 10 mg, diphenhydramine, 25 mg) 1 hour before anesthesia ± corticosteroids (eg, prednisone, 40–60 mg, 13, 7, and 1 hour before anesthesia) at the discretion of the anesthetist. This is extrapolated from the regimen used in patients with contrast media allergies. The value of adding an H_2 blocker (eg, ranitidine 1 hour before anesthesia) remains unknown.[3] To prevent anxiety-triggered mast cell degranulation, premedication with sedatives, such as benzodiazepines, should be considered.

Tryptase

Tryptase is a serine protease predominantly retained in the granules of mast cells and released after their activation and degranulation. An increase from baseline level during allergic symptoms is suggestive of IgE-mediated mast cell activation and correlates with the clinical severity of the reaction.[21]

Serum tryptase peaks at 30 to 90 minutes after the onset of symptoms and decreases in a few hours. Total serum tryptase level greater than 11.4 µg/L is consistent with systemic anaphylaxis.[22] Thus, it is important to measure tryptase value in all patients immediately after a reaction to confirm mast cell activation, and also to compare the acute value with the basal tryptase value, which should be measured several days after full recovery of the patient.

Anesthesia in Childhood Mastocytosis

Anaphylaxis in children with pediatric-onset mastocytosis is rare and probably over-stated. Even with these patients, however, the anesthetist should be aware of the clinical conditions of the patient and should have a thorough understanding of mastocytosis and its manifestations.[18,19]

So far, there is no evidence of a higher risk of reactions in patients with pediatric-onset mastocytosis. Although a range of equally effective drugs is available, those with minimal histamine release should be selected (eg, fentanyl and vecuronium instead of morphine and atracurium or mivacurium). Medications and equipment to treat perioperative anaphylaxis should be readily available.

Anesthesia in Adult Patients with Mastocytosis

The risk of anaphylaxis seems to be higher in adults with mastocytosis than in children, but it is not currently possible to clarify whether the severity of the reaction during anesthesia is a consequence of a higher mast cell load and if the frequency of reactions is higher compared with the general population. Randomized, controlled trials regarding the safety of anesthetic drugs in patients with mastocytosis are not available; thus, the indications for their use can be based only on case reports and case series, or on the use of those drugs considered safer in the general population (**Table 1**).

In general, histamine-releasing drugs (ie, certain opioids and neuromuscular blocking agents) should be avoided if possible or administered slowly. Induction agents are generally considered to be well tolerated (thiopental is associated with the highest number of reports). Inhalant anesthetics of the fluran family have not been associated with anaphylaxis.[17,23]

Muscle relaxants with the highest unspecific histamine release are atracurium and mivacurium. Rocuronium and succinylcholin have been described as being associated with the highest number of allergic reactions.[23] Vecuronium, pancuronium, and cisatracurium have not been reported to cause a high number of reactions perioperatively.

Opioids, such as morphine and codeine, should be avoided if possible because they have been associated with mast cell activation in patients with mastocytosis. Fentanyl and related agents remifentanyl, sufentanyl, and alfentanyl do not seem related to a high risk of reactions.[23]

Local Anesthesia

There are not enough data to support an increased risk for mastocytosis in patients with local anesthesia. A recent retrospective study on mastocytosis in pregnancy reported good tolerance to epidural amide-type local anesthesia, and reported mild symptoms of mast cell mediators release (generalized erythema and flushing) in 5 (11%) out of 45 patients only.[20] Moreover, labor induction was carried out in nine vaginal deliveries using oxytocine (N = 8) and dinoprostone (N = 1) without any symptom. At the discretion of the anesthetist, prophylactic antiallergic therapy was given in 38% of cases, using different combinations of antihistamines and corticosteroids.

Table 1
Perioperative drugs associated with a lower or higher risk of reactions during surgical procedures in mastocytosis

Perioperative Drugs	Low Risk	Avoid[a]
Intravenous analgesics		
Opioids	Fentanyl	Morphine
	Sulfentanyl	Codeine
	Remifentanyl	
	Alfentanyl	
Analgesic	Paracetamol (acetaminophen)	
General anesthetics		
Hypnotics	Propofol	Thiopental
	Etomidate	
	Ketamine	
Benzodiazepine	Midazolam	
Halogenated gases	Desflurane	
and nitrous oxide	Isoflurane	
	Sevoflurane	
	Nitrous oxide	
Neuromuscular blocking agents		
Depolarizing neuromuscular		Succinylcholine
blocking agents		
Nondepolarizing steroidal	Pancuronium	Rocuronium
neuromuscular blocking agents	Vecuronium	
Nondepolarizing benzylisoquinolin	Cis-atracurium	Atracurium
neuromuscular blocking agents		Mivacurium
Anticholinergic	Atropine	
Plasma substitutes	Cristalloids	Gelatin
	Albumin	
Local anesthetics	Amide-type	

[a] If other agents can be used that are equally effective.

General recommendations for anesthesia

1. Children have a low risk of anaphylaxis during anesthesia, except for those with extensive skin disease and especially active disease-forming blisters. The latter group of children should be anesthetized with caution (the same as with adults).
2. Patients with previous reactions during anesthesia or toward other drugs should be considered for allergy assessment before surgery to identify responsible allergens.
3. The anesthetist must be informed about the form of mastocytosis, basal serum tryptase levels as a marker of the total mast cell load, and previous anaphylactic episodes.
4. Any regular maintenance medication taken to maintain mast cell stability and limit the effects of mast cell mediators should be continued during the operation.
5. Emergency medications and equipment to treat anaphylaxis should be immediately available and the anesthetist should monitor the patient closely during surgical procedures.
6. Where possible, prudence recommends administration of incremental dose infusion rather than single boluses of needed drugs (opioids, muscle relaxants) known to activate mast cells.

7. Potential physical trigger factors and stress should be avoided and premedication with sedatives, such as benzodiazepines, should be considered.
8. When possible, anesthesiology records from previous surgeries tolerated in the recent past should be obtained.
9. If the patient has no history of general anesthesia, most experts recommend administration of safer drugs as mentioned previously along with premedication with an H_1 antihistamine.

MCD AND USE OF RCM

Anaphylaxis triggered by RCM in patients with mastocytosis is mainly reported in some case reports, along with a few cases in large studies on patients with mastocytosis, mainly adults as a consequence, perhaps, of greater RCM exposure.[1,2,5,9]

In a Spanish study on patients with anaphylaxis and other mast cell–mediator release symptoms, drug reactions were triggers of severe systemic reactions in 19% of patients but none were RCM.[12] Very limited data have been published about subjects with systemic reactions to RCM in the general population who subsequently underwent specific evaluation for mastocytosis. In an Italian study on patients with food and drug anaphylaxis only 8.1% of patients with drug hypersensitivity had high tryptase values (>11.4 μg/L), one of whom was allergic to RCM in absence of MCD.[11] In a large European multicenter study performed in patients with adverse reactions to RCM, no patients were diagnosed with SM.[24]

Because of the limited data available, it is not possible to assess the risk of anaphylactic reactions in patients with mastocytosis or mast cell activation syndrome who have been exposed to RCM, compared with the general population. No specific recommendations have been proposed to prevent anaphylaxis in patients with mastocytosis and previous drug anaphylaxis.[3,25] Although many groups suggest giving premedication to prevent or reduce severity of possible reactions, the use of premedication has to be established.

Therefore, because RCM may induce in the general population severe reactions, sometimes fatal, and even with nonionic RCM, it seems reasonable to take a cautious approach in patients with mastocytosis by performing premedication in selected cases and alerting medical staff about the management of possible severe reactions.

OTHER DRUGS
Antibiotics

There are a few reports on anaphylaxis triggered by antibiotics, especially β-lactams (amoxicillin, ampicillin, penicillin V), but also with aminoglicosides.[1,2,26] A case of anaphylaxis has been recently described that occurred during penicillin skin testing, which was nevertheless negative, in a suspected β-lactam–allergic woman with high levels of basal tryptase.[27]

NSAIDs

There are some reports of adverse reactions to NSAIDs in patients with mastocytosis, mostly to aspirin and pyrazolones but also to different NSAIDs (diclofenac, ibuprofen, naproxen).[1,2] Moreover, the case of anaphylaxis elicited by ingestion of carrots together with acetylsalicylic acid, 500 mg, in a young man with mastocytosis, but not when taken separately, underlines that even in patients suffering from MCD sometimes cofactors (eg, aspirin or alcohol) are needed to provoke anaphylaxis.[2,28]

In general, only a small proportion of patients with mastocytosis seem to develop idiosyncratic reactions to NSAIDs, even if they may develop into very severe reactions.[29] Because most adult patients have a history of exposure to acetylsalicylic acid or other NSAIDs in their lifetime, the tolerance of these medications can be easily obtained through patient history. In a patient who has been taking NSAIDs without any allergic or other adverse reactions, there would not be any need to discontinue it specifically from a mastocytosis standpoint. In contrast, in patients with a history of NSAID reactions, the consequences could be very severe and even fatal. Therefore, all NSAIDs (including parenteral forms, such as ketorolac) should be strictly avoided in these patients. These patients should also consider wearing a medic alert bracelet.

Opioids

Opioids are known as histamine-releasing drugs. In vitro studies have demonstrated that morphine and buprenorphine have a concentration-dependent capacity to induce histamine and tryptase release from mast cells.[30] Other authors observed mast cell activation with codeine and meperidine.[31] Moreover, some clinical reports confirm these data by describing adverse reactions after intake of codeine and morphine.[2,32] Anecdotal experience suggests that fentanyl and derivatives are generally well tolerated.

General Considerations

Considering the overly limited data on tolerance or on the hazards of antibiotic and analgesic drugs for patients with MCD, it is not possible to give general recommendations that apply to all patients. As a general consideration, medications previously and continuously tolerated by the patient are allowed. Moreover, if the tolerance of an analgesic, NSAID, or antibiotic drug is unknown, a graded provocation test can be performed. Finally, it is important to refer all patients with adverse reactions to drugs to an allergy specialist, especially patients with mastocytosis, for appropriate counseling and testing (eg, skin testing, provocation test) at a specialized center under close supervision.

SUMMARY

Drug-induced anaphylaxis might occur in patients with mastocytosis; however, the association between mastocytosis and drug anaphylaxis does not seem to be as strong as it is with Hymenoptera sting anaphylaxis. In patients with mastocytosis, anaphylactic reactions triggered by different drugs, such as anesthetics, RCM, antibiotics, NSAIDs, codeine, and narcotics, have been reported. Therefore, in case of anaphylaxis, MCD should be considered in the differential diagnosis; the level of serum tryptase during acute reaction and at baseline and an accurate skin examination might provide useful clues for a differential diagnosis. Patients with mastocytosis with previous drug anaphylaxis may have a greater risk of new reactions to drugs and they should be considered for allergy evaluation.

Regarding general anesthesia, based on data available in patients with mastocytosis, it can be concluded that the risk for children with pediatric-onset mastocytosis seems limited and prophylactic antiallergic premedication may not be obligatory. It is, however, important to continue chronic antimediator therapies in children and adults. Severe reactions have been reported in some adults with mastocytosis. Anesthetic agents to be administered to adult patients need to be carefully selected. The anesthetist should be informed of the diagnosis of mastocytosis and prepared for an emergency treatment of anaphylaxis and should try to avoid possible trigger factors. There is no evidence of the efficacy of premedication before anesthesia or RCM administration to prevent or reduce severity of reactions; however, there is no evidence to the contrary and in practice it should be considered, depending on the risk of the individual patient.

Finally, given the current limited information available regarding safety of antibiotics and NSAIDs, it is not possible to state clear indications, but it is reasonable to suggest that patients take medications previously and continuously tolerated or, otherwise, to perform drug provocation tests under medical supervision.

REFERENCES

1. Gonzalez de Olano D, de la Hoz Caballer B, Nunez Lopez R, et al. Prevalence of allergy and anaphylactic symptoms in 210 adult and pediatric patients with mastocytosis in Spain: a study of the Spanish Network on Mastocytosis (REMA). Clin Exp Allergy 2007;37:1547–55.
2. Brockow K, Jofer C, Behrendt H, et al. Anaphylaxis in patients with mastocytosis: a study on history, clinical features and risk factors in 120 patients. Allergy 2008; 63:226–32.
3. Brockow B. Drug allergy in mast cell disease. Curr Opin Allergy Clin Immunol 2011;12:354–60.
4. Brockow K, Romano A, Blanca M, et al. General considerations for skin test procedures in the diagnosis of drug hyper-sensitivity. Allergy 2002;57:45–51.
5. Valabij J, Robinson S, Johnston D, et al. Unexplained loss of consciousness: systemic mastocytosis. J R Soc Med 2000;91:141–2.
6. Renauld V, Goudet V, Mouton-Faivre C, et al. Case report: perioperative immediate hypersensitivity involves not only allergy but also mastocytosis. Can J Anaesth 2011;58:456–9.
7. Bilo MB, Frontini F, Massaccesi C, et al. Mast cell diseases and the severity and course of intraoperative anaphylaxis. Ann Allergy Asthma Immunol 2009;103: 175–6.
8. Goldfinger MM, Sandadi J. Undiagnosed systemic mastocytosis in a teenager revealed during general anesthesia. Paediatr Anaesth 2010;20:290–1.
9. Weingarten TN, Volcheck GW, Sprung J. Anaphylactoid reaction to intravenous contrast in patient with systemic mastocytosis. Anaesth Intensive Care 2009; 37:646–9.
10. Bonadonna P, Perbellini O, Passalacqua G, et al. Clonal mast cell disorders in patients with systemic reactions to Hymenoptera stings and increased serum tryptase levels. J Allergy Clin Immunol 2009;123:680–6.
11. Bonadonna P, Zanotti R, Pagani M, et al. How much specific is the association between Hymenoptera venom allergy and mastocytosis? Allergy 2009;64: 1379–82.
12. Alvarez-Twose I, González de Olano D, Sánchez-Muñoz L, et al. Clinical, biological, and molecular characteristics of clonal mast cell disorders presenting with systemic mast cell activation symptoms. J Allergy Clin Immunol 2010;125: 1269–78.
13. Gurrieri C, Weingarten TN, Martin DP, et al. Allergic reactions during anesthesia at a large United States referral center. Anesth Analg 2011;113:1202–12.
14. Lobera T, Audicana MT, Pozo MD, et al. Study of hypersensitivity reactions and anaphylaxis during anesthesia in Spain. J Investig Allergol Clin Immunol 2008; 18:350–6.
15. Dewachter P, Laroche D, Mouton-Faivre C, et al. Immediate reactions following iodinated contrast media injection: a study of 38 cases. Eur J Radiol 2011;77: 495–501.

16. Dybendal T, Guttormsen AB, Elsayed S, et al. Screening for mast cell tryptase and serum IgE antibodies in 18 patients with anaphylactic shock during general anaesthesia. Acta Anaesthesiol Scand 2003;47:1211–8.
17. Dewachter P, Castells MC, Hepner DL, et al. Perioperative management of patients with mastocytosis. Anesthesiology 2013;120:753–9.
18. Carter MC, Uzzaman A, Scott LM, et al. Pediatric mastocytosis: routine anesthetic management for a complex disease. Anesth Analg 2008;107:422–7.
19. Ahmad N, Evans P, Lloyd-Thomas AR. Anesthesia in children with mastocytosis: a case based review. Paediatr Anaesth 2009;19:97–107.
20. Matito A, Alvarez-Twose I, Morgado JM, et al. Clinical impact of pregnancy in mastocytosis: a study of the Spanish Network on Mastocytosis (REMA) in 45 cases. Int Arch Allergy Immunol 2011;156:104–11.
21. Van der Linden PW, Hack CE, Poortman J, et al. Insect sting challenge in 138 patients: relation between clinical severity of anaphylaxis an mast cell activation. J Allergy Clin Immunol 1992;90:110–8.
22. Schwartz LB. Diagnostic value of tryptase in anaphylaxis and mastocytosis. Immunol Allergy Clin North Am 2006;26:451–63.
23. Mertes PM, Malinovsky JM, Jouffroy L, et al. Reducing the risk of anaphylaxis during anesthesia: 2011 updated guidelines for clinical practice. J Investig Allergol Clin Immunol 2011;21:442–53.
24. Brockow K, Romano A, Aberer W, et al. Skin testing in patients with hypersensitivity reactions to iodinated contrast media: a European multicenter study. Allergy 2009;64:234–41.
25. Brockow K, Christiansen C, Kanny G, et al. Management of hypersensitivity reactions to iodinated contrast media. Allergy 2005;60:150–8.
26. Schwartz LB, Metcalfe DD, Miller JS, et al. Tryptase levels as an indicator of mast cell activation in systemic anaphylaxis and mastocytosis. N Engl J Med 1987;316:1622–6.
27. Alonso Diaz De Durana MD, Fernandez-Rivas M, Casas ML, et al. Anaphylaxis during negative penicilline skin prick testing confirmed by elevated serum tryptase. Allergy 2003;58:159.
28. Pfeffer I, Fischer J, Biedermann T. Acetylsalicylic acid dependent anaphylaxis to carrots in a patient with mastocytosis. J Dtsch Dermatol Ges 2011;9:230–1.
29. Brockow K, Metcalfe DD. Mastocytosis. Chem Immunol Allergy 2010;95:110–24.
30. Stellato C, Cirillo R, Amato P, et al. Human basophil/mast cell releasability. Anesthesiology 1992;77:932–40.
31. Blunk JA, Schmelz M, Zeck S, et al. Opioid-induced mast cell activation and vascular responses is not mediated by mu-opioid receptor: an in vivo microdyalisis study in human skin. Anesth Analg 2004;98:364–70.
32. Vaughan ST, Jones NG. Systemic mastocytosis presenting as profound collapse during anaesthesia. Anaesthesia 1998;53:804–7.

Neuropsychological Features of Adult Mastocytosis

Daniela S. Moura, PhD[a,b,c,d,e],
Sophie Georgin-Lavialle, MD, PhD[a,b,c,d,e,f],
Raphaël Gaillard, MD, PhD[g,h], Olivier Hermine, MD, PhD[a,b,c,d,e],*

KEYWORDS

- Mastocytosis • Mast cell • Kit • Depression • Anxiety • Cognitive impairment
- Headache

KEY POINTS

- Mastocytosis is associated with several and disabling general and neuropsychological symptoms, including pain, headache, anxiety, depression, and cognitive impairment.
- Cognitive impairment in mastocytosis is not linked to depression.
- Anxious and depression symptoms may improve after treatments by tyrosine kinase inhibitors aiming at reducing mast cell activation.

FUTURE CONSIDERATIONS

Neurologic and psychiatric symptoms should be evaluated prospectively on large cohorts of patients. In addition, they should be evaluated in children populations, which are poorly studied in this respect.

New research is needed to better understand the pathophysiology of these manifestations. The results of this research could point out the role of mast cells in neurologic and psychiatric disorders outside mastocytosis.

[a] INSERM UMR 1163, Laboratory of Cellular and Molecular Mechanisms of Hematological Disorders and Therapeutical Implications, Paris, France; [b] Paris Descartes – Sorbonne Paris Cité University, Imagine Institute, Paris, France; [c] CNRS ERL 8254, Paris, France; [d] Laboratory of Excellence GR-Ex, Paris, France; [e] Service d'Hématologie clinique, Assistance Publique-Hôpitaux de Paris, Hôpital Necker, Paris, France; [f] Service de médecine Interne, Hôpital Tenon, Assistance Publique-Hôpitaux de Paris, Université Pierre et Marie Curie, 4 rue de la chine, Paris 75020, France; [g] Laboratoire de "Physiopathologie des maladies Psychiatriques", Centre de Psychiatrie et Neurosciences, U894, INSERM, Université Paris Descartes, Sorbonne Paris Cité, Paris, France; [h] Service de Psychiatrie, Faculté de Médecine Paris Descartes, Centre Hospitalier Sainte-Anne, Université Paris Descartes, Sorbonne Paris Cité, Paris, France

* Corresponding author. Service d'Hématologie Adultes et centre de référence sur les mastocytoses, Hôpital Necker-Enfants Malades, 161 Rue des Sèvres, Paris 75743 Cedex 15, France.
E-mail address: ohermine@gmail.com

Immunol Allergy Clin N Am 34 (2014) 407–422
http://dx.doi.org/10.1016/j.iac.2014.02.001   immunology.theclinics.com

INTRODUCTION

Mastocytosis is defined as an excessive accumulation of mast cells in several organs or tissues. In most cases, the disease is indolent and does not reduce life expectancy. The disease is associated, however, with an underestimated chronic disability, presumably linked to the release of mast cell mediators by abnormal mast cells that includes flushes and the well-defined gastrointestinal symptoms, cardiovascular instability, and skin involvement, in particular pruritus and esthetic concerns. In addition, it is well recognized that in almost one-third of the patients, general symptoms, including fatigue and musculoskeletal pain, could also have a major impact on the quality of life. Although less recognized and less attributed to mediators released from abnormal mast cells, symptoms, such as headache, anxiety, mood, and cognitive impairment, are frequent and should be specifically evaluated because they may require specific therapies and are associated with significant impairment of social life and professional activities. In this review, in addition to the authors' studies on psychiatric and neurologic disorders, the major recent findings concerning neuropsychological symptoms in mastocytosis are reviewed and data supporting the hypothesis that abnormal mast cell activation and to a less extent mast cell accumulation are involved in these disorders are discussed.

EPIDEMIOLOGY
Neurologic Features

Few studies are focused on neurologic symptoms associated with mastocytosis (**Table 1**). In earlier studies of a large cohort of patients, some investigators reported frequent acute or chronic headache; more rarely, syncope and acute-onset back pain; and, in a few cases, clinical and radiological features resembling or allowing a diagnosis of multiple sclerosis.[1–3] In addition, several case reports discussed rare associations between mastocytosis and various neurologic conditions, including chorea, encephalopathy, and strokes.[4–8] From these studies, it is difficult, however, to link these neurologic manifestations with abnormal mast cell activation and they may have been more fortuitous than causal. Two recent studies, however, reported neurologic symptoms on large cohorts of adult patients with mastocytosis.[2,3] First, they investigated the occurrence of headache by sending questionnaires to 171 patients with systemic mastocytosis. They received 64 responses, and 36 patients (56.2%) complained of headache.[3] These patients displayed headaches, which were classified as migraines (37.5%) or tension-type headaches (17.2%). Second, they tried to identify which complication of the disease could have an impact on the nervous system in a retrospective study of 223 adult patients with mastocytosis.[3] The most frequent symptoms they found were headache (n = 78; 35%), followed by syncope (n = 12; 5.4%), acute back

Table 1		
Main neuropsychological features in mastocytosis		
Neuropsychological Features	Percentage (%)	Reference
Depression and anxiety	40–60	Moura et al,[25] 2011
Headache	35–56	Smith et al,[3] 2011
Including migraine	37.5	Smith et al,[2] 2011
Cognitive impairment	38.6	Moura et al,[32] 2012
Syncope	5	Smith et al,[2] 2011
Back pain	4	Smith et al,[2] 2011
Multiple sclerosis	1.3	Smith et al,[2] 2011

pain (n = 9; 4%), and clinical and radiological features, allowing a diagnosis of multiple sclerosis (n = 3; 1.3%). The frequency of all these symptoms seems higher than might be expected in the general population of the country in which the study was performed (0.1%), suggesting that mast cell activation may be involved in these disorders.

Depression

In mastocytosis, although mood disorders are clinically observed and are one of the main complaints of patients, specific descriptive literature reports are rare[9–12] and concern small number of patients. Quantitative and qualitative descriptions of these symptoms in larger cohorts are still missing. In a seminal study by Rogers and colleagues in 1986,[9] depression frequency and features were investigated. In this study, depression was diagnosed after psychiatric interview in 40% of patients (n = 10). In 2008, the authors further reported a prevalence of 75% of depression symptoms among 88 patients with indolent mastocytosis, including cutaneous and systemic forms of the disease.[13] The authors' first descriptive study looked at a large sample of 288 subjects. The results of this first study showed a prevalence of depression in mastocytosis at approximately 60%, which confirmed the results of previous studies of a smaller number of patients.[9] The higher prevalence reported in the authors' study could be explained by the different methods of assessment and largely by the choice of a low cut-point of the Hamilton depression rating scale used to consider patients as depressed.

Cognitive Impairment

Soter and colleagues[12] were the first to report cognitive impairment in mastocytosis in the 1970s. In this study, they reported neuropsychiatric symptoms among patients with mastocytosis as "attention and concentration disorders, irritability, fatigue, headache, socio-relational difficulties and poor motivation" in 5 patients of 8.[12] Complaints about memory impairment in mastocytosis have only been specifically studied in 1986 in 10 patients with an old version of the clinical Wechsler Memory Scale.[9] According to the investigators, most patients presented disorders of cognition affecting memory and attention that fluctuated with the disease and were in some cases improved by histamine antagonists used to control the activity of mast cells. The authors have confirmed these results and shown in 57 patients with mastocytosis that cognitive impairment is a common symptom (38.6%). The prevalence of memory impairment in the authors' sample was high but not as much as suggested by Rogers and colleagues (70% in a sample of 10 patients). In addition, the authors' study provided evidence that memory impairment in mastocytosis was not related to age or level of education of patients (mean age 42 years and high level of education [32%] in the group with disorders). The prevalence of cognitive impairment in the authors' sample was significantly higher than reported in the literature in younger populations (45–59 years) suffering from chronic diseases, such as diabetes, or in the elderly (65 years and over) where the prevalence of cognitive impairment without dementia is approximately 15% to 40%.[14–17] The prevalence of cognitive impairment in the authors' sample was similar to that observed in multiple sclerosis, an inflammatory disease in which mast cell activation (without mastocytosis) may play a role and in which the prevalence of cognitive impairment is estimated between 40% and 60%.[18–20]

CLINICAL SYMPTOMS
Neurologic Symptoms

Neurologic symptoms can be acute, related to mast cell mediator release, such as headache and syncope, or permanent, related to mast cell infiltration, such as back pain, in cases of vertebral infiltration with or without fracture. Headaches were frequently reported in 35% of patients in a large cohort of 223 patients.[3] In a second study by the same group based on a smaller number of patients (36 patients) using a questionnaire, it was shown[2] that 25% of patients displayed chronic daily headache, 37.5% presented migraine, and 17.2% complained of tension-type headache, mostly episodic. Among the patients with migraine, two-thirds reported an associated aura, most frequently visual. Typical aura could be reported with or without migraine among 39% of the patients of the cohort. Symptoms that are clearly associated with abnormal mast cell activity, such as flushes, pruritus, and/or diarrhea, were more common in patients with either tension-type headache or migraine than in patients not reporting headache. Beurey and colleagues[21] reported syncope as early as in 1971, and this symptom has been more extensively reported by Smith and colleagues[3] in 12 patients of 223 with mastocytosis.[22] The patients reported by Smith and colleagues had been referred to a neurologist for indeterminate spells with episodic loss of consciousness. When performed, cerebral MRI, electroencephalograms (EEGs), and cardiac evaluations were considered normal. When reported, the spells evolved over the course of several minutes, culminating with a brief syncopal episode. The most commonly associated symptoms were loose stools, abdominal cramps, nausea, hot flushing, light-headedness, palpitations, and diaphoresis, suggesting a role of acute mast cell mediator release. Smith and colleagues[3] identified 3 patients with clinical and radiological features compatible with the diagnosis of multiple sclerosis. In this report, 1 man 25 years old and 2 women 57 and 64 years old, respectively, met the revised McDonald clinical criteria for multiple sclerosis. Finally, several case reports were published reporting rare neurologic features associated with mastocytosis, including chorea (n = 2), encephalopathy (n = 2), cerebral infarction (n = 1), coma (n = 1), and strokes with cervical artery dissection (n = 2).[4–8,23,24] Such isolated case reports may be fortuitous associations and were not confirmed on the large cohort of Smith and colleagues in 2011.

Psychological Symptoms

Depression characteristics and assessment

Although psychological symptoms (depression and disorders of attention and memory) are part of chronic manifestations of mastocytosis, patients suffering from mastocytosis and concerned by these disorders express great suffering linked to the misunderstanding and lack of recognition of their symptoms by themselves but also by physicians or relatives. As discussed previously, no reports in the literature have studied extensively depression characteristics in a large group of patients with mastocytosis. In an attempt to better characterize depression based on a questionnaire, the authors performed, in a large cohort, a detailed analysis of symptoms in patients complaining of mood disorders. The data suggest that depression associated with mastocytosis comprises mainly affective-cognitive aspects (depressed mood, guilt, feelings of failure, and poor motivation [loss of interest in the work and activities]) and anxiosomatic aspects (somatic and psychic anxiety and middle and late insomnia).[25] Symptoms like psychomotor slowing and insight problems are rare and are considered atypical symptoms in this population. It is also important to consider the limitation of depression assessment using questionnaires instead of a structured interview diagnosis based on *Diagnostic and Statistical Manual of Mental Disorders* criteria.[26] Although the Hamilton Depression Rating Scale is still the gold standard for evaluating depression in clinical trials, it may not be the best choice for mastocytosis patients because of the over-representation of somatic items that may overlap with symptoms of the disease.[27–29] By studying in detail the Hamilton score, however, the authors could demonstrate that a high-level score was associated with core depression symptoms, such as sadness and loss of motivation. The use of a more accurate clinical depression scale, the Beck Depression Rating Scale, led to similar results but with a slightly lower rate of depression.[30,31] The use of more than one scale and/or scales less biased by somatic symptoms should be preferred to screen for depression in mastocytosis. Regardless of the type of questionnaires used, however, it is also important to complete the assessment of patients presenting with more severe symptomatology detected by questionnaires using a psychiatric interview to confirm diagnosis and provide, if necessary, proper medications.

Cognitive impairment characteristics and assessment

Among mastocytosis patients, cognitive symptoms were mostly characterized by attention impairment.[9,32] Due to their characteristics, cognitive impairment in mastocytosis seems to meet the criteria for an "unspecified cognitive disorder" as described in the *DSM* (Fourth Edition).[26] These disorders were not linked to depression, age, level of education, or clinical subcategories. Moreover, no correlation was found between these cognitive disorders and the provision of antihistaminic drugs. In addition to cognitive impairment, lack of motivation is an important symptom to consider in this group of patients. Although difficult to quantify, this symptom shares some links with fatigue and could help understand the primary pathways and mechanisms involved with cognition impairment. Fatigue is a complex symptom composed of both psychic (motivational) and somatic dimensions. The psychic dimension of fatigue is often associated with symptoms, such as pain and affective and cognitive alterations, and is more difficult to characterize.[33,34] Its behavioral expression (motivation and reward responsiveness), however, has a specific neural circuit involving dopaminergic subcortical structures, such as putamen and anterior cingulate cortex, that could be implicated in difficulties to sustain attention and/or to engage in even simple actions among these patients.[35] Assessment of cognitive impairment in mastocytosis should be more systematic in patients with complaints and should focus on attention and auditory memory and executive functions as well.

PATHOPHYSIOLOGY

Although the pathophysiology of infiltrative complications, such as spinal cord compression, is easy to understand by a mechanical role of mast cell infiltration of vertebral bone, the pathophysiology of fatigue, cognitive dysfunction, psychiatric symptoms, and headache remains unclear (**Fig. 1**).

Mast Cells in the Brain

Mast cells are present in variable quantities in all tissues and organs, especially along vessels, including the brain, which is rich in mast cells. In this organ, they are preferentially located near blood vessels at the level of the blood-brain barrier and also at the nerve endings of sensory and sympathetic fibers.[36] In addition, mast cells are found particularly and in high density in certain structures of the diencephalon, especially in the hypothalamus, which is involved in systems of stress response, emotion, and cognition, and also in amygdales, in the ventral portion of the median eminence, near the pituitary gland at these anterior and posterior sides as well as in the hippocampal formation and surrounding leptomeninges and meningeal spaces at the level of the olfactory bulb.[37–43] A large number of mast cells reside in the thalamus, which lesions or stimulation of the dorsomedial portion and earlier kernels have been associated with changes in emotional reactivity and pain.[38,44–47]

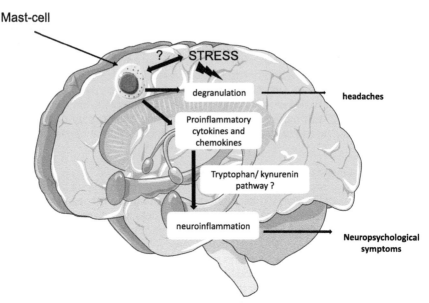

Fig. 1. How mast-cells might be involved in the etiology of neuropsychiatric symptoms associated to mastocytosis? (*Adapted from* Selvier Medical Art.)

Mast Cells, Stress Response, Cognition, and Emotionality

Because of their particular distribution and density in related brain structures, mast cells' overactivity may interfere with brain function and adversely affect stress response, cognition, and emotionality.[37,42,48–57] In a previous work, the authors showed that patients with mastocytosis displayed high levels of perceived stress linked to lower telomere length.[31] Perceived stress results from cognitive and emotional evaluation of situations by individuals. The brain structures involved in physiological stress response are also implicated in cognitive appraisal as well as emotion and behavioural responses to adversity. In mastocytosis, in line with other studies in the field of stress, chronic hyperactivation of the stress response system has been hypothesized to explain the high prevalence of neuropsychological symptoms as well as a high tendency to perceive stress in conventional situations.[31,58–61] The pathologic variation of the number and the activation of mast cells in the brain could lead to a dysfunction of these systems. In line with these observations, negative emotion expressed in mastocytosis could also result from conditioning process involving responses to stress. Mast cells could be recruited through aversive conditioning. Once conditioning is obtained, psychological cues could lead to mast cell activation,[62–64] which could maintain aberrant responses to stress.

Mast Cell Neuroinflammation and Depression

The cytoplasm of mast cells contains many granulations of preformed mediators, such as histamine, tryptase, serotonin, cytokines, and chemokines (interleukin [IL]-3, IL-4, IL-5, IL-6, IL-8, granulocyte macrophage–colony-stimulating factor, and TNF-α),[23,30,31] which, in cases of abnormal release, may explain part of all the symptoms found in patients with mastocytosis, including olfactory hypersensitivity, headache and migraines, pain, and probably mood, anxiety, and cognitive disorders. Histamine has a modulator effect in some mnemonic systems, but its exact function in memory remains controversial.[65–67] In their study of memory disorders in mastocytosis, Roger and colleagues[9] suggested that histamine might be responsible for memory disorders in mastocytosis. Their hypothesis was based on the fact that their patients improved their neuropsychiatric symptomatology with antihistamine drugs. Serotonin produced by mast cells contributes to hippocampal function.[68] In mastocytosis, Kushnir-Sukhov and colleagues[69,70] have shown that patients displaying gastrointestinal and neuropsychological symptoms presented low levels of serum serotonin. In line with these studies, it could be hypothesized that an abnormal deviation of the metabolism of the serotonin produced by mast cells may interfere with normal function of the hippocampus and may be involved in the memory loss observed in patients with mastocytosis. In addition, it is not excluded that inflammatory mast cell cytokines, like TNF-α, could also trigger depression in mastocytosis.[56,71–76] Several studies have shown that inflammation related to mediator release by mast cells is linked to depression.[34,73,77–84] Moreover, inflammation could lead to activation of indoleamine 2,3-dioxygenase (IDO), which breaks down tryptophan into kynurenine, explaining fatigue[35,85] and cognitive impairment[86] through accumulation of kynurenic acid and quinolinic acid and possibly the reduced levels of serotonin in mastocytosis patients.[70]

Mast Cells and Headache

In migraine, mast cells might be involved through their interactions with peptidergic and cholinergic neurons.[87] At this level, presynaptic endings may capture mediator release by mast cell granules.[44,88–90] In agreement with this hypothesis, some studies have suggested a direct role of mast cell degranulation in headache[91] and found that symptoms reflective of mast cell activity were significantly greater in individuals reporting headaches.[2] Vascular instability in periphery may result in poor perfusion of the brain but could also be related to prostaglandin and histamine release at the brain level.[3]

Mast Cells and Multiple Sclerosis

The role of mast cells in the pathophysiology of multiple sclerosis is extensively suggested in the literature. Mast cells are detected in human multiple sclerosis lesions and increase mast cell activity, as assessed by a high level of tryptase, is detectable in the cerebrospinal fluid of patients with active multiple sclerosis.[92–95] Furthermore, several studies have found an association between mast cell burden and susceptibility to experimental autoimmune encephalitis.[3,96]

DIAGNOSIS

Neuropsychiatric symptoms are thus frequently associated with mastocytosis and may present as various clinical features. Clinicians may face 2 situations.

Mastocytosis Was Not Previously Diagnosed

In patients with cognitive and/or mood complaints in which mastocytosis was not previously diagnosed, associated clinical symptoms and signs in favor of this diagnosis should be looked for. In the presence of skin lesions, the diagnosis of mastocytosis is easy and a usual clinical investigation should be made that may include skin biopsies, bone marrow aspiration and biopsy, and measurement of tryptase levels. Tryptase levels and eventually bone marrow aspiration and biopsies should be performed in cases of the presence of unusual psychiatric features or symptoms compatible with mast cell activation, including mainly gastrointestinal symptoms, flushes, pruritus, bone and musculoskeletal pains, and osteoporosis. In these cases, a diagnosis of mastocytosis could be made following the standard World Health Organization criteria but in some cases no evidence of mast infiltration may be found and the diagnosis of mast cell activation syndrome could be proposed. Mast cell activation syndrome has recently been described and diagnostic criteria have been written and include patients presenting with symptoms suggesting mast cell degranulation without any diagnostic criteria for a specific entity.[97] The absence of a clonal mast cell population suggests that in this entity, mast cells are quantitatively normal but qualitatively abnormal, probably with a lower threshold of activation. Some studies suggest that this not well-defined entity is genetically determined. Overall, stabilizing mast cells or inhibiting effects of mast cell degranulation with therapeutics, such as antihistamine or cromolyn sodium, is effective for some symptoms, such as pruritus or GI tract disturbances, but, except for a few case reports,[9] their impact on psychiatric symptoms is not known.

Mastocytosis Was Previously Diagnosed

When a diagnosis of mastocytosis is already known, because of their high frequency, neuropsychiatric symptoms should be systematically investigated. Unfortunately, both by patients and physicians, they are still not linked to mastocytosis in a significant number of cases. When confronted with neurologic and psychiatric symptoms, specialists in neurology and psychiatry should perform a specific and extensive workup. Then, in some cases, more specific examinations should be performed, including cerebral scan or MRI. In cases of neurologic deficits and/or headaches, cardiac testing with ECG and Holter ECG rule out cardiac rhythm dysfunction; neurologic assessment with EEG to eliminate seizure in case of syncope should be performed. Acute back pain should prompt neuroimaging of the spine to look for vertebral fracture with the risk of spinal cord compression. If a diagnosis of multiple sclerosis is suspected, cerebrospinal MRI and lumbar puncture should be performed.

TREATMENT

Treatment of indolent mastocytosis aims to relieve symptoms and requires a therapeutic adjustment tailored to each patient profile. Therefore, the treatment is essentially symptomatic.[98] Until recently, the treatment was intended mainly to prevent and limit degranulation and/or its consequences. Only in aggressive forms does the treatment aim to control the proliferation of tumor mast cells. New therapeutic approaches are being developed, including tyrosine kinase inhibitors, aimed at blocking the tyrosine kinase activity of KIT or other kinases involved in mast cell activation, like Lyn. Aspirin has been thought efficacious in the prophylaxis against syncope in mastocytosis.[1]

Psychotherapeutic Interventions

Although depression symptoms in mastocytosis seem related to systemic aspects of the disease, the implication of mast cells in stress response, behavior, and emotion regulation has been suggested by several studies.[68] Health psychology focuses on the impact of physical illness on emotions and cognitions. The concept of *emotional adjustment* is often used to understand how an individual negotiates emotionally with the impact of physical illness and its symptoms. In this process of psychological adaptation to the disease, patients may develop specific cognitions that reflect the way they build their understanding of what is happening to them. The concept of "sense of coherence," developed by Antonovsky in the 1970s, describes an understanding of events by individuals (sense of comprehensibility), feeling that they can manage (sense of manageability) and feeling they have a sense (sense of meaningfulness). The sense of coherence promotes better emotional adjustment to disease.[99–103] Therefore, a cognitive-behavioral approach with pragmatic strategies and information to improve understanding of the disease and the development of personal emotional management strategies of certain symptoms may be of greater benefit to these patients than psychodynamic approachs. Besides this general approach to psychological consequences of the disease, methods focusing on emotion and stress management, such as mindfulness meditation,[104] could also promote better cognitive and psychological adjustment. They might even contribute to interrupting the stress–mast cell activation interplay by reducing both psychological stress as a mast cell activation promoter and biologic stress as a mast cell activation consequence.

Psychotropic Drugs

According to general guidelines,[105] patients with a formal diagnosis of moderate to severe depression should benefit from an antidepressant prescription with well-tolerated antidepressants, such as selective serotonin reuptake inhibitors (SSRIs). Moreover, it has been shown that SSRIs can reduce endotoxin-induced fatigue[106] and even prevent depression induced by high-dose interferon-alpha, another condition related to inflammation.[107] Considering noradrenaline and dopamine involvement in motivation and lack of energy,[108,109] other classes of antidepressants, such as monoamine oxidase inhibitors, the noradrenaline and dopamine reuptake inhibitor bupropion, and serotonin-norepinephrine reuptake inhibitors or tricyclics, could also be prescribed. In another condition with debilitating fatigue, multiple sclerosis (MS), amantadine has shown efficacy in approximately one-third of patients.[110] The wake-promoting agent modafinil could also be prescribed if required. Alternatively, antidepressants with hypnotic properties, such as mianserin or mirtazapine, alone or in association, could target insomnia and decrease central histamine effects. Finally, in line with antihistamine drugs use, further studies could assess the benefits of blockade of mediators released by mast cells. Neurokinine-1 antagonists, such as aprepitant, showed promise in animal studies and early clinical trials as novel antidepressants.[111] Even if larger clinical trials did not confirm this property, aprepitant might target cognitive impairment and/or depression in mastocytosis or in patients with mast cell activation. Similarly, the tumor necrosis factor antagonist infliximab has been recently shown to improve depressive symptoms in patients with high baseline inflammatory biomarkers[112] and could target fatigue[78] in other conditions. Finally, ketamine or other N-methyl-D-aspartate (NMDA) receptors antagonists, such as memantine, might be useful to treat depression[113] and fatigue through blockade of NMDA stimulation by quinolinic acid after IDO activity increase.[85]

Tyrosine Kinase Inhibitor Therapy

KIT (CD117) is the receptor for the stem cell factor that is the main cytokine involved in mastocytopoiesis. Adult patients with systemic mastocytosis usually have mutations in c-Kit (D816V), which allows abnormal survival, proliferation, and activation of these cells.[98] The only kinase inhibitor that has been investigated for the effect of mast cell inhibition on neuropsychiatric symptoms is masitinib. Masitinib is an oral inhibitor selectively blocking c-Kit wild-type, platelet-derived growth factor receptor, and Lyn kinase activities. When tested in vivo in symptomatic patients with systemic mastocytosis, masitinib was able to decrease clinical symptoms linked to the release of mast cell mediators.[13] Among these symptoms, psychiatric symptoms, including depression, cognitive impairment, and anxiety, were significantly improved. The authors showed, in a sample of 35 patients, that masitinib treatment was associated (50%–67% of cases) with a significant improvement in depression (independently), with 25% to 75% remission, depending on the criteria chosen for depression. Treatment with masitinib was associated with a significant reduction of the scores of the dimension involving the mental depression symptoms, such as depressive mood anxiety and guilt. This result suggests that the improvement of depression may be influenced by the inhibitory effect of masitinib on the activation of mast cells and is consistent with the probable systemic nature of depression in this disease. Although these results do not definitively demonstrate the role of mast cells in the depression in mastocytosis, it highlights their probable contribution.

SUMMARY

Neuropsychological symptoms in matocytosis are not rare. Neurologic features are dominated by headache but various neurologic symptoms car occur. Urticaria pigmentosa and unexplained recurrent episodes of flushing, palpitations, abdominal pain, and loss of consciousness with spontaneous recovery may alert a neurologist to a possible systemic mastocytosis diagnosis. Depression and cognitive impairment (attention and memory) are 2 common symptoms in mastocytosis that are not linked causally. Patients with mastocytosis have increased sensitivity to stress that has been associated with peripheral leukocyte shorter telomeres[31] and may participate in diseases associated with mastocytosis. Further work is warranted to assess whether or not cardiovascular diseases, cancer, and aging are more frequent in mastocytosis than in other systemic diseases. Alternatively, mast cells could be the link between reactive stress and anxiety and shortening telomere.[114] This hypersensitivity to stress could suggest a hyperactivation of the response to stress through the mast cells in this pathology. This hyperactivation could be linked to the high prevalence of depression among these patients. Finally, if the entanglement of biologic and psychological factors in this disease seems important, the role of emotional regulation mechanisms, including difficulties in identifying emotions in the holding of depressive symptomatology, is not excluded, and this aspect of the emotional functioning of these patients can be an attractive therapeutic target for those with more severe depressive symptomatology. In addition, drugs that specifically inhibit release of mast cells and/or that reduce their number may be attractive to improve these symptoms and in extension could be useful in some psychiatric and neurologic disorders, as recently suggested with kinase inhibitors in multiple sclerosis[115] and Alzheimer disease.[71]

REFERENCES

1. Castells M, Austen KF. Mastocytosis: mediator-related signs and symptoms. Int Arch Allergy Immunol 2002;127(2):147–52.
2. Smith JH, Butterfield JH, Pardanani A, et al. Neurologic symptoms and diagnosis in adults with mast cell disease. Clin Neurol Neurosurg 2011;113(7):570–4.
3. Smith JH, Butterfield JH, Cutrer FM. Primary headache syndromes in systemic mastocytosis. Cephalalgia 2011;31(15):1522–31.
4. Frijns CJ, Troost J. Generalized mastocytosis and neurological complications in a 71-year-old patient. Clin Neurol Neurosurg 1992;94(3):257–60.
5. Iriarte LM, Mateu J, Cruz G, et al. Chorea: a new manifestation of mastocytosis. J Neurol Neurosurg Psychiatry 1988;51(11):1457–8.
6. Kanekura T, Sekiyama M, Mochitomi Y, et al. A case of mastocytosis with chorea. J Dermatol 2001;28(8):451–2.

7. Larroche C, Chadenat ML, Chaunu MP, et al. Strokes associated with cervical artery dissection, and systemic mastocytosis: an unfortuitous association? A report of two cases. Rev Med Interne 2005;26(10):820–3 [in French].
8. Tajima Y, Hamada K, Houzenn H, et al. Sequential magnetic resonance features of encephalopathy induced by systemic mastocytosis. Intern Med 1994;33(1): 23–6.
9. Rogers MP, Bloomingdale K, Murawski BJ, et al. Mixed organic brain syndrome as a manifestation of systemic mastocytosis. Psychosom Med 1986;48(6):437–47.
10. Casassus P, Caillat-Vigneron N, Martin A, et al. Treatment of adult systemic mastocytosis with interferon-α: results of a multicentre phase II trial on 20 patients. Br J Haematol 2002;119(4):1090–7.
11. Lortholary O, Casassus P, Laroche L, et al. Systemic mastocytosis and malignant mastocytosis. Presse Med 1990;19(3):125–8 [in French].
12. Soter NA, Austen KF, Wasserman SI. Oral disodium cromoglycate in the treatment of systemic mastocytosis. N Engl J Med 1979;301(9):465–9.
13. Hermine O, Lortholary O, Leventhal PS, et al. Case-control cohort study of patients' perceptions of disability in mastocytosis. PLoS One 2008;3(5):e2266 [Research Support, Non-U.S. Gov't].
14. Flicker C, Ferris SH, Reisberg B. Mild cognitive impairment in the elderly: predictors of dementia. Neurology 1991;41(7):1006–9.
15. Petersen RC, Smith GE, Waring SC, et al. Mild cognitive impairment: clinical characterization and outcome. Arch Neurol 1999;56(3):303–8.
16. Creavin ST, Gallacher J, Bayer A, et al. Metabolic syndrome, diabetes, poor cognition, and dementia in the Caerphilly Prospective Study. J Alzheimers Dis 2012;28(4):931–9.
17. Peltz CB, Corrada MM, Berlau DJ, et al. Cognitive impairment in nondemented oldest-old: prevalence and relationship to cardiovascular risk factors. Alzheimers Dement 2012;8(2):87–94.
18. Rao SM, Leo GJ, Ellington L, et al. Cognitive dysfunction in multiple sclerosis. II. Impact on employment and social functioning. Neurology 1991;41(5):692–6 [Research Support, U.S. Gov't, P.H.S.].
19. Bobholz JA, Rao SM. Cognitive dysfunction in multiple sclerosis: a review of recent developments [review]. Curr Opin Neurol 2003;16(3):283–8.
20. Caceres F, Vanotti S, Rao S. Epidemiological characteristics of cognitive impairment of multiple sclerosis patients in a Latin American country. J Clin Exp Neuropsychol 2012;33(10):1094–8.
21. Beurey J, Arnould G, Webir M, et al. Mastocytoses: formes syncopales. Bull Sot Fr Dermatol Syph 1971;78:601–4.
22. Arnould G, Beurey J, Weber M, et al. Formes syncopales des mastocytoses. Presse Med 1971;79:1345–6.
23. Boncoraglio GB, Brucato A, Carriero MR, et al. Systemic mastocytosis: a potential neurologic emergency. Neurology 2005;65(2):332–3.
24. Jost E, Michaux L, Vanden Abeele M, et al. Complex karyotype and absence of mutation in the c-kit receptor in aggressive mastocytosis presenting with pelvic osteolysis, eosinophilia and brain damage. Ann Hematol 2001;80(5):302–7.
25. Moura DS, Sultan S, Georgin-Lavialle S, et al. Depression in patients with mastocytosis: prevalence, features and effects of masitinib therapy. PLoS One 2011; 6(10):e26375 [Clinical Trial, Phase I Clinical Trial, Phase II Multicenter Study Research Support, Non-U.S. Gov't].
26. Diagnostic and statistical manual of mental disorders. 4th edition. Washington, DC: American Psychiatric Association (APA); 1994.

27. Moritz S, Meier B, Hand I, et al. Dimensional structure of the Hamilton depression rating scale in patients with obsessive-compulsive disorder. Psychiatry Res 2004;125(2):171–80.

28. Wasteson E, Brenne E, Higginson IJ, et al. Depression assessment and classification in palliative cancer patients: a systematic literature review. Palliat Med 2009;23(8):739–53.

29. Zimmerman M, Posternak MA, Chelminski I. Is the cutoff to define remission on the Hamilton rating scale for depression too high? J Nerv Ment Dis 2005;193(3): 170–5.

30. Beck AT, Steer RA, Brown GK. Beck depression inventory—second edition (BDI-II). San Antonio (TX): The Psychological Corporation; 1996.

31. Georgin-Lavialle S, Moura DS, Bruneau J, et al. Leukocyte telomere length in mastocytosis: correlations with depression and perceived stress. Brain Behav Immun 2013;35:51–7.

32. Moura DS, Sultan S, Georgin-Lavialle S, et al. Evidence for cognitive impairment in mastocytosis: prevalence, features and correlations to depression. PLoS One 2012;7(6):e39468 [Research Support, Non-U.S. Gov't].

33. Chaudhuri A, Behan PO. Fatigue and basal ganglia. J Neurol Sci 2000; 179(S1–2):34–42.

34. Capuron L, Pagnoni G, Demetrashvili MF, et al. Basal ganglia hypermetabolism and symptoms of fatigue during interferon-alpha therapy. Neuropsychopharmacology 2007;32(11):2384–92.

35. Dantzer R, Heijnen CJ, Kavelaars A, et al. The neuroimmune basis of fatigue. Trends Neurosci 2013;37(1):39–46.

36. Khalil M, Ronda J, Weintraub M, et al. Brain mast cell relationship to neurovasculature during development. Brain Res 2007;1171:18–29.

37. Edvinsson L, Cervos-Navarro J, Larsson LI, et al. Regional distribution of mast cells containing histamine, dopamine, or 5-hydroxytryptamine in the mammalian brain. Neurology 1977;27(9):878–83.

38. Matsumoto I, Inoue Y, Shimada T, et al. Brain mast cells act as an immune gate to the hypothalamic-pituitary-adrenal axis in dogs. J Exp Med 2001;194(1):71–8.

39. Goldschmidt RC, Hough LB, Glick SD, et al. Mast cells in rat thalamus: nuclear localization, sex difference and left-right asymetry. Brain Res 1984;323:2096217.

40. Taiwo OB, Kovacs KJ, Sun Y, et al. Unilateral spinal nerve ligation leads to an asymmetrical distribution of mast cells in the thalamus of female but not male mice. Pain 2005;114(1–2):131–40.

41. Marshall PS, Colon EA. Effects of allergy season on mood and cognitive function. Ann Allergy 1993;71(3):251–8.

42. Marathias K, Lambracht-Hall M, Savala J, et al. Endogenous regulation of rat brain mast cell serotonin release. Int Arch Allergy Appl Immunol 1991;95(4): 332–40.

43. Kovacs KJ, Larson AA. Mast cells accumulate in the anogenital region of somatosensory thalamic nuclei during estrus in female mice. Brain Res 2006; 1114(1):85–97.

44. Paus R, Theoharides TC, Arck PC. Neuroimmunoendocrine circuitry of the 'brain-skin connection'. Trends Immunol 2006;27(1):32–9.

45. Campbell DJ, Kernan JA. Mast cells in the central nervous system. Nature 1966; 210(5037):756–7.

46. Cirulli F, Pistillo L, de Acetis L, et al. Increased number of mast cells in the central nervous system of adult male mice following chronic subordination stress. Brain Behav Immun 1998;12(2):123–33.

47. Ng WX, Lau IY, Graham S, et al. Neurobiological evidence for thalamic, hippocampal and related glutamatergic abnormalities in bipolar disorder: a review and synthesis. Neurosci Biobehav Rev 2009;33(3):336–54.

48. Theoharides TC, Konstantinidou AD. Corticotropin-releasing hormone and the blood-brain-barrier. Front Biosci 2007;12:1615–28.

49. Silverman AJ, Asarian L, Khalil M, et al. GnRH, brain mast cells and behavior. Progress in brain research. Elsevier; 2002. p. 315–25.

50. Nautiyal KM, Ribeiro AC, Pfaff DW, et al. Brain mast cells link the immune system to anxiety-like behavior. Proc Natl Acad Sci U S A 2008;105(46):18053–7.

51. Esposito P, Gheorghe D, Kandere K, et al. Acute stress increases permeability of the blood-brain-barrier through activation of brain mast cells. Brain Res 2001; 888(1):117–27.

52. Esposito P, Chandler N, Kandere K, et al. Corticotropin-releasing hormone and brain mast cells regulate blood-brain-barrier permeability induced by acute stress. J Pharmacol Exp Ther 2002;303(3):1061–6.

53. Bugajski AJ, Chlap Z, Gadek M, et al. Effect of isolation stress on brain mast cells and brain histamine levels in rats. Agents Actions 1994;41(Spec No):C75–6.

54. Theoharides TC, Spanos C, Pang X, et al. Stress-induced intracranial mast cell degranulation: a corticotropin-releasing hormone-mediated effect. Endocrinology 1995;136(12):5745–50.

55. Theoharides TC, Rozniecki JJ, Sahagian G, et al. Impact of stress and mast cells on brain metastases. J Neuroimmunol 2008;205(1–2):1–7.

56. Theoharides TC, Cochrane DE. Critical role of mast cells in inflammatory diseases and the effect of acute stress. J Neuroimmunol 2004;146(1–2):1–12.

57. Theoharides TC. Mast cells and stress–a psychoneuroimmunological perspective. J Clin Psychopharmacol 2002;22(2):103–8.

58. Lazarus RS, Folkman S. Stress, coping and adaptation. New York: Springer; 1984.

59. Kalogeromitros D, Syrigou EK, Makris M, et al. Nasal provocation of patients with allergic rhinitis and the hypothalamic-pituitary-adrenal axis. Ann Allergy Asthma Immunol 2007;98(3):269–73.

60. Han KS. Perceived stress, mood state, and symptoms of stress of the patient with chronic illness. Taehan Kanho Hakhoe Chi 2003;33(1):87–94 [in Korean].

61. Gui XY. Mast cells: a possible link between psychological stress, enteric infection, food allergy and gut hypersensitivity in the irritable bowel syndrome. J Gastroenterol Hepatol 1998;13(10):980–9.

62. MacQueen G, Marshall J, Perdue M, et al. Pavlovian conditioning of rat mucosal mast cells to secrete rat mast cell protease II. Science 1989;243(4887):83–5.

63. Gauci M, Husband AJ, Saxarra H, et al. Pavlovian conditioning of nasal tryptase release in human subjects with allergic rhinitis. Physiol Behav 1994;55(5):823–5.

64. Kumagai M, Nagano M, Suzuki H, et al. Effects of stress memory by fear conditioning on nerve-mast cell circuit in skin. J Dermatol 2011;38(6):553–61.

65. Van Ruitenbeek P, Vermeeren A, Riedel WJ. Histamine H1-receptor blockade in humans affects psychomotor performance but not memory. J Psychopharmacol 2008;22(6):663–72.

66. Tsujii T, Yamamoto E, Ohira T, et al. Effects of sedative and non-sedative H1 antagonists on cognitive tasks: behavioral and near-infrared spectroscopy (NIRS) examinations. Psychopharmacology (Berl) 2007;194(1):83–91.

67. Tashiro M, Mochizuki H, Iwabuchi K, et al. Roles of histamine in regulation of arousal and cognition: functional neuroimaging of histamine H1 receptors in human brain. Life Sci 2002;72(4–5):409–14.

68. Nautiyal KM, Dailey CA, Jahn JL, et al. Serotonin of mast cell origin contributes to hippocampal function. Eur J Neurosci 2012;36(3):2347–59.

69. Kushnir-Sukhov NM, Brown JM, Wu Y, et al. Human mast cells are capable of serotonin synthesis and release. J Allergy Clin Immunol 2007;119(2):498–9.

70. Kushnir-Sukhov NM, Brittain E, Scott L, et al. Clinical correlates of blood serotonin levels in patients with mastocytosis. Eur J Clin Invest 2008;38(12): 953–8.

71. Piette F, Belmin J, Vincent H, et al. Masitinib as an adjunct therapy for mild-to-moderate Alzheimer's disease: a randomised, placebo-controlled phase 2 trial. Alzheimers Res Ther 2011;3(2):16.

72. Metcalfe DD. Mast cells and mastocytosis. Blood 2008;112(4):946–56 [Research Support, N.I.H., Intramural Review].

73. Haroon E, Raison CL, Miller AH. Psychoneuroimmunology meets neuropsychopharmacology: translational implications of the impact of inflammation on behavior. Neuropsychopharmacology 2012;37(1):137–62.

74. Chavarria A, Alcocer-Varela J. Is damage in central nervous system due to inflammation? Autoimmun Rev 2004;3(4):251–60.

75. Cao J, Boucher W, Kempuraj D, et al. Acute stress and intravesical corticotropin-releasing hormone induces mast cell dependent vascular endothelial growth factor release from mouse bladder explants. J Urol 2006;176(3): 1208–13.

76. Bienenstock J, Tomioka M, Matsuda H, et al. The role of mast cells in inflammatory processes: evidence for nerve/mast cell interactions. Int Arch Allergy Appl Immunol 1987;82(3–4):238–43.

77. Harrison NA, Brydon L, Walker C, et al. Neural origins of human sickness in interoceptive responses to inflammation. Biol Psychiatry 2009;66(5):415–22.

78. Monk JP, Phillips G, Waite R, et al. Assessment of tumor necrosis factor alpha blockade as an intervention to improve tolerability of dose-intensive chemotherapy in cancer patients. J Clin Oncol 2006;24(12):1852–9.

79. Maes M, Berk M, Goehler L, et al. Depression and sickness behavior are Janus-faced responses to shared inflammatory pathways. BMC Med 2012;10:66.

80. Capuron L, Fornwalt FB, Knight BT, et al. Does cytokine-induced depression differ from idiopathic major depression in medically healthy individuals? J Affect Disord 2009;119:181–5.

81. Raison CL, Borisov AS, Broadwell SD, et al. Depression during pegylated interferon-alpha plus ribavirin therapy: prevalence and prediction. J Clin Psychiatry 2005;66(1):41–8.

82. Raison CL, Borisov AS, Majer M, et al. Activation of central nervous system inflammatory pathways by interferon-alpha: relationship to monoamines and depression. Biol Psychiatry 2009;65(4):296–303.

83. Raison CL, Borisov AS, Woolwine BJ, et al. Interferon-alpha effects on diurnal hypothalamic-pituitary-adrenal axis activity: relationship with proinflammatory cytokines and behavior. Mol Psychiatry 2010;15(5):535–47.

84. Capuron L, Miller AH. Immune system to brain signaling: neuropsychopharmacological implications. Pharmacol Ther 2011;130(2):226–38.

85. Morimoto T, Sunagawa Y, Katanasaka Y, et al. Drinkable preparation of Theracurmin exhibits high absorption efficiency–a single-dose, double-blind, 4-way crossover study. Biol Pharm Bull 2012;36(11):1708–14.

86. Forrest CM, Mackay GM, Oxford L, et al. Kynurenine metabolism predicts cognitive function in patients following cardiac bypass and thoracic surgery. J Neurochem 2011;119(1):136–52.

87. Theoharides TC, Donelan J, Kandere-Grzybowska K, et al. The role of mast cells in migraine pathophysiology. Brain Res Brain Res Rev 2005;49(1):65–76.
88. Johnson D, Krenger W. Interactions of mast cells with the nervous system–recent advances. Neurochem Res 1992;17(9):939–51 [Research Support, Non-U.S. Gov't Research Support, U.S. Gov't, P.H.S. Review].
89. Bienenstock J. Relationships between mast cells and the nervous system. Revue Française d'Allergologie et d'Immunologie Clinique 2002;42:11–5.
90. Wilhelm M, Silver R, Silverman AJ. Central nervous system neurons acquire mast cell products via transgranulation. Eur J Neurosci 2005;22(9):2238–48.
91. Levy D, Burstein R, Kainz V, et al. Mast cell degranulation activates a pain pathway underlying migraine headache. Pain 2007;130(1–2):166–76.
92. Ibrahim MZ, Reder AT, Lawand R, et al. The mast cells of the multiple sclerosis brain. J Neuroimmunol 1996;70(2):131–8.
93. Kruger PG. Mast cells and multiple sclerosis: a quantitative analysis. Neuropathol Appl Neurobiol 2001;27(4):275–80.
94. Rozniecki JJ, Hauser SL, Stein M, et al. Elevated mast cell tryptase in cerebrospinal fluid of multiple sclerosis patients. Ann Neurol 1995;37(1):63–6.
95. Couturier N, Zappulla JP, Lauwers-Cances V, et al. Mast cell transcripts are increased within and outside multiple sclerosis lesions. J Neuroimmunol 2008; 195(1–2):176–85.
96. Secor VH, Secor WE, Gutekunst CA, et al. Mast cells are essential for early onset and severe disease in a murine model of multiple sclerosis. J Exp Med 2000; 191(5):813–22.
97. Valent P, Akin C, Arock M, et al. Definitions, criteria and global classification of mast cell disorders with special reference to mast cell activation syndromes: a consensus proposal. Int Arch Allergy Immunol 2011;157(3):215–25.
98. Georgin-Lavialle S, Barete S, Suarez F, et al. Current concepts and treatment advances in systemic mastocytosis. Rev Med Interne 2008;30(1):25–34 [in French].
99. Wiesmann U, Dezutter J, Hannich HJ. Sense of coherence and pain experience in older age. Int Psychogeriatr 2013;26(1):123–33.
100. Apers S, Moons P, Goossens E, et al. Sense of coherence and perceived physical health explain the better quality of life in adolescents with congenital heart disease. Eur J Cardiovasc Nurs 2013;12(5):475–83.
101. Barthelsson C, Nordstrom G, Norberg A. Sense of coherence and other predictors of pain and health following laparoscopic cholecystectomy. Scand J Caring Sci 2010;25(1):143–50.
102. Gustavsson-Lilius M, Julkunen J, Keskivaara P, et al. Predictors of distress in cancer patients and their partners: the role of optimism in the sense of coherence construct. Psychol Health 2011;27(2):178–95.
103. Haukkala A, Konttinen H, Lehto E, et al. Sense of coherence, depressive symptoms, cardiovascular diseases, and all-cause mortality. Psychosom Med 2013; 75(4):429–35.
104. Rosenkranz MA, Davidson RJ, Maccoon DG, et al. A comparison of mindfulness-based stress reduction and an active control in modulation of neurogenic inflammation. Brain Behav Immun 2012;27(1):174–84.
105. Association AP. Practice guideline for the treatment of patients with major depressive disorder. 3rd edition. Washington, DC: APA; 2010 [updated 2010; cited]. Available at: http://psychiatryonline.org/content.aspx?bookid=28&sectionid=1667485.
106. Hannestad J, DellaGioia N, Ortiz N, et al. Citalopram reduces endotoxin-induced fatigue. Brain Behav Immun 2011;25(2):256–9.

107. Musselman DL, Lawson DH, Gumnick JF, et al. Paroxetine for the prevention of depression induced by high-dose interferon alfa. N Engl J Med 2001;344(13): 961–6.

108. Treadway MT, Zald DH. Reconsidering anhedonia in depression: lessons from translational neuroscience. Neurosci Biobehav Rev 2011;35(3):537–55.

109. Gaillard R, Gourion D, Llorca PM. Anhedonia in depression. Encephale 2013; 39(4):296–305 [in French].

110. Rosenberg JH, Shafor R. Fatigue in multiple sclerosis: a rational approach to evaluation and treatment. Curr Neurol Neurosci Rep 2005;5(2):140–6.

111. Hafizi S, Chandra P, Cowen J. Neurokinin-1 receptor antagonists as novel antidepressants: trials and tribulations. Br J Psychiatry 2007;191:282–4.

112. Raison CL, Rutherford RE, Woolwine BJ, et al. A randomized controlled trial of the tumor necrosis factor antagonist infliximab for treatment-resistant depression: the role of baseline inflammatory biomarkers. JAMA Psychiatry 2013; 70(1):31–41.

113. Naughton M, Clarke G, O'Leary OF, et al. A review of ketamine in affective disorders: current evidence of clinical efficacy, limitations of use and pre-clinical evidence on proposed mechanisms of action. J Affect Disord 2014;156:24–35.

114. Epel ES, Blackburn EH, Lin J, et al. Accelerated telomere shortening in response to life stress. Proc Natl Acad Sci U S A 2004;101(49):17312–5.

115. Vermersch P, Benrabah R, Schmidt N, et al. Masitinib treatment in patients with progressive multiple sclerosis: a randomized pilot study. BMC Neurol 2012;12:36.

Mast Cell Sarcoma: Clinical Management

Catherine R. Weiler, MD, PhD, Joseph Butterfield, MD*

KEYWORDS

- Mast cell sarcoma • Mastocytosis • Clinical presentation of mast cell sarcoma
- Treatment of mast cell sarcoma • Prognosis of mast cell sarcoma

KEY POINTS

- Mast cell sarcoma is the rarest mast cell disorder.
- Prognosis of mast cell sarcoma is poor.
- Mast cell sarcoma affects both genders.
- Mast cell sarcoma is more common in canine, murine, and bovine species.

INTRODUCTION

Special stains for mast cells were described by Paul Ehrlich around the late 1800s and early 1900s. He studied dyes that stain tissues, cells, and infectious organisms. In 1908 he shared the highest scientific distinction, the Nobel Prize, with Metchnikoff, for this work. Mast cells have been described and named by him. Since then, they were identified in different tissues in many species.[1] The earliest report of mast cell sarcoma using different electronic computer searches dates back to 1948.[1] The species affected was dogs.

The disorders affecting mast cells have been described under the terms "cutaneous mastocytosis," "systemic mastocytosis," "mast cell leukemia," and "mast cell sarcoma" (**Table 1**).[2–5]

CLINICAL PRESENTATION AND PROGNOSIS

Human mast cell sarcoma is a very rare disorder of mast cells. There are 17 reported cases in the literature between 1997 and 2013.[6–18] In addition, included are 3 unpublished reports of patients diagnosed at the authors' institution (**Table 2**). The disorder

The authors have no disclosures and no conflicts of interest. Dr J. Butterfield and Dr C.R. Weiler are funded by Mayo Clinic Rochester.

Program of Excellence in Mast Cell and Eosinophil Disorders, Division of Allergic Disease, Department of Internal Medicine, W-15 Mayo Building, 200 First Street Southwest, Rochester, MN 55905, USA
* Corresponding author.
E-mail address: Butterfield.joseph@mayo.edu

Immunol Allergy Clin N Am 34 (2014) 423–432
http://dx.doi.org/10.1016/j.iac.2014.01.004
0889-8561/14/$ – see front matter © 2014 Elsevier Inc. All rights reserved.

Table 1
Classification of mast cell disorders

Groups of Mast Cell Disorders	Suggested Subgroups
Cutaneous mastocytosis	Urticaria pigmentosa Telangiectasia eruptiva perstans Bullous cutaneous mastocytosis Diffuse cutaneous mastocytosis
Systemic mastocytosis	Indolent Smoldering Aggressive Mastocytosis with an associated hematologic non-mast cell disorder
Mast cell leukemia	Aleukemic mast cell leukemia Leukemic mast cell leukemia
Mast cell sarcoma	

is difficult to diagnose because the mast cells in the tumor occasionally lose some of their surface diagnostic markers.

Organs Affected

Mast cell sarcoma can affect any part of the body. The reported affected areas are outlined in **Table 2**. Those include the following:

- Larynx
- Colon
- Small bowel
- Bones (tibia and temporal bone in 2 different patients)
- Buccal mucosa with invasion of the mandible and the external auditory canal

Occasionally mast cell sarcoma becomes metastatic, and in one report, the tumor was identified after it became metastatic. On other occasions mast cell sarcoma was associated with systemic mastocytosis and mast cell leukemia.

Age Groups Affected

The reports of mast cell sarcoma span from infants to elderly patients. The youngest patient was diagnosed at age 8 months and the oldest was diagnosed at 77 years. The median age of the patients was 39 years.

Survival

Patients who develop mast cell sarcoma have a short life expectancy (see **Table 2**), likely because of the lack of effective therapeutic measures, and the aggressiveness of the disorder. The survival ranged from 2 months to 8 years. Two patients had the longest survival because the tumor expressed c-kit without a mutation that is resistant to imatinib mesylate. Those 2 patients responded to imatinib mesylate therapy after surgical excision and radiation therapy. A third patient with uterine mast cell sarcoma was reported to achieve complete remission after surgery, radiation, and therapy with imatinib mesylate. This last patient's tumor did not express the Asp816Val c-kit mutation. The median survival of the patients for whom survival data was reported is 6 months.

Table 2
Patients reported in the literature and identified in clinical electronic records

Number Assigned to Patients	Gender	Age at Onset	Age at Death	Site(s) of Mast Cell Sarcoma and Associated Disorders	References
1	F	71	76	Larynx, then metastatic	8
2	M	64	64	Metastatic	18
3	M	63	63	Metastatic with systemic mastocytosis	23
4	F	32	34	Colon, subsequent metastasis	21
5	F	8	8	Cerebral	7
6	M	44	Alive 2013	Left buttock, systemic mastocytosis with negative c-kit mutation and eosinophilia. Rx imatinib mesylate	Mayo Clinic Rochester records
7	M	4	4	Left tibia and aleukemic mast cell leukemia	9
8	M	71	72	Initial CMML, then developed small intestine mast cell sarcoma	Mayo Clinic Rochester records
9	M	61	Last contact 2012	Buccal mucosa extending into the mandible, surgery, chemotherapy, and radiation therapy	Mayo Clinic Rochester records
10	F	39	Complete remission	Uterus with ascites, negative c-kit, Rx imatinib mesylate	22
11	M	Elderly	After 4.5 mo of the diagnosis	Small intestine	10
12	F	63	N/A	Scalp with systemic mastocytosis Novel Kit mutation	23
13	F	15	N/A	Temporal bone	17
14	M	0	2	Right external auditory canal	16
15	M	39	41	Cutaneous mast cell sarcoma with a history of cutaneous mastocytosis and a mastocytoma	11
16	M	25	25	Thoracic mast cell sarcoma with mediastinal adenopathy and metastasis known familial indolent mastocytosis	13
17	M	42	42	Splenomegaly, mediastinal mast cell sarcoma with adenopathy	13
18	F	12	Alive in 2013	Left middle ear	18
19	M	19	Alive in 2013	Lip	18
20	F	77	77	Pelvis	18

Abbreviations: F, female; M, male; N/A, not available; Rx, therapy.

Clinical Presentation

The presentation of each of the patients reported has been unique. Mast cell sarcoma can affect any organ. It generally presents as a mass with relatively rapid growth. The symptoms depend on the site of the mass. All the patients' reports in the literature and those found in the electronic medical records are summarized in **Table 2**.

The first patient,[8] a woman aged 71, presented with a mass in the larynx that was first diagnosed as Wegener granulomatosis and treated with high-dose corticosteroids. Subsequent biopsies, about a year later, demonstrated the diagnosis of mast cell sarcoma, which became metastatic soon after the diagnosis, and she died at age 76.

The second patient,[19] a man aged 62, presented with systemic disease and died within 3 weeks of diagnosis.

The third patient,[20] a man aged 63, was known to have a history of systemic mastocytosis. He presented with metastatic mast cell sarcoma at the age of 63 and died within 5 weeks of the diagnosis.

The fourth patient,[21] a woman aged 32, presented with a colonic mast cell sarcoma involving retroperitoneal lymph nodes. Within 2 years, she developed metastatic disease involving the lymphatics and died at age 34.

The fifth patient,[7] a girl aged 8, presented with cerebral mast cell sarcoma and died the same year of presentation.

The sixth patient (seen at Mayo Clinic Rochester) was a 44-year-old man. He presented with worsening pain and visible skin induration of the left buttock in 2005. He was found to have mast cell sarcoma of the buttock. A concomitant bone marrow biopsy test result showed the presence of systemic mastocytosis. C-kit analysis was negative for the Asp816Val mutation. He was last contacted, and was doing well, in 2013.

The seventh patient,[9] a 4-year old boy, presented with a painful mass of his left tibia that was shown to be mast cell sarcoma. Because of subsequent elevation of serum tryptase and the development of a rash, he underwent a sternal bone marrow biopsy test. Study of the bone marrow and peripheral blood showed the presence of aleukemic mast cell leukemia. He died the year of diagnosis.

The eighth patient (seen at the Mayo Clinic Rochester) was a 71-year-old man with known chronic myelomonocytic leukemia (CMML). He developed gastroenterologic symptoms for which surgical intervention was required. The surgery showed an area of small intestinal thickening, which was resected. The pathology testing identified the presence of small intestine mast cell sarcoma from which he died the following year.

The ninth patient (seen at Mayo Clinic Rochester) was a 61-year-old man. He presented with a mass in the buccal mucosa in 2009. The mass subsequently enlarged and invaded the mandible. He underwent multiple therapeutic modalities. The last contact with him was in 2012 at which time he was asymptomatic. Imaging studies available included computed tomographic (CT) scan of the jaw, positron emission tomography scan of the head, and bone scan (**Fig. 1**).

The tenth patient,[22] a 39-year-old woman, presented with a uterine mass associated with massive ascites. The biopsy specimen showed mast cell sarcoma that expressed c-kit. The Kit Asp816Val mutation was absent. After multiple therapeutic modalities, the authors considered her in complete remission.

The eleventh patient[10] was referred to as an "elderly man." He was found to have small intestinal mast cell sarcoma from which he died within 4.5 months.

The twelfth patient,[23] a 63-year-old woman, presented with a mass in her scalp causing headaches. The biopsy specimen showed mast cell sarcoma and a bone

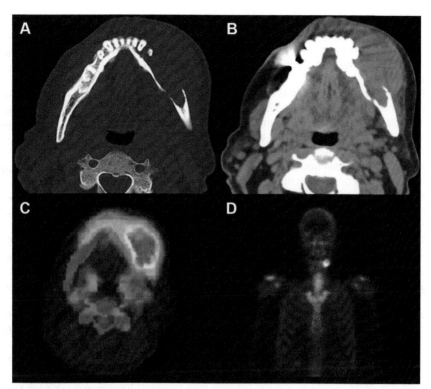

Fig. 1. (*A*) Patient #9-Axial noncontrast CT of the face, bone window, shows an expansile and lytic lesion of the left mandibular body, with associated cortical destruction laterally. (*B*) Axial contrast-enhanced CT, soft tissue window, shows an associated heterogenously attenuating and enhancing soft tissue mass of the left lower face with the associated lytic involvement of the adjacent mandible. (*C*) Axial F-18 FDG positron emission tomography/ CT image shows associated hypermetabolism of the soft tissue and lytic mass of the left mandible. (*D*) Coronal nuclear medicine Technetium-99m bone scan shows uptake in the left mandible corresponding to the mass noted on CT.

marrow biopsy test demonstrated existing systemic mastocytosis with c-kit D816V mutation. The authors did not mention the age at death of this patient.

The thirteenth patient[17] was a 15-year-old girl who was found to have mast cell sarcoma of the temporal bone. The age of death of this patient was not reported in this article.

The fourteenth patient reported[16] was a male infant who developed a mass in the right external auditory canal. Biopsies showed the mass to be mast cell sarcoma. Despite multiple therapeutic modalities, he died at age 2.

The fifteenth patient[11] was a 39-year-old man. He had a long-term history of cutaneous mastocytosis. He developed a mastocytoma that transformed into mast cell sarcoma. Despite therapeutic intervention, he died within 26 months.

The sixteenth patient[13] was a 25-year-old man with familial indolent mastocytosis and urticaria pigmentosa. He presented with inguinal adenopathy and reduced lower extremity mobility. Further work-up revealed multiple lesions compressing the lower spinal cord and a large lesion compressing the thoracic spinal cord.

The seventeenth patient[13] was a 42-year-old man. He presented with fever, sweats, rash, and cytopenias. He had a history of unexplained splenomegaly. At presentation he was found to have a mediastinal mass, generalized lymphadenopathy, multiple bone lytic lesions, and back muscle infiltration. He died within 1 to 2 months of presentation.

The eighteenth patient[18] was a 12-year-old girl who presented with a large left middle ear mass, initially diagnosed as Langerhans cell histiocytosis, that proved resistant to multiple courses of chemotherapy as well as to local debulking surgery. The correct diagnosis was made only after 2 additional pathology reviews.

The nineteenth patient[18] was a 19-year-old man who presented with a progressively enlarging submucosal nodule on the right lower lip. This patient also had a history of childhood-onset cutaneous mastocytosis that had resolved. An initial diagnosis was of ALK-negative anaplastic large cell lymphoma. Despite imatinib therapy and excision, the tumor recurred after 19 months.

The twentieth patient[18] was a 77-year-old woman with right hip and groin pain who subsequently was found to have a pelvic mass. She declined bone marrow biopsy testing and died under hospice care after 4 months.

THERAPEUTIC MODALITIES

Multiple chemotherapeutic agents and tyrosine kinase antagonists have been tried and failed. The only 2 patients whose therapy seemed to be successful responded to a combination of multiple modalities including surgical debulking, radiation therapy, and combination chemotherapeutic agents including imatinib mesylate, a tyrosine kinase inhibitor.

Over the years during which the disease was reported the following agents were used.

In May 1970, the first patient, a 71-year-old woman, was misdiagnosed as having laryngeal Wegener granulomatosis and treated with surgical resection and high-dose systemic steroids. Steroids were continued until March 1972 at which point she was found to have a recurrence of the subglottic mass and what appeared to be metastatic disease with lymphadenopathy, which resulted in repeated pathologic evaluation revealing the diagnosis of mast cell sarcoma. She was treated with high-dose bleomycin over 6 weeks. The metastatic and primary lesion continued to grow. Bleomycin was replaced with high-dose radiation therapy, which resulted in transient remission. By December 1973, the metastatic disease recurred. Chemotherapy according to a modified "De Vita" regimen was successful transiently. She had recurrence of the metastatic disease and hepatosplenomegaly resulting in her demise in May 1974.[8]

The second patient[19] report did not review the therapeutic intervention.

The third patient[20] report did not review the therapeutic intervention.

The fourth patient[21] was a 32-year-old woman with mast cell sarcoma infiltrating the colon. She first underwent surgical resection of the lesion. After 2 years, she presented with a large abdominal mass and lymphadenopathy. Subsequent treatment included prednisone and radiation therapy. Despite the therapy, she died at age 34 from metastatic disease.

The fifth patient was an 8-year old girl who presented in 2001 with severe headaches and was found to have intracranial mast cell sarcoma. At first, she was treated with prednisolone and then surgical resection. This treatment was followed by radiation therapy, subcutaneous interferon α2b, and cytarabine intrathecally. The tumor continued to proliferate instead of regress. She was treated with the regimen for myelogenous leukemia/sarcoma in childhood. Interferon was discontinued and she received cytosine arabinoside, etoposide, idarubicin, and prednisolone. This regimen did not result in a remission and was therefore changed. Prednisolone was continued; thioguanine, vincristine, and Adriamycin were added. This regimen was followed by a combination of arabinoside and mitoxantrone and subsequently followed by arabinoside and etoposide. This regimen resulted in a partial remission. However, the tumor recurred 5 weeks after the discontinuation of the chemotherapy. The parents declined additional therapy and the child died within 6 weeks of the recurrence.[7]

The sixth patient (from the Mayo Clinic records) was a 44-year old man. He presented in 2005 with left buttock pain and infiltration of the skin with hardening. Imaging studies showed a mass in the left gluteal area. He was treated with aggressive surgical resection, which was followed by imatinib mesylate therapy. The patient was still alive when contacted in 2013.

The seventh patient, according to a report published 2007,[9] was a 4-year old boy that was hospitalized for an 8-month history of pain, edema, and deformation of his right tibia, which was diagnosed as mast cell sarcoma with destructive bone invasion. A sternal bone marrow biopsy test revealed the presence of associated aleukemic mast cell leukemia. Despite aggressive surgical resection and chemotherapy (not specified in the case report), he died 10 months after hospitalization.

The eighth patient (seen at Mayo Clinic Rochester) was a 32-year old man. He was known to have CMML, which was under observation. After he developed abdominal pain and hemoptysis, thickening of the wall of the small bowel was identified. He underwent a diagnostic laparoscopy that revealed a mast cell sarcoma infiltrating the small bowel wall. He underwent surgical resection with end-to-end anastomosis. He initially did well but was subsequently found to have metastatic disease. He was treated with imatinib mesylate. Despite the therapy, he died within a year.

The ninth patient (seen at the Mayo Clinic Rochester) was a 61-year-old man. He was first seen in 2009 for a buccal lesion, which had been found to extend into and invade the mandible. He underwent aggressive surgical resection and radiation therapy, followed by imatinib mesylate therapy. He was last contacted in 2012 and was doing well on imatinib therapy.

The tenth patient[22] was a 39-year-old woman who was found to have mast cell sarcoma of the uterus. She underwent total hysterectomy and bilateral oophorectomy. Treatment with imatinib mesylate was added. The authors report that she achieved total remission.

The eleventh patient was an elderly male patient with small intestinal mast cell sarcoma, reported in 2011.[10] He underwent a diagnostic and therapeutic surgical resection with end-to-end anastomosis. Reverse transcription-polymerase chain reaction was used to study c-kit. He had an unusual mutation at c-kit Asn822Lys. He was initially treated with 40 mg prednisolone followed by 400 mg imatinib mesylate. He experienced what was a partial remission after 2 months of therapy. At the third month, however, the disease recurred. Therapy with interferon α2b was instituted and resulted in an apparent resolution of the sarcoma after 6 months of interferon therapy. However, 2 months later, he was again started on therapy with imatinib mesylate. He died within 4 to 5 months of the diagnosis.

For the twelfth patient, therapy and prognosis were not discussed in the article.[23]

Regarding the thirteenth patient, a report of a 15-year-old girl was published in March 2013.[17] She presented with a headache and was found to have mast cell sarcoma of the temporal bone. It expressed c-kit, and mutation analysis revealed L799F mutation. The initial diagnosis and therapy followed a protocol for Langerhans cell histiocytosis 3. Subsequent evaluation showed tumor progression. The therapies tried included vinblastine, dexamethasone, cladribine, clofarabine, multiple combination chemotherapeutic agents combined with tyrosine kinase antagonists, radiation therapy, and multiple surgical resections. Despite that, the tumor did not regress. No additional information about the patient was provided.

In May 2013, another report of an infant, the fourteenth patient, with mast cell sarcoma was published.[16] The child presented with purulent otorrhea at 4 months of age. After treatment of the infection, a small mass was identified in the auditory canal that grew and invaded the bone by the age of 8 months. It was initially diagnosed as Langerhans cell histiocytosis. At the age of 11 months, the mass enlarged and serum tryptase was found to be elevated (34 ng/mL, with normal level <11.5 ng/mL). C-kit Asp816Val mutation was absent. The child was treated with surgical debulking and the experimental drug PKC412 for 1 year. This treatment reduced the tumor size and allowed for further debulking. At the time of the report, the child was 2 years of age.

Another report published in 2012[11] reviewed the clinical history of a 40-year-old man, the fifteenth patient, with known persistent cutaneous mastocytosis. He experienced a malignant transformation of a cutaneous mastocytoma into mast cell sarcoma. Surgical excision, radiation therapy, and imatinib therapy failed to induce a remission. The patient died within a few months.

A publication in February 2013[13] reported 2 patients. The first (sixteenth) was of a 25-year-old man with a history of familial indolent systemic mastocytosis and urticaria pigmentosa. He was found to have a large thoracic mast cell sarcoma with metastasis to the lymph nodes and the bones. He failed therapy of 1 month with dasatinib and corticosteroids. After failed dasatinib therapy, cytosine arabinoside in combination with cyclophosphamide was tried but failed. When the tumor invaded the sphenoid sinus, therapy with cladribine was started but also failed and he died within a few days.

The second (seventeenth) patient was a 42-year-old man with a history of unexplained splenomegaly. He developed mast cell B symptoms, which include fever, night sweats, leukopenias, anemia, and hepatosplenomegaly. A CT scan of the chest and abdomen revealed the presence of mediastinal and retroperitoneal lymphadenopathy. It also showed a muscular dorsal mass with lytic bone lesions. After an erroneous initial diagnosis (anaplastic lymphoma), positive stains for c-kit, tryptase, and CD30 suggested the diagnosis of mast cell sarcoma. C-kit mutation analysis showed Val560Gly mutation. Therapy with corticosteroids and dasatinib was started but failed. The patient died within 10 days.

Patient 18, a 12-year-old girl, did not respond to therapy with 2CDA/Ara-C, ICE, clofarabine, ALCL 99, idarubicin/Velcade/Ara-C, and decitabine. Subsequently she was given radiation treatment and imatinib mesylate and scheduled for allogeneic stem cell transplantation. She is alive with persistent disease 45 months following initial presentation.

Patient 19, a 19-year-old man, experienced recurrent tumor 19 months after excision and treatment with imatinib 400 mg daily.

Patient 20 died 4 months following diagnosis after treatment with pamidronate and radiotherapy.

SUMMARY

Mast cell sarcoma is the rarest and most difficult of mast cell neoplasms to treat. Mast cell sarcoma might occur in any age group and could initially present in various organs. It tends to metastasize. An approach using combined surgical debulking, radiation therapy, and newer chemotherapeutic agents targeting mutated c-kit (tyrosine kinase inhibitors) seems to have the best chance to induce remission. The authors' data revealed an almost 2:1 male-to-female ratio. Furthermore, 4 of the 20 patients with mast cell sarcoma had underlying systemic or cutaneous mastocytosis.

REFERENCES

1. Mulligan RM. Neoplastic diseases of dogs; mast cell sarcoma, lymphosarcoma, histiocytoma. Arch Pathol (Chic) 1948;46(5):477–92.
2. Sandes AF, Medeiros RS, Rizzatti EG. Diagnosis and treatment of mast cell disorders: practical recommendations. Sao Paulo Med J 2013;131(4):264–74.
3. Valent P, Arock M, Akin C, et al. The classification of systemic mastocytosis should include mast cell leukemia (MCL) and systemic mastocytosis with a clonal hematologic non-mast cell lineage disease (SM-AHNMD). Blood 2010;116(5):850–1.
4. Valent P, Akin C, Sperr WR, et al. Mast cell proliferative disorders: current view on variants recognized by the World Health Organization. Hematol Oncol Clin North Am 2003;17(5):1227–41.
5. Pardanani A. Systemic mastocytosis in adults: 2013 update on diagnosis, risk stratification, and management. Am J Hematol 2013;88(7):612–24.
6. Galanis E, Li CY, Phyliky R. Mast cell disease mimicking granulocytic sarcoma. Am J Hematol 1997;56(3):194–5.
7. Guenther PP, Huebner A, Sobottka SB, et al. Temporary response of localized intracranial mast cell sarcoma to combination chemotherapy. J Pediatr Hematol Oncol 2001;23(2):134–8.
8. Horny HP, Parwaresch MR, Kaiserling E, et al. Mast cell sarcoma of the larynx. J Clin Pathol 1986;39(6):596–602.
9. Brcic L, Vuletic LB, Stepan J, et al. Mast-cell sarcoma of the tibia. J Clin Pathol 2007;60(4):424–5.
10. Bugalia A, Abraham A, Balasubramanian P, et al. Mast cell sarcoma of the small intestine: a case report. J Clin Pathol 2011;64(11):1035–7.
11. Auquit-Auckbur I, Lazar C, Deneuve S, et al. Malignant transformation of mastocytoma developed on skin mastocytosis into cutaneous mast cell sarcoma. Am J Surg Pathol 2012;36(5):779–82.
12. Georgin-Lavialle S, Aguilar C, Guieze R, et al. Mast cell sarcoma in an infant: a case report and review of the literature. J Pediatr Hematol Oncol 2013;35(4):315–20 doi:310.1097/MPH.1090b1013e318279e318392.
13. Georgin-Lavialle S, Aguilar C, Guieze R, et al. Mast cell sarcoma: a rare and aggressive entity–report of two cases and review of the literature. J Clin Oncol 2013;31(6):e90–7.
14. Chott A, Guenther P, Huebner A, et al. Morphologic and immunophenotypic properties of neoplastic cells in a case of mast cell sarcoma. Am J Surg Pathol 2003;27(7):1013–9.
15. Krauth MT, Fodinger M, Rebuzzi L, et al. Aggressive systemic mastocytosis with sarcoma-like growth in the skeleton, leukemic progression, and partial loss of mast cell differentiation antigens. Haematologica 2007;92(12):e126–9.
16. Bautista-Quach MA, Booth CL, Kheradpour A, et al. Mast cell sarcoma in an infant: a case report and review of the literature. J Pediatr Hematol Oncol 2013;35(4):315–20.
17. Kim YS, Wu H, Pawlowska AB, et al. Pediatric mast cell sarcoma of temporal bone with novel L799F (2395 C>T) KIT mutation, mimicking histiocytic neoplasm. Am J Surg Pathol 2013;37(3):453–8.

18. Ryan RJ, Akin C, Castells M, et al. Mast cell sarcoma: a rare and potentially under-recognized diagnostic entity with specific therapeutic implications. Mod Pathol 2013;26:533–43.
19. Horny HP, Kaiserling E, Sillaber C, et al. Bone marrow mastocytosis associated with an undifferentiated extramedullary tumor of hemopoietic origin. Arch Pathol Lab Med 1997;121(4):423–6.
20. Sotlar K, Horny HP, Lebherz J, et al. Assoziation einer Knochenmarksmastozytose mit extrem unreifem extramedullarem Mastzellsarkom. Pathologe 1997; 18(3):252–6.
21. Kojima M, Nakamura S, Itoh H, et al. Mast cell sarcoma with tissue eosinophilia arising in the ascending colon. Mod Pathol 1999;12(7):739–43.
22. Ma HB, Xu X, Liu WP, et al. Successful treatment of mast cell sarcoma of the uterus with imatinib. Int J Hematol 2011;94(5):491–4.
23. Falleti J, Borgia L, Lalinga A, et al. Mast cell sarcoma of the scalp: the first sign of undisclosed systemic mastocytosis? Pathol Res Pract 2012;208(11):683–6. http://dx.doi.org/10.1016/j.prp.2012.1006.1010.

Treatment Strategies in Mastocytosis

Frank Siebenhaar, MD[a],*, Cem Akin, MD, PhD[b],
Carsten Bindslev-Jensen, MD, PhD, DMSc[c], Marcus Maurer, MD[a],
Sigurd Broesby-Olsen, MD[c]

KEYWORDS

- Mastocytosis • Antimediator therapy • Mediator-related symptoms • Antihistamine
- Platelet-activating factor • Anti-IgE

KEY POINTS

- Most patients with mastocytosis suffer from the indolent form.
- Mediator-related symptoms and comorbidities significantly affect the quality of life.
- Available treatment options include antihistamines and other drugs directed against the effects of mast cells and their mediators.
- All of these drugs are off label.
- The recommendation to use these drugs is almost exclusively based on expert opinion; controlled clinical trials need to be performed.
- A better understanding of mechanisms in mastocytosis will allow for the identification of future targets for effective treatments.

INTRODUCTION

Mastocytosis is a heterogeneous group of diseases with an increased number of mast cells (MCs) in 1 or multiple organs, ranging from indolent to very rare aggressive forms with fatal outcome.[1] The current World Health Organization classification differentiates between 7 mastocytosis subtypes (**Table 1**), dividing cutaneous from systemic

Disclosure: Dr Akin has a consultancy agreement with Novartis. Drs Siebenhaar and Maurer received honorarium for consultancy and lectures as well as study support from Uriach. Drs Broesby-Olsen and Bindslev-Jensen have nothing to disclose.
[a] Department of Dermatology and Allergy, Interdisciplinary Mastocytosis Center Charité, Charité-Universitätsmedizin Berlin, Charitéplatz 1, Berlin 10117, Germany; [b] Division of Rheumatology, Allergy, Immunology, Mastocytosis Center, Harvard Medical School, Brigham and Women's Hospital, 1 Jimmy Fund Way, Room 626B, Boston, MA 02115, USA; [c] Department of Dermatology, Allergy Centre, Mastocytosis Centre Odense University Hospital, MastOUH, Odense University Hospital, Sdr. Boulevard 29, Entrance 142, 5000 Odense C, Denmark
* Corresponding author. Department of Dermatology and Allergy, Allergie-Centrum-Charite/ECARF, Charité-Universitätsmedizin Berlin, Charitéplatz 1, Berlin 10117, Germany.
E-mail address: frank.siebenhaar@charite.de

Immunol Allergy Clin N Am 34 (2014) 433–447
http://dx.doi.org/10.1016/j.iac.2014.01.012
0889-8561/14/$ – see front matter © 2014 Elsevier Inc. All rights reserved.
immunology.theclinics.com

Table 1			
World Health Organization classification of mastocytosis			
Category	**Frequency (%)**	**Prognosis**	**Therapeutic Options**
CM ISM	>80	Good	Antimediator therapy, ultraviolet or topical treatments, emergency medication, osteoporosis treatment
SM-AHNMD	10	Variable	Plus treatment of AHNMD
ASM	5	Poor	Plus cytoreductive therapy
MCL MSC	<5	Poor	Plus cytoreductive therapy, bone marrow transplantation (MCL)
ECM	<1	Good	Plus surgical excision (if applicable)

Abbreviations: ASM, aggressive systemic mastocytosis; CM, cutaneous mastocytosis; ECM, extracutaneous mastocytoma; ISM, indolent systemic mastocytosis; MCL, MC leukemia; MSC, MC sarcoma; SM-AHNMD, systemic mastocytosis with associated hematologic non-MC disease.
Data from Valent P, Horny HP, Escribano L, et al. Diagnostic criteria and classification of mastocytosis: a consensus proposal. Leuk Res 2001;25(7):603–25; and Cardet JC, Akin C, Lee MJ. Mastocytosis: update on pharmacotherapy and future directions. Expert Opin Pharmacother 2013;14(15):2033–45.

forms.[2,3] Patients with systemic mastocytosis frequently also exhibit cutaneous lesions which is specified as mastocytosis in the skin (MIS), whereas cutaneous mastocytosis (CM) excludes systemic involvement. Mastocytosis is classified as a rare disease with an estimated prevalence of around 1 per 10.000[4]; however, epidemiologic studies are lacking, and the disease is probably underdiagnosed. Pathogenic mechanisms involve the presence of somatic, activating c-kit-mutations, most commonly the Kit D816V point mutation, which is present in more than 95% of adults and 40% of children with mastocytosis.[5]

The signs and symptoms in mastocytosis result either from effects of MC mediators or from organ impairment caused by MC infiltration. Of these signs and symptoms, mediator-related symptoms are prevalent and occur in all types of mastocytosis, whereas problems caused by infiltrating MCs are seen only in the rare, aggressive forms of mastocytosis.[6]

Mediator-related signs and symptoms are diverse. They may be acute, related to a sudden MC degranulation, or chronic and involve the skin (pruritus, flushing, and cosmetic complaints), the gastrointestinal tract (reflux, ulcers, cramping, and diarrhea), and the central nervous system (depression, moods, and cognitive symptoms) and musculoskeletal pain. Anaphylactic episodes occur in around 30% to 40% of patients and may be unpredictable, recurring, and non–IgE mediated.[7–10] In addition, disease-associated comorbidities like osteoporosis or associated hematologic disorders are seen.

No curative therapy for mastocytosis exists, and the most important overall aim of treatment is the control of symptoms. Patients with cutaneous mastocytosis (CM) and indolent systemic mastocytosis (ISM) (ie, most patients with mastocytosis) have a normal, or near normal, life expectancy compared with the general population,[11] which underlines that the focus of disease management should be on symptom control.

Treatment recommendations for mastocytosis are based mostly on expert opinion rather than evidence obtained from controlled clinical trials. In this article, current treatment options available in mastocytosis are presented, with a focus on the control of mediator-related symptoms in patients with indolent disease.

GENERAL CONSIDERATIONS

In general, mastocytosis is best handled by a coordinated, multidisciplinary approach by centers with experience in managing the disease. The focus should be on individualized, tailored treatment and follow-up depending on symptoms and disease manifestations.

Overall, treatment strategies are divided into antimediator therapy aimed at MC mediators and cytoreductive therapies aiming at reduction of neoplastic MC burden. The latter should be reserved for patients with aggressive disease or severely affected patients with ISM because of potential side effects.

All patients benefit from thorough information and counseling tailored to the individual, bearing in mind that many patients go on the Internet for information, which may vary greatly in quality and relevance given the rarity and heterogeneity of the disease and thus may result in misinformation and unnecessary concerns.

Further, it is important to clarify relevant triggers for MC degranulation in order to avoid these. Even although some MC triggers are common (heat, alcohol, insect stings, spicy foods, certain drugs), general advice to avoid a long list of potential triggers is not helpful, but must be individualized and relevant to the patient's experiences. Information must be given on potential risk situations (eg, general anesthesia, contrast media), and it is advisable to provide written information on the disease to the patient and relevant health care professionals (eg a disease passport).

In general, most mastocytosis centers equip all adult patients with mastocytosis with an adrenaline autoinjector for use in case of anaphylaxis (**Fig. 1**). In children with mastocytosis, the risk of anaphylaxis is lower than in adults, and there is no consensus whether to prescribe an adrenaline autoinjector for all children or only in children with severe disease/bullous skin lesions/basal tryptase levels higher than 100 µg/L or a previous anaphylactic episode.[7,9,12]

CM IN CHILDREN

The skin lesions in mastocytosis differ depending on the age of disease onset.[13] In children, mastocytosis is mainly limited to skin; the most common type is the solitary mastocytoma. Other childhood-onset forms include maculopapular, nodular, xanthelasmoid, or pachydermatous lesions, as well as diffuse CM with the involvement of the entire integument.[14] Up to the age of 3 years, some children suffer from blistering in affected areas, mostly as a result of mechanical irritation. Childhood-onset CM has a high chance of spontaneous remission, and treatment should be

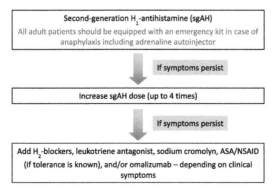

Fig. 1. Proposed therapeutic algorithm for antimediator treatment in mastocytosis.

based on symptoms. Clinically symptomatic mastocytomas may be treated with short-term high-potency topical corticosteroids or injected with crystalline steroid solutions. In single cases, the use of topical pimecrolimus has been reported to result in the remission of lesions.[15] Mastocytomas accompanied by systemic symptoms (ie, recurrent anaphylaxis) may warrant surgical excision, depending on the location of the tumor.[16]

SKIN LESIONS IN ADULTS

In 80% to 90% of patients with adult-onset ISM, the skin is affected. The cutaneous manifestation typically presents with maculopapular skin lesions (historically called urticaria pigmentosa) with a positive Darier sign (whealing and flushing on mechanical irritation). The clinical picture ranges from only a few lesions, which are easy to miss in a routine diagnostic workup, to widespread lesions that cover up to 80% of the skin compartment. About 60% of patients complain about recurrent pruritic episodes or whealing, especially when exposed to triggers of MC activation, whereas some patients do not have any subjective symptoms at the skin. The number and distribution of the cutaneous lesions show individual variations but are of a chronic-stable nature. A major issue in many patients is cosmetic complaints, especially in youth. The challenge here is that the skin lesions are caused by MC infiltration, so an effective treatment demands reduction of this infiltration. The disappearance of cutaneous lesions in mastocytosis has been reported with the use of cytoreductive drugs, like tyrosine kinase inhibitors (TKIs) and cladribine in patients with advanced cases of systemic mastocytosis (SM)[17,18]; however, the use of these potentially toxic drugs is obsolete in purely cutaneous or indolent forms of mastocytosis. So, therapeutic options to interfere with the clinical appearance of the skin lesions are virtually absent and limited to phototherapy, including UVA$_1$, narrow-band UVB, and UVA plus psoralen. There is well-reported efficacy of phototherapy in CM and MIS in regard to the mediator-related skin symptoms, including pruritus; however, complete or permanent disappearance of the lesions is not reported, and the overall period of symptom reduction is short.[19] The immediate response may be improved by combining phototherapy with short-term high-potent topical steroids under occlusion; however, this does not influence the long-term efficacy outcome of the treatment. Thus, given the potential side effects of recurrent ultraviolet phototherapy, a calculated use of this treatment modality should be considered. Single case studies report about the successful use of neodymium-doped yttrium aluminum garnet laser therapy, which is certainly not an option for all patients, because of the different intensity and distribution of lesions, but is potentially useful for some patients (eg, with skin lesions in the face).[20,21]

SKIN SYMPTOMS

Recurring episodes of pruritus, whealing, and flushing can be controlled by first-generation and second-generation H$_1$ antihistamines (sgAH).[22] However, many patients may need increased doses of antihistamines to completely control symptoms.[23,24] During the last 2 decades, only 1 single controlled clinical trial showing efficacy of sgAH in the treatment of mastocytosis has been performed.[22] In this trial, the sgAH rupatadine has been shown to significantly reduce mediator-related symptoms and improve patients' quality of life. Despite missing further evidence for mastocytosis, treatment regimens and guidelines for other MC-driven diseases (ie, chronic spontaneous urticaria), it can be considered to increase the dose up to 4-fold the usual daily dose.[25] In most countries, antihistamines are not licensed to be used in patients younger than 2 years. However, the pharmacologic profile of most sgAH may allow for their use during pregnancy and infancy. Sodium cromolyn has been reported to be effective in both children and adults to relieve cutaneous symptoms, used topically as well as perorally.[26,27] The mechanism of action is not clear, because enteric absorption of sodium cromolyn is minimal[28] and its effects on human MCs unclear.[29] The use of topical steroids may be valuable to reduce skin symptoms as short-term use; however, long-term use must be avoided because of side effects, taking into account the chronicity of the disease. In addition, other substances, including polidocanol and topical antihistamines, have been reported to support relief of pruritus in CM. Further treatment considerations for skin symptoms besides sgAH include efforts to block additional mediators that are involved in symptom formation (ie, leukotrienes, platelet-activating factor, or prostaglandins).[22,30–33]

GASTROINTESTINAL SYMPTOMS

Gastrointestinal manifestations in patients with mastocytosis are highly prevalent and may be severe.[34,35] About 30% of patients with mastocytosis have gastrointestinal symptoms, including bloating, abdominal pain, nausea, and diarrhea. Patients with mastocytosis also show a significantly higher incidence of duodenal ulcers. The gastrointestinal symptoms of mastocytosis are not disease specific, and differential diagnoses must be considered and ruled out (ie, *Helicobacter pylori*–associated ulcers, celiac disease, inflammatory bowel disease, irritable bowel syndrome, or malignant disease). Patients with moderate or severe symptoms should be referred to a gastroenterologist. Histologic analyses of duodenal biopsies may show increased numbers of neoplastic MCs, but this does not correlate clearly with the clinical symptoms. Moreover, histologic findings are nonspecific and may lead to misinterpretation in the absence of other clinical signs for mastocytosis.[35] Treatment options for gastrointestinal symptoms include continued use of sgAH up to 4-fold of daily recommended dose, H_2-blockers, proton pump inhibitors, and oral sodium cromolyn, which has been shown to be effective in the control of diarrhea in many patients. Further, triggers that may provoke gastrointestinal symptoms in the individual patient must be identified and avoided, including the subgroup of patients with IgE-mediated food allergy. In the rare aggressive forms of mastocytosis, malabsorption caused by profound MC infiltration of the gastrointestinal tract may be seen, and warrant further aggressive therapies or glucocorticoid use.[36,37]

OTHER MC MEDIATOR–RELATED SYMPTOMS

Neuropsychiatric symptoms, which include headache, loss of concentration/memory problems, fatigue and depressive symptoms, are prevalent and seen in approximately one-third of adults with mastocytosis.[8,38–40] In about 10% of patients, symptoms are severe and have tremendous impact on daily life. The pathogenesis and mechanisms involved are not clear but probably involve MC mediator effects in the central nervous system. Hormonal factors in women may also be involved. Further, secondary causes may play an important role, bearing in mind that mastocytosis is a chronic disease, with heterogeneous, often severe symptoms, which in many cases are not easy to cope with. Management should include a thorough workup for differential diagnoses depending on symptoms and severity involving psychiatric or neurologic workup. Treatment options include sgAH (often updosed), leukotriene antagonists, antidepressants, and psychological support. Sodium cromolyn reportedly also may have a slow-onset beneficial effect on this type of symptoms[41]; however, the mechanism of action is not clear, especially because of the aforementioned lack of absorption of the drug from the gastrointestinal tract, and other studies have not been able to document a similar effect.[42,43]

Poorly localized pain from soft tissue and bone is a frequent finding in mastocytosis[44] and may be related to MC prostaglandin synthesis, but mechanisms are poorly understood. Differential diagnoses, mainly rheumatic, must be considered. Treatment options include nonsteroidal antiinflammatory drugs (NSAIDs)/aspirin if tolerated, sgAH, leukotriene antagonist, and sodium cromolyn, in addition to low-potency analgesics and nonpharmacologic measurements recommending exercise and physiotherapy.[42,45–47] Bisphosphonates have been reported to relieve bone pain, in patients with mastocytosis treated for osteoporosis.[48] Symptoms may sometimes be severe and influence daily functions; however, opioids should be generally avoided in most of these cases because of side effects and chronicity of symptoms, and further because they are a frequent trigger of MC degranulation. If these symptoms, associated with mastocytosis, are provoked by MC mediator release (possible because of unidentified or multiple factors), more general approaches of inhibiting MC functions may result in better symptom control. Such approaches are either missing or infrequently used because of lacking evidence. Recent reports have promised potential beneficial effects using omalizumab, a humanized anti-IgE antibody, in the treatment of mastocytosis.[49–51] Omalizumab is labeled for the therapy for severe allergic asthma and has been recently shown to be effective in symptom control of a variety of MC-mediated diseases, including urticaria, mastocytosis, and idiopathic anaphylaxis.[49–53] A controlled clinical trial to investigate the efficacy of omalizumab in the treatment of mastocytosis is ongoing.

BONE DISEASE AND OSTEOPOROSIS

Bone manifestations are a frequent finding in adult patients with mastocytosis, most commonly osteoporosis or osteopenia and more rarely, osteolytic lesions or osteosclerosis.[54–56] Around half of adults with SM have osteopenia or osteoporosis, which may go undetected because of lack of symptoms. It is in general advisable to screen all adult patients by dual-energy X-ray absorptiometry (DXA) as well as checking vitamin D levels and supplement if low, including sufficient daily calcium intake.

Further workup and radiologic examinations depend on clinical presentation, including presence of focal skeletal symptoms or bone pain.

The pathogenic mechanisms involved in the bone manifestations of mastocytosis are not clear but may involve an effect of MC mediators such as histamine, heparin, and interleukin 6 or MC-derived cytokines such as Receptor Activator of NF-κB Ligand (RANKL), which influence balance of bone formation and resorption.[57,58]

Controlled clinical trials investigating effect of specific treatments in mastocytosis-associated osteoporosis are lacking, and it is advisable to follow general guidelines for osteoporosis concerning treatment and follow-up in these patients, including treatment with bisphosphonates and vitamin D plus calcium supplements. Patients with severe osteoporosis and osteoporotic fractures and young individuals should be evaluated by specialists in osteoporosis.

The lack of knowledge regarding the pathologic mechanisms involved limit present disease-specific treatments. It may be speculated that an effective antimediator or MC stabilizing treatment may prevent development of osteoporosis in mastocytosis, but data are lacking. Further, the effectiveness of newer drugs such as denosumab remains to be elucidated. MC burden itself does not seem to increase frequency of osteoporosis,[8,59] and cytoreductive treatments are in general not warranted. As opposed to the rarely encountered large, osteolytic bone lesions, osteoporosis/osteoporotic fractures should not be considered a C-finding and sign of aggressive disease.

ANAPHYLAXIS

Anaphylaxis is defined as an acute, suddenly occurring, severe systemic hypersensitivity reaction in at least 2 organ systems, often including skin symptoms, consisting of wheal-and-flare–type reactions, pruritus and flushing, respiratory compromise, or cardiovascular responses, including decreased blood pressure with or without the loss of consciousness.[60,61]

Epidemiologic data on the incidence of anaphylaxis in the normal population vary because of diversity in study designs and definitions of anaphylaxis from 8 to 50 per 100,000 person years.[62–66] The lifetime prevalence of anaphylaxis has been calculated to be approximately 0.05% to 2.0%.[67] The results of previous studies and clinical observations indicate an increased risk of anaphylaxis in mastocytosis with a reported prevalence of about 35% to 50% in adult patients with various subtypes of mastocytosis.[7,68,69] The most prominent cause of anaphylaxis in mastocytosis is Hymenoptera sting in up to 50% of cases.[70] Drugs, including antibiotics, opioids, NSAIDs, radio contrast media, and muscle relaxants are also common reported causes of anaphylaxis in mastocytosis, whereas more infrequent triggers include IgE-mediated food allergy. The incidence of IgE-mediated food allergy in mastocytosis is not known to be greater than that of the general population, but the symptoms of food allergy may be more severe if the patient has both conditions. Isolated exposure to more general triggers like heat, cold, physical stress, exercise, alcohol, and spicy foods is rarely related to severe anaphylactic reactions, but may act combined. Despite described elicitation factors, the rate of anaphylaxis of unknown cause (ie, idiopathic anaphylaxis) is reported to be very high in mastocytosis and to occur in about 35% of cases.[70] Although the overall rate of type I IgE-mediated sensitizations in mastocytosis and the prevalence of atopy are suggested to not differ from the general population, patients with mastocytosis may be more prone to react to unusual triggers (eg, Diptera bites).[10,71] It has been reported that the risk for severe anaphylactic reactions in mastocytosis is not correlated with the MC burden,[8] or may even be inversely correlated,[72] and patients without skin lesions tend to show more frequent anaphylactic reactions with unique features.[9,70,73] Therefore, anaphylactic episodes are frequently the first sign that lead to further investigation and result in the diagnosis of a previous undetected SM in patients with anaphylaxis. No predicting factors are available allowing for the exact risk estimation of anaphylaxis in mastocytosis.[74] Therefore, the meticulous management of patients with mastocytosis to prevent unpredictable and potentially life-threatening anaphylactic episodes is of major importance. Equipment with emergency medication and treatment strategies targeting the elicitation factor should also be considered in patients with mastocytosis. Patients with Hymenoptera allergy are eligible for specific immunotherapy (SIT) to bee or wasp venom or both and should be given lifelong treatment.[75] In cases of severe bee sting anaphylaxis, a dose adjustment should be considered to better protect the patient from recurrent anaphylactic episodes.[76] However, patients with mastocytosis are also at higher risk of experiencing severe side effects to venom injections, and thus, SIT is not tolerated by all patients. Because SIT in Hymenoptera anaphylaxis is the only available treatment option that reduces the risk of life-threatening anaphylactic episodes, strategies to improve the tolerability of SIT in patients with mastocytosis are of great value. In recent years, numerous case studies have reported major success in simultaneously treating patients with omalizumab. It has been reported in many patients that the treatment of omalizumab resulted in increased tolerability of SIT and mediated solid protection from anaphylactic episodes in patients with mastocytosis.[77–81]

KIT-TARGETING THERAPIES

Somatic Kit-mutations have been recognized as one of the major pathogenic factors in mastocytosis. KIT (CD117) is a transmembrane receptor tyrosine kinase that is involved in MC survival, differentiation, and activation under the control of its ligand stem cell factor (SCF).[82] More than 95% of patients are detected to carry the D816V Kit-mutation, a point mutation with substitution of valine for aspartate in codon 816 of exon 17.[5] This gain-of-function mutation leads to an autoactivation of the receptor kinase, resulting in SCF-independent signaling. Besides the occurrence of Kit-mutations, other incidences (eg, secondary mutations of TET2 or epigenetic factors) are suggested to be involved in the determination of the disease category and intensity of symptoms.[83–86] However, during recent years, Kit-targeting agents have been in the research focus as a novel therapeutic strategy in mastocytosis. Imatinib is the only TKI that has received approval from the US Food and Drug Administration (FDA) for the treatment of aggressive SM. Patients carrying the D816V mutation are resistant to imatinib, and therefore, its use is restricted to non-D816V mutations, which excludes most patients with mastocytosis. However, imatinib has been reported to be effective in selected patient populations.[87] Second-generation TKIs, including dasatinib and nilotinib, so far have shown limited overall clinical efficacy. The protein kinase C inhibitor midostaurin is under investigation for efficacy in advanced types of mastocytosis. Preliminary data analyses show efficacy in terms of a reduced MC burden in a subset of patients.[88] The wild type Kit inhibitor masitinib was tested in patients with indolent mastocytosis and showed effects on symptom improvement in some patients but did not result in a significant reduction of the MC burden.[89] No Kit-targeting therapy has been approved for the use in D816V-positive patients with mastocytosis, and the use of TKIs is an option in selected cases of severely affected patients with advanced forms of mastocytosis. The results of ongoing and future studies will show their value for use in indolent types of mastocytosis.

FUTURE PERSPECTIVES

A true revival of MC research is under way. Because of the tremendous progress made during recent years, the field now has the tools to translate newly acquired knowledge of MC biology to novel therapies and measures of disease control.

Downregulation of MC function and survival is warranted in mastocytosis treatment. Human MCs have recently been reported to express receptors that could allow for the induction of apoptosis and inhibition of activation, like the Tumor Necrosis Factor Related Apoptosis Inducing Ligand receptor (TRAIL-R) and the inhibitory receptors CD300a and Siglec-8.[90–92] TRAIL-R is the only death receptor known so far to be expressed on human MCs and, therefore, exhibit an interesting therapeutic target. The newly described inhibitory receptors, CD300a and Siglec-8, showed potential downregulatory properties on MC activation and survival in vivo.[93] A selective targeting of these receptors could lead to a potential innovative treatment strategy in mastocytosis.[90]

MCs express a variety of other receptors allowing for the modulation of both activating or inhibiting pathways, which might serve as novel therapeutic targets in disease control. Although with some of those targets we are close to developing drugs, for others, further basic studies on their functions are required. For example, BH3-only proteins, a group of proapoptotic factors, have been described to modulate MC survival in vitro and in vivo.[94–99] Agents, like calcineurin inhibitors or dimethylfumarate, have been reported to induce apoptosis in MCs and in disease models of mastocytosis.[100–102] Other substances were tested for their efficacy in pilot clinical trials, like the raft modulator miltefosine. Miltefosine has been shown to reduce the release of histamine, tumor necrosis factor, and prostaglandin D_2 from MCs on IgE-mediated and non-IgE–mediated activation. In addition, topical administration of miltefosine showed a reduction of histamine-induced wheal-and-flare–type skin reactions in vivo. In a randomized, placebo-controlled, double-blind clinical trial, topical miltefosine has been shown to inhibit MC activation in patients with CM.[103–106]

The recent creation of mouse models carrying the Kit D816V mutation and its mouse homologue Kit D814V, respectively, will allow more insight in the pathologic features of disease development and the associated alteration in MC function.[107] Physiologically, skin MCs are found in close anatomic vicinity to blood vessels and sensory nerves, which has been shown to be relevant in various inflammatory conditions.[108,109] In which sense such intense immunologic interactions are affected by mastocytosis to contribute to the elicitation of symptoms is unknown, but they may harbor additional targets for innovative treatment options.

Taken together, there is increasing evidence for MC mediators and receptors as well as other drugable targets to have a strong potential for therapeutic intervention. However, a more detailed understanding of their pathophysiologic functions is required to develop effective therapeutic strategies free from side effects in future. The first controlled clinical trials have already shown that cutaneous SM and ISM are diseases suitable for study of new drugs that can be tested for efficacy and safety.

ACKNOWLEDGMENTS

The authors wish to thank the strategic funding of the COST Action BM1007: mast cells and basophils-targets for innovative therapies.

REFERENCES

1. Metcalfe DD. Mast cells and mastocytosis. Blood 2008;112(4):946–56.
2. Valent P, Akin C, Escribano L, et al. Standards and standardization in mastocytosis: consensus statements on diagnostics, treatment recommendations and response criteria. Eur J Clin Invest 2007;37(6):435–53.
3. Valent P, Horny HP, Escribano L, et al. Diagnostic criteria and classification of mastocytosis: a consensus proposal. Leuk Res 2001;25(7):603–25.
4. van Doormaal JJ, Arends S, Brunekreeft KL, et al. Prevalence of indolent systemic mastocytosis in a Dutch region. J Allergy Clin Immunol 2013;131(5): 1429–31.e1.
5. Cardet JC, Akin C, Lee MJ. Mastocytosis: update on pharmacotherapy and future directions. Expert Opin Pharmacother 2013;14(15):2033–45.
6. Carter MC, Metcalfe DD, Komarow HD. Mastocytosis. Immunol Allergy Clin North Am 2014;34(1):181–96.
7. Brockow K, Jofer C, Behrendt H, et al. Anaphylaxis in patients with mastocytosis: a study on history, clinical features and risk factors in 120 patients. Allergy 2008;63(2):226–32.
8. Broesby-Olsen S, Kristensen T, Vestergaard H, et al. KIT D816V mutation burden does not correlate to clinical manifestations of indolent systemic mastocytosis. J Allergy Clin Immunol 2013;132(3):723–8.
9. Alvarez-Twose I, Zanotti R, Gonzalez-de-Olano D, et al. Nonaggressive systemic mastocytosis (SM) without skin lesions associated with insect-induced anaphylaxis shows unique features versus other indolent SM. 2014;133(2):520–8.
10. Reiter N, Reiter M, Altrichter S, et al. Anaphylaxis caused by mosquito allergy in systemic mastocytosis. Lancet 2013;382(9901):1380.

11. Lim KH, Tefferi A, Lasho TL, et al. Systemic mastocytosis in 342 consecutive adults: survival studies and prognostic factors. Blood 2009;113(23):5727–36.

12. Fried AJ, Akin C. Primary mast cell disorders in children. Curr Allergy Asthma Rep 2013;13(6):693–701.

13. Siebenhaar F, Weller K, Blume-Peytavi U, et al. Childhood-onset mastocytosis. Hautarzt 2012;63(2):104–9 [in German].

14. Hartmann K, Henz BM. Cutaneous mastocytosis–clinical heterogeneity. Int Arch Allergy Immunol 2002;127(2):143–6.

15. Correia O, Duarte AF, Quirino P, et al. Cutaneous mastocytosis: two pediatric cases treated with topical pimecrolimus. Dermatol Online J 2010;16(5):8.

16. Hartmann K, Metcalfe DD. Pediatric mastocytosis. Hematol Oncol Clin North Am 2000;14(3):625–40.

17. Bennett M, Chubar Y. Response of urticaria pigmentosa to cladribine in a patient with systemic mastocytosis. Br J Haematol 2013;160(4):420.

18. Ustun C, DeRemer DL, Akin C. Tyrosine kinase inhibitors in the treatment of systemic mastocytosis. Leuk Res 2011;35(9):1143–52.

19. Guhl S, Hartmann K, Tapkenhinrichs S, et al. Ultraviolet irradiation induces apoptosis in human immature, but not in skin mast cells. J Invest Dermatol 2003;121(4):837–44.

20. Bedlow AJ, Gharrie S, Harland CC. The treatment of urticaria pigmentosa with the frequency-doubled Q-switch Nd:YAG laser. J Cutan Laser Ther 2000;2(1):45–7.

21. Resh B, Jones E, Glaser DA. The cosmetic treatment of urticaria pigmentosa with Nd:YAG laser at 532 nanometers. J Cosmet Dermatol 2005;4(2):78–82.

22. Siebenhaar F, Fortsch A, Krause K, et al. Rupatadine improves quality of life in mastocytosis: a randomized, double-blind, placebo-controlled trial. Allergy 2013;68(7):949–52.

23. Siebenhaar F, Degener F, Zuberbier T, et al. High-dose desloratadine decreases wheal volume and improves cold provocation thresholds compared with standard-dose treatment in patients with acquired cold urticaria: a randomized, placebo-controlled, crossover study. J Allergy Clin Immunol 2009;123(3):672–9.

24. Weller K, Ziege C, Staubach P, et al. H1-antihistamine up-dosing in chronic spontaneous urticaria: patients' perspective of effectiveness and side effects– a retrospective survey study. PloS One 2011;6(9):e23931.

25. Zuberbier T, Asero R, Bindslev-Jensen C, et al. EAACI/GA(2)LEN/EDF/WAO guideline: management of urticaria. Allergy 2009;64(10):1427–43.

26. Edwards AM, Capkova S. Oral and topical sodium cromoglicate in the treatment of diffuse cutaneous mastocytosis in an infant. BMJ Case Rep 2011. http://dx.doi.org/10.1136/bcr.02.2011.3910. Accessed June 29, 2011.

27. Vieira Dos Santos R, Magerl M, Martus P, et al. Topical sodium cromoglicate relieves allergen- and histamine-induced dermal pruritus. Br J Dermatol 2010; 162(3):674–6.

28. Yoshimi A, Hashizume H, Kitagawa M, et al. Absorption mechanism of 1,3-bis(2-ethoxycarbonylchromon-5-yloxy)-2-((S)-lysyloxy)propane dihydrochloride (N-556), a prodrug for the oral delivery of disodium cromoglycate. Biol Pharm Bull 1993; 16(4):375–8.

29. Okayama Y, Benyon RC, Rees PH, et al. Inhibition profiles of sodium cromoglycate and nedocromil sodium on mediator release from mast cells of human skin, lung, tonsil, adenoid and intestine. Clin Exp Allergy 1992;22(3):401–9.

30. Castells M. Mast cell mediators in allergic inflammation and mastocytosis. Immunol Allergy Clin North Am 2006;26(3):465–85.

31. Guinot P, Summerhayes C, Berdah L, et al. Treatment of adult systemic mastocytosis with a PAF-acether antagonist BN52063. Lancet 1988;2(8602):114.

32. Macpherson JL, Kemp A, Rogers M, et al. Occurrence of platelet-activating factor (PAF) and an endogenous inhibitor of platelet aggregation in diffuse cutaneous mastocytosis. Clin Exp Immunol 1989;77(3):391–6.

33. Turner PJ, Kemp AS, Rogers M, et al. Refractory symptoms successfully treated with leukotriene inhibition in a child with systemic mastocytosis. Pediatr Dermatol 2012;29(2):222–3.

34. Jensen RT. Gastrointestinal abnormalities and involvement in systemic mastocytosis. Hematol Oncol Clin North Am 2000;14(3):579–623.

35. Sokol H, Georgin-Lavialle S, Canioni D, et al. Gastrointestinal manifestations in mastocytosis: a study of 83 patients. J Allergy Clin Immunol 2013;132(4):866–73.e1–3.

36. Escribano L, Akin C, Castells M, et al. Current options in the treatment of mast cell mediator-related symptoms in mastocytosis. Inflamm Allergy Drug Targets 2006;5(1):61–77.

37. Metcalfe DD, Akin C. Mastocytosis: molecular mechanisms and clinical disease heterogeneity. Leuk Res 2001;25(7):577–82.

38. Moura DS, Sultan S, Georgin-Lavialle S, et al. Evidence for cognitive impairment in mastocytosis: prevalence, features and correlations to depression. PloS One 2012;7(6):e39468.

39. Moura DS, Sultan S, Georgin-Lavialle S, et al. Depression in patients with mastocytosis: prevalence, features and effects of masitinib therapy. PloS One 2011;6(10):e26375.

40. Rogers MP, Bloomingdale K, Murawski BJ, et al. Mixed organic brain syndrome as a manifestation of systemic mastocytosis. Psychosom Med 1986;48(6):437–47.

41. Soter NA, Austen KF, Wasserman SI. Oral disodium cromoglycate in the treatment of systemic mastocytosis. N Engl J Med 1979;301(9):465–9.

42. Horan RF, Sheffer AL, Austen KF. Cromolyn sodium in the management of systemic mastocytosis. J Allergy Clin Immunol 1990;85(5):852–5.

43. Mallet AI, Norris P, Rendell NB, et al. The effect of disodium cromoglycate and ketotifen on the excretion of histamine and N tau-methylimidazole acetic acid in urine of patients with mastocytosis. Br J Clin Pharmacol 1989;27(1):88–91.

44. Johnstone PA, Mican JM, Metcalfe DD, et al. Radiotherapy of refractory bone pain due to systemic mast cell disease. Am J Clin Oncol 1994;17(4):328–30.

45. Butterfield JH. Survey of aspirin administration in systemic mastocytosis. Prostaglandins Other Lipid Mediat 2009;88(3–4):122–4.

46. Worobec AS. Treatment of systemic mast cell disorders. Hematol Oncol Clin North Am 2000;14(3):659–87, vii.

47. Worobec AS, Metcalfe DD. Mastocytosis: current treatment concepts. Int Arch Allergy Immunol 2002;127(2):153–5.

48. Lim AY, Ostor AJ, Love S, et al. Systemic mastocytosis: a rare cause of osteoporosis and its response to bisphosphonate treatment. Ann Rheum Dis 2005;64(6):965–6.

49. Douglass JA, Carroll K, Voskamp A, et al. Omalizumab is effective in treating systemic mastocytosis in a nonatopic patient. Allergy 2010;65(7):926–7.

50. Matito A, Blazquez-Goni C, Morgado JM, et al. Short-term omalizumab treatment in an adolescent with cutaneous mastocytosis. Ann Allergy Asthma Immunol 2013;111(5):425–6.

51. Siebenhaar F, Kuhn W, Zuberbier T, et al. Successful treatment of cutaneous mastocytosis and Meniere disease with anti-IgE therapy. J Allergy Clin Immunol 2007;120(1):213–5.
52. Maurer M, Rosen K, Hsieh HJ, et al. Omalizumab for the treatment of chronic idiopathic or spontaneous urticaria. N Engl J Med 2013;368(10):924–35.
53. Pitt TJ, Cisneros N, Kalicinsky C, et al. Successful treatment of idiopathic anaphylaxis in an adolescent. J Allergy Clin Immunol 2010;126(2):415–6 [author reply: 6].
54. Guillaume N, Desoutter J, Chandesris O, et al. Bone complications of mastocytosis: a link between clinical and biological characteristics. Am J Med 2013; 126(1):75.e1–7.
55. Rossini M, Zanotti R, Bonadonna P, et al. Bone mineral density, bone turnover markers and fractures in patients with indolent systemic mastocytosis. Bone 2011;49(4):880–5.
56. van der Veer E, van der Goot W, de Monchy JG, et al. High prevalence of fractures and osteoporosis in patients with indolent systemic mastocytosis. Allergy 2012;67(3):431–8.
57. Hartmann K, Wagner N, Rabenhorst A, et al. Serum IL-31 levels are increased in a subset of patients with mastocytosis and correlate with disease severity in adult patients. J Allergy Clin Immunol 2013;132(1):232–5.
58. Rabenhorst A, Christopeit B, Leja S, et al. Serum levels of bone cytokines are increased in indolent systemic mastocytosis associated with osteopenia or osteoporosis. J Allergy Clin Immunol 2013;132(5):1234–7.e7.
59. Kushnir-Sukhov NM, Brittain E, Reynolds JC, et al. Elevated tryptase levels are associated with greater bone density in a cohort of patients with mastocytosis. Int Arch Allergy Immunol 2006;139(3):265–70.
60. Dhami S, Panesar SS, Roberts G, et al. Management of anaphylaxis: a systematic review. Allergy 2013;69(2):168–75.
61. Sampson HA, Munoz-Furlong A, Campbell RL, et al. Second symposium on the definition and management of anaphylaxis: summary report–Second National Institute of Allergy and Infectious Disease/Food Allergy and Anaphylaxis Network symposium. J Allergy Clin Immunol 2006;117(2):391–7.
62. Moneret-Vautrin DA, Morisset M, Flabbee J, et al. Epidemiology of life-threatening and lethal anaphylaxis: a review. Allergy 2005;60(4):443–51.
63. Bohlke K, Davis RL, DeStefano F, et al. Epidemiology of anaphylaxis among children and adolescents enrolled in a health maintenance organization. J Allergy Clin Immunol 2004;113(3):536–42.
64. Decker WW, Campbell RL, Manivannan V, et al. The etiology and incidence of anaphylaxis in Rochester, Minnesota: a report from the Rochester Epidemiology Project. J Allergy Clin Immunol 2008;122(6):1161–5.
65. Helbling A, Hurni T, Mueller UR, et al. Incidence of anaphylaxis with circulatory symptoms: a study over a 3-year period comprising 940,000 inhabitants of the Swiss Canton Bern. Clin Exp Allergy 2004;34(2):285–90.
66. Yocum MW, Butterfield JH, Klein JS, et al. Epidemiology of anaphylaxis in Olmsted County: a population-based study. J Allergy Clin Immunol 1999; 104(2 Pt 1):452–6.
67. Lieberman P, Camargo CA Jr, Bohlke K, et al. Epidemiology of anaphylaxis: findings of the American College of Allergy, Asthma and Immunology Epidemiology of Anaphylaxis Working Group. Ann Allergy Asthma Immunol 2006;97(5):596–602.
68. Florian S, Krauth MT, Simonitsch-Klupp I, et al. Indolent systemic mastocytosis with elevated serum tryptase, absence of skin lesions, and recurrent severe anaphylactoid episodes. Int Arch Allergy Immunol 2005;136(3):273–80.

69. Gonzalez de Olano D, de la Hoz Caballer B, Nunez Lopez R, et al. Prevalence of allergy and anaphylactic symptoms in 210 adult and pediatric patients with mastocytosis in Spain: a study of the Spanish network on mastocytosis (REMA). Clin Exp Allergy 2007;37(10):1547–55.
70. Gulen T, Hagglund H, Dahlen B, et al. High prevalence of anaphylaxis in patients with systemic mastocytosis–a single-center experience. Clin Exp Allergy 2013;44(1):121–9.
71. Matito A, Bartolome-Zavala B, Alvarez-Twose I, et al. IgE-mediated anaphylaxis to *Hippobosca equina* in a patient with systemic mastocytosis. Allergy 2010; 65(8):1058–9.
72. van Anrooij B, van der Veer E, de Monchy JG, et al. Higher mast cell load decreases the risk of Hymenoptera venom-induced anaphylaxis in patients with mastocytosis. J Allergy Clin Immunol 2013;132(1):125–30.
73. Alvarez-Twose I, Bonadonna P, Matito A, et al. Systemic mastocytosis as a risk factor for severe Hymenoptera sting-induced anaphylaxis. J Allergy Clin Immunol 2013;131(2):614–5.
74. Biedermann T, Rueff F, Sander CA, et al. Mastocytosis associated with severe wasp sting anaphylaxis detected by elevated serum mast cell tryptase levels. Br J Dermatol 1999;141(6):1110–2.
75. Dugas-Breit S, Przybilla B, Dugas M, et al. Serum concentration of baseline mast cell tryptase: evidence for a decline during long-term immunotherapy for Hymenoptera venom allergy. Clin Exp Allergy 2010;40(4):643–9.
76. Przybilla B, Rueff F. Insect stings: clinical features and management. Dtsch Arztebl Int 2012;109(13):238–48.
77. Bonadonna P, Zanotti R, Muller U. Mastocytosis and insect venom allergy. Curr Opin Allergy Clin Immunol 2010;10(4):347–53.
78. Carter MC, Robyn JA, Bressler PB, et al. Omalizumab for the treatment of unprovoked anaphylaxis in patients with systemic mastocytosis. J Allergy Clin Immunol 2007;119(6):1550–1.
79. Kontou-Fili K. High omalizumab dose controls recurrent reactions to venom immunotherapy in indolent systemic mastocytosis. Allergy 2008;63(3): 376–8.
80. Kontou-Fili K, Filis CI. Prolonged high-dose omalizumab is required to control reactions to venom immunotherapy in mastocytosis. Allergy 2009;64(9):1384–5.
81. Kontou-Fili K, Filis CI, Voulgari C, et al. Omalizumab monotherapy for bee sting and unprovoked "anaphylaxis" in a patient with systemic mastocytosis and undetectable specific IgE. Ann Allergy Asthma Immunol 2010;104(6): 537–9.
82. Boissan M, Feger F, Guillosson JJ, et al. c-Kit and c-kit mutations in mastocytosis and other hematological diseases. J Leukoc Biol 2000;67(2):135–48.
83. Schwaab J, Schnittger S, Sotlar K, et al. Comprehensive mutational profiling in advanced systemic mastocytosis. Blood 2013;122(14):2460–6.
84. Soucie E, Hanssens K, Mercher T, et al. In aggressive forms of mastocytosis, TET2 loss cooperates with c-KITD816V to transform mast cells. Blood 2012; 120(24):4846–9.
85. Tefferi A, Levine RL, Lim KH, et al. Frequent TET2 mutations in systemic mastocytosis: clinical, KITD816V and FIP1L1-PDGFRA correlates. Leukemia 2009; 23(5):900–4.
86. Traina F, Visconte V, Jankowska AM, et al. Single nucleotide polymorphism array lesions, TET2, DNMT3A, ASXL1 and CBL mutations are present in systemic mastocytosis. PloS One 2012;7(8):e43090.

87. Alvarez-Twose I, Gonzalez P, Morgado JM, et al. Complete response after imatinib mesylate therapy in a patient with well-differentiated systemic mastocytosis. J Clin Oncol 2012;30(12):e126–9.

88. Gotlib J, Kluin-Nelemans HC, George TI, et al. KIT inhibitor midostaurin in patients with advanced systemic mastocytosis: results of a planned interim analysis of the global CPKC412D2201 trial. Blood 2012;120:799.

89. Paul C, Sans B, Suarez F, et al. Masitinib for the treatment of systemic and cutaneous mastocytosis with handicap: a phase 2a study. Am J Hematol 2010; 85(12):921–5.

90. Karra L, Berent-Maoz B, Ben-Zimra M, et al. Are we ready to downregulate mast cells? Curr Opin Immunol 2009;21(6):708–14.

91. Karra L, Levi-Schaffer F. Down-regulation of mast cell responses through ITIM containing inhibitory receptors. Adv Exp Med Biol 2011;716:143–59.

92. Migalovich-Sheikhet H, Friedman S, Mankuta D, et al. Novel identified receptors on mast cells. Front Immunol 2012;3:238.

93. Berent-Maoz B, Salemi S, Mankuta D, et al. Human mast cells express intracellular TRAIL. Cell Immunol 2010;262(2):80–3.

94. Aichberger KJ, Gleixner KV, Mirkina I, et al. Identification of proapoptotic Bim as a tumor suppressor in neoplastic mast cells: role of KIT D816V and effects of various targeted drugs. Blood 2009;114(26):5342–51.

95. Alfredsson J, Puthalakath H, Martin H, et al. Proapoptotic Bcl-2 family member Bim is involved in the control of mast cell survival and is induced together with Bcl-XL upon IgE-receptor activation. Cell Death Differ 2005;12(2):136–44.

96. Ekoff M, Kaufmann T, Engstrom M, et al. The BH3-only protein Puma plays an essential role in cytokine deprivation induced apoptosis of mast cells. Blood 2007;110(9):3209–17.

97. Hartmann K, Artuc M, Baldus SE, et al. Expression of Bcl-2 and Bcl-xL in cutaneous and bone marrow lesions of mastocytosis. Am J Pathol 2003;163(3): 819–26.

98. Karlberg M, Ekoff M, Huang DC, et al. The BH3-mimetic ABT-737 induces mast cell apoptosis in vitro and in vivo: potential for therapeutics. J Immunol 2010; 185(4):2555–62.

99. Peter B, Cerny-Reiterer S, Hadzijusufovic E, et al. The pan-Bcl-2 blocker obatoclax promotes the expression of Puma, Noxa, and Bim mRNA and induces apoptosis in neoplastic mast cells. J Leukoc Biol 2013;95(1):95–104.

100. Forster A, Preussner LM, Seeger JM, et al. Dimethylfumarate induces apoptosis in human mast cells. Exp Dermatol 2013;22(11):719–24.

101. Ma Z, Jiao Z. Mast cells as targets of pimecrolimus. Curr Pharm Des 2011; 17(34):3823–9.

102. Ma Z, Tovar JP, Kwong KY, et al. Pimecrolimus induces apoptosis of mast cells in a murine model of cutaneous mastocytosis. Int Arch Allergy Immunol 2010; 153(4):413–8.

103. Magerl M, Rother M, Bieber T, et al. Randomized, double-blind, placebo-controlled study of safety and efficacy of miltefosine in antihistamine-resistant chronic spontaneous urticaria. J Eur Acad Dermatol Venereol 2012;27(3): e363–9.

104. Maurer M, Magerl M, Metz M, et al. Miltefosine: a novel treatment option for mast cell-mediated diseases. J Dermatolog Treat 2013;24(4):244–9.

105. Weller K, Artuc M, Jennings G, et al. Miltefosine inhibits human mast cell activation and mediator release both in vitro and in vivo. J Invest Dermatol 2009; 129(2):496–8.

106. Hartmann K, Siebenhaar F, Belloni B, et al. Effects of topical treatment with the raft modulator miltefosine and clobetasol in cutaneous mastocytosis: a randomized, double-blind, placebo-controlled trial. Br J Dermatol 2010;162(1):185–90.
107. Gerbaulet A, Wickenhauser C, Scholten J, et al. Mast cell hyperplasia, B-cell malignancy, and intestinal inflammation in mice with conditional expression of a constitutively active kit. Blood 2011;117(6):2012–21.
108. Metz M, Siebenhaar F, Maurer M. Mast cell functions in the innate skin immune system. Immunobiology 2008;213(3–4):251–60.
109. Siebenhaar F, Magerl M, Peters EM, et al. Mast cell-driven skin inflammation is impaired in the absence of sensory nerves. J Allergy Clin Immunol 2008;121(4): 955–61.

Index

Note: Page numbers of article titles are in **boldface** type.

A

Activation markers, in mast cells, 304
Adaptive immune system, CD30 in, 346
Age factors, in mastocytosis, 284
Aggressive systemic mastocytosis, 213, 242
    diagnosis of, 211
    epidemiology of, 285
    flow cytometry for, 305–306
    KIT mutations in, 246
    liver involvement in, 330
    prognosis for, 288–289
AHNMD. *See* Associated hematologic non-mast cell clonal disease (AHNMD).
Alendronate, for bone disorders, 393
Alkaline phosphatase, in bone disorders, 387
Allergic rhinitis, mast cell-eosinophil pair in, 358–359
Allergy
    CD30 action in, 344–345
    drug, **397–405**
    Hymenoptera venom, **365–381**
Amantadine, 415
Amygdales, mast cells in, 411
Anaphylaxis, 209, 223
    bleeding in, 274
    epidemiology of, 439
    in anesthesia, 398–402
    in drug allergy, **397–405**
    in Hymenoptera venom allergy, 366–377
    prevalence of, 284
    risk factors for, 291
    treatment of, 371–377, 439
Anesthesia, in mastocytosis, 398–402
Antibiotics, allergy to, 402
Anticoagulants, mast cell tryptases as, **263–281**
Antihistamines, 399, 436–437
Apoptosis, CD30 in, 346
Aprepitant, 415
Ascitic fluid, mast cell identification in, 307–308
Aspirin, allergy to, 402–403
Associated hematologic non-mast cell clonal disease (AHNMD), 242–243
    definition of, 208
    diagnosis of, 213
    epidemiology of, 286

Immunol Allergy Clin N Am 34 (2014) 449–460
http://dx.doi.org/10.1016/S0889-8561(14)00028-9
0889-8561/14/$ – see front matter © 2014 Elsevier Inc. All rights reserved.
immunology.theclinics.com

Moving?

Make sure your subscription moves with you!

To notify us of your new address, find your **Clinics Account Number** (located on your mailing label above your name), and contact customer service at:

Email: journalscustomerservice-usa@elsevier.com

800-654-2452 (subscribers in the U.S. & Canada)
314-447-8871 (subscribers outside of the U.S. & Canada)

Fax number: 314-447-8029

Elsevier Health Sciences Division
Subscription Customer Service
3251 Riverport Lane
Maryland Heights, MO 63043

*To ensure uninterrupted delivery of your subscription, please notify us at least 4 weeks in advance of move.